Jochen A. Werner · R. Kim Davis · (Eds.)

Metastases in Head and Neck Cancer

Jochen A. Werner
R. Kim Davis · (Eds.)

Metastases in Head and Neck Cancer

With 106 Figures and 21 Tables

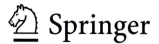 Springer

ISBN 3-540-20507-1
Springer Berlin Heidelberg New York

Jochen A. Werner M.D.
Professor and Chairman
Department of Otolaryngology,
Head and Neck Surgery
Philipps University of Marburg
Deutschhausstrasse 3
35037 Marburg
Germany

R. Kim Davis M.D.
Grant H. and Mildred Burrows
Beckstrand Professor of Surgical Oncology
Chief, Division of Otolaryngology,
Head and Neck Surgery
University of Utah, School of Medicine
3C 120 University Health Sciences Center
Salt Lake City, Utah, 84132–2301
USA

Library of Congress Control Number: 2004105240

Springer is a part of Springer Science + Business Media

springeronline.com

© Springer-Verlag Berlin Heidelberg 2004
Printed in Germany

Editor: Ute Heilmann, Heidelberg
Desk editor: Dörthe Mennecke-Bühler, Heidelberg
Production editor: Bernd Wieland, Heidelberg
Illustrations: R. Henkel, Heidelberg
Cover design: F. Steinen, ᵉStudio Calamar, Spain
Typesetting: AM-productions, Wiesloch
Printing and bookbinding: Stürtz AG, Würzburg

21/3150 – 5 4 3 2 1 0
Printed on acid-free paper

Preface

Our intent in writing the book "Metastases in Head and Neck Cancer" is to provide the reader with a comprehensive and cohesive presentation of this very important topic. As we have shared a common treatment philosophy over many years, it has been a pleasure to relate our experiences with this important topic.

This book is unique in that it supplies an in-depth discussion of lymphology and pathology that provides a strong basic science background to help the reader understand this disease process. The intent of the book is not to be a "how to do it" manual. Rather, it is to develop the necessary basic science background blended with our experiences in order to provide a framework of thinking about why metastasis occurs, where it occurs, and what the treatment options are.

While neck dissection is covered in great detail, the chapters on diagnosis and radiation therapy provide in-depth discussions of modern techniques at the "cutting edge". In this regard the descriptions of IMRT elaborate a treatment technique that has the potential to significantly change how radiation therapy is delivered to head and neck cancer. The diagnosis chapter provides a detailed discussion of ultrasonography, something which American head and neck surgeons use less frequently than their colleagues in Europe and elsewhere, who have significant experience with this technique from which all can benefit.

The authors wish to give special thanks to Dr. Anja Dünne for the vast amount of work she has performed in helping to compile this book. We also want to especially thank our secretaries, Susanne Zapf and Leora Loy, for their patience in transcribing and revising these chapters on numerous occasions. We finally express our love and thanks to our families for their constant understanding, support, love, and patience in helping such a project to proceed.

JOCHEN A. WERNER
R. KIM DAVIS

Contents

Contributors

VILIJA AVIZONIS M.D.
Radiation Oncologist
LDS Hospital
Eighth Avenue & C Street
Salt Lake City, Utah, 84143
USA

R. KIM DAVIS M.D.
Grant H. and Mildred Burrows
Beckstrand Professor of Surgical Oncology
Chief, Division of Otolaryngology,
Head and Neck Surgery
University of Utah, School of Medicine
3C 120 University Health Sciences Center
Salt Lake City, Utah, 84132–2301
USA

BURKARD M. LIPPERT M.D.
Department of Otolaryngology,
Head and Neck Surgery
Philipps University of Marburg
Deutschhausstrasse 3
35037 Marburg
Germany

ROLAND MOLL M.D.
Institute of Pathology
Philipps University of Marburg
Baldingerstrasse
35043 Marburg
Germany

JOCHEN A. WERNER M.D.
Professor and Chairman
Department of Otolaryngology,
Head and Neck Surgery
Philipps University of Marburg
Deutschhausstrasse 3
35037 Marburg
Germany

Basics of Lymphology

1.1 Embryology and Anatomy

1.1.1 Lymph Vessels

1.1.1.1 History

Lymph vessels were first described after the other parts of the vascular system were already known. The reason for this delay was undoubtedly their delicate and transparent appearance. Hippocrates (460–377 B.C.) and Aristotle (384–322 B.C.), as well as the outstanding anatomists of the Alexandrian school, Herophilus (about 300 B.C.) and Erasistratos (about 310–250 B.C.), knew about parts of the lymphatic system. Their notes indicate "white blood" vessels with "transparent liquid" and "intestinal arteries containing milky liquid." Aristotle noted that there were veins in the human body which were very small and which he assumed were responsible for transport of the nutritional processes of the stomach to other parts of the body. Hippocrates had previously observed that vessels of the stomach were very difficult to identify, and that they had different structures from arteries and veins. These vessels of the stomach, he said, transported a turbid liquid. Erasistratos, often credited as the father of physiology, also described numerous vessels in the area of the mesentery transporting milky liquid. The significance of the lymph vessels as independent from the vascular system, however, apparently was not understood by these scientists. As a result, their observations went unnoticed for centuries.

Up until the second half of the fifteenth century no significant progress in the anatomy of the lymphatic system was made. With the development of more so-phisticated techniques for sectioning organs, im-proved technical equipment – especially magnifying lenses – and, finally, improved injection techniques, reliable identification of lymph vessels became possible.

Maasa described the lymph vessels of the kidney in 1532 [1]. The ductus thoracicus of the horse was mentioned in 1563 by Eustachius (1520–1574). At the time, Eustachius held a chair for anatomy in Rome. His description of the ductus thoracicus also identified the outlet of the thoracic duct into the left subclavian vein. The inferior connections of the thoracic duct, however, were not described. It is not surprising therefore that Eustachius was not able to clarify the function of this anatomic structure.

During the vivisection of a well-nurtured dog in Milan on 23 July 1622, Gaspare Asellius, professor of anatomy and surgery in Pavia, Italy (▶ Fig. 1.1), accidentally discovered the extraordinarily delicate and beautiful white strands in the intestines which surprisingly contained a milky liquid. He recognized that these milky vessels could not be the already known intestinal nerves [2–4]. Asellius called the lymph vessels "venae albae et lacteae." The term "lacteae" referred not to lac, milk, but to lactis, the enteron. Asellius followed the lymphatic vessels up to a large gland (pancreas Aselli). He assumed that from there the lymph vessels would drain to the liver. Asellius realized the absorbing function of the "venae albae." The differentiation between lymph vessels and veins should thus be attributed to Asellius. He also described lymph vessels in other animal species, including the cat, sheep, cow, pig and horse. However, he did not manage to identify human lymph vessels. The reason for this was likely the restrictions in the republic of Pavia around 1600 on human anatomy sections. Although Asellius had no access to human material, he imagined that lymph vessels also occurred in humans. In 1628, shortly after Asellius published his manuscript entitled, "De lactibus sive lacteis venis," the first descriptions of human lymph vessels were made by Brechet. Six years later, Johann Vesling from Padua also verified human lymph vessels. It was he, who, in 1653, first published illustrations of human lymph vessels.

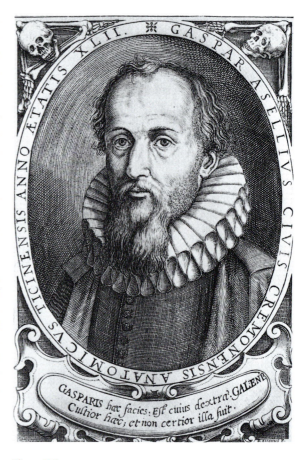

Figure 1.1

Gaspare Asellius, Professor of Anatomy and Surgery in Pavia, Italy

With the discovery of blood circulation by William Harvey (1578–1657), came a renewed interest in the "Venae lacteae" of Asellius, which, during subsequent decades, had been confirmed to be an independent vascular system. Acceptance of Asellius's observations was facilitated by the rejection of the liver as a blood producing organ and collector of the lymph vessels.

Already in 1653 the Swede, Olaf Rudbeck, knew about lymphatic valves, a discovery that, over half of a century later, Ruysch claimed to have made himself. Rudbeck, who started his anatomic examinations of lymph vessels in 1650, was able to prove that lymph vessels occur in different parts of the human body, including the rectum, esophagus, leg and the backside of the sternum. In 1653, Rudbeck's famous opponent, the anatomist Thomas Bartholin (1616–1680) from Copenhagen, Denmark, gave the milky vessels the name still used today, "vasa lymphatica."

Bartholin's publications on the lymphatic system contributed significantly to a better understanding of lymph vessels. His earliest manuscript, published in 1652, was entitled "De lacteis thoracices in homine brutisque" [5, 6]. Bartholin and Rudbeck independently described the anatomy of the lymphatic system [5, 6]. Because nerves at that time were considered to be a third vascular type, Bartholin and Rudbeck designated lymph vessels the fourth vascular type.

In 1661, Jean Pecquet identified the cisterna chyli (in dogs) and the thoracic duct traversing the liver. He called it "ductus chyliferus." He described both the thoracic duct and the right lymphatic duct, including their inflow into the confluence of the internal jugular and subclavian vein on both sides [7, 8]. It was also Pecquet who identified the relationship between the cisterna chyli and the inferior vena cava. Injection trials led him to conclude that these connections were the first lympho-venous anastomoses.

In 1665, Frederick Ruysch (1638–1731) published a manuscript entitled, "Dilucidatio valvularum," in which he described and brilliantly illustrated the morphology and function of the lymphatic valves. Understandably, the lymphatic valves were compared to those of the veins. As a result of his contributions, and those of his colleagues, the existence of lymph vessels became largely accepted toward the end of the seventeenth century [9].

After Nuck's description in 1692 of mercury injections into lymph vessels, the careful preparations of Mascagni, nearly a century later, crowned the anatomic research on lymphatics. His twenty-seven large copper engravings entitled, "Vasorum Lymphaticorum Corporis Humani Historia et Ichnographia" (1787) brilliantly illustrated the complete lymphatic system, a feat not overshadowed even today by current lymphography in completeness and beauty.

Paolo Mascagni, professor of anatomy in Siena, Italy, demonstrated that the beginnings of the lymphatic system have no direct connection to the blood vessels in the interstitial region [10]. It was the anatomist William Hunter (1718–1783), however, who, working in London, identified the significance of the lymphatic system in the absorption of these interstitial liquids.

By furthering our understanding of regional lymphatic drainage and lymphatic topography, William Cruikshank (1745–1800), also made significant contributions to our understanding of human lymph vessels. At last the lymphatic system was established as such and viewed as a system of branched, absorbing lymph vessels. This recognition enabled William Hunter to hypothesize that lymph vessels had an absorbing function in all parts of the body. He described lymph vessels as forming an extended vascular system together with the thoracic duct [11].

During the end of the eighteenth, and the beginning of the nineteenth, century, several illustrations of notable quality were made of the topography of the human lymphatic system. Here especially the illustrations by Andrew Fyfe that were published in 1800 are worth mentioning. His drawings were based on cadaver dissections and mercury injections performed by Alexander Monroe II [12].

In Paris in 1847, a professor of anatomy named Sappey began an intensive investigation of the lymphatic system. His results were published 27 years later in an extraordinary atlas [13]. In 1862, Von Recklinghausen (1833–1910) identified the lymphatic endothelial cells using the black dye, silver nitrate [14].

In 1821, Fohmann described the direct relationship between peripheral veins and lymph vessels in various subjects, including in birds, seals, otters, cats, dogs, horses, cows and humans [15]. His notes, however, were controversial and have remained so up to the present from the viewpoint of scientists who dispute the validity of physiologic anastomoses between lymph vessels and veins.

The nineteenth century witnessed another significant contribution to lymphology. Carl Ludwig [11] and Ernest Starling [16] proved that lymphatic liquid emerges in tissue as a filtration product of blood, and, furthermore, that mobile cells existing in the interstitium can recirculate via lymph vessels into the

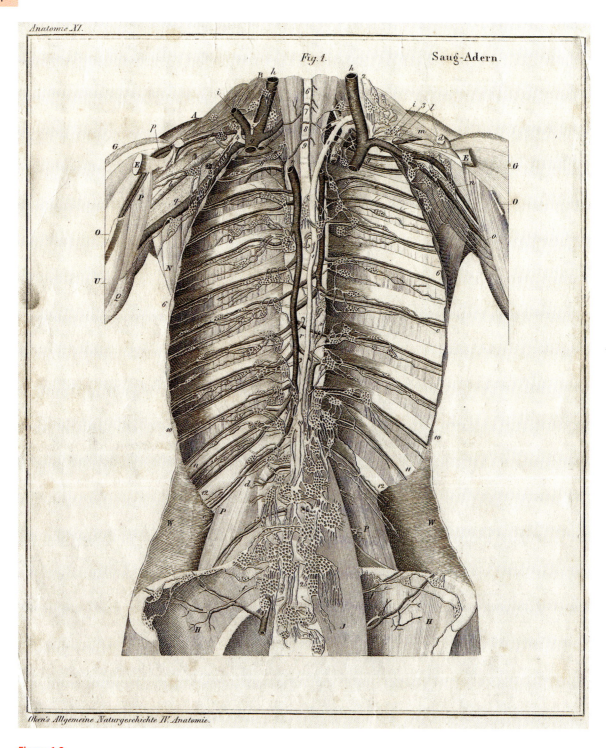

Figure 1.2

Image of the lymphatic system of the torso, called suction system

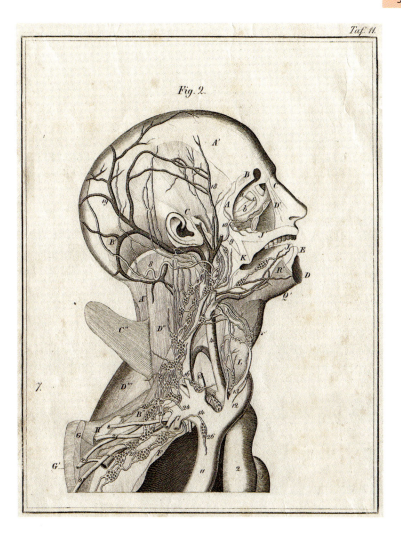

Figure 1.3

Image of the lymphatic system of the head and neck

vascular blood system (▶ Figs. 1.2, 1.3). The selective lymphogenic absorption of large molecules that cannot directly be reabsorbed in the vascular system was described by Field [17] and Yoffey [18].

Although Le Dran (1685–1770) was the first to describe the extension of carcinomas via lymph vessels (a observation that was verified by John Hunter, who stressed its significance as vehicle of possible lymphogenic metastatic spread), it was Astley Cooper who, in 1840, applied the knowledge of the lymphogenic metastatic process to breast cancer. He examined the lymph vessels of the breast with injection techniques thereby establishing the modern concept of surgery of the associated lymphatic drainage [19]. Virchow (1860) added to Cooper's observations in reference to tumor dissemination and described the significant role of the lymph nodes as a defense mechanism.

1.1.1.2 Embryology

In the fifth embryonic week, about two weeks after the beginning development of the blood vascular system, the lymphatic system develops in a similar way. The venous and lymphatic systems are thus connected to one another relatively early. Initially, six so-called primary lymphatic saccules arise, including both jugular lymph saccules, both iliac lymph sacs, the retroperitoneal lymph sac and the chylocyst. From there, the lymph vessels develop alongside the major venous trunks. From the jugular lymph saccules, the lymphatic vessels grow to the head and neck, as well as to the upper extremity; from the iliac lymphatic saccules, the lymphatic vessels grow to the legs and the lower part of the body; and from the retroperitoneal lymph sac and the chylocyst, they grow to the intestine and other abdominal organs. Two large lymphatic trunks, known as the right and the left thoracic ducts, also develop in the area of the thorax. The final thoracic duct develops from the caudal part of the right thoracic duct, the transverse anastomosis between the two original lymphatic trunks and the cranial part of the left thoracic duct. This accounts for the various origins and courses of the thoracic duct in adults [20].

1.1.1.3 Morphology

The lymphatic system begins with finger-shaped initial lymph vessels that consist of wide vascular lumens having a diameter of about 30–50 μm. The network of initial lymph vessels consists of two parts. First, there are the valveless lymphatic capillaries, sometimes called lymph sinuses, and second, there are the valvular precollectors.

The term lymphatic capillaries implies a structural relationship to the blood capillaries which, however, is controversial, due to several morphological and functional differences between the two. The initial lymphatic system can increase its diameter up to 100 μm – fifty-fold, compared to its condition at rest. For this reason some investigators favor the term, lymphatic sinus. [21, 22].

Near the adventitia of a hollow viscous, near the capsule of the parenchyma of an organ or at the border of the dermis to the subcutaneous tissues of the skin, the precollectors become the so-called collectors. The proximal part of a collector is determined by its initial range and the first lymph node station as a peripheral collector. The postnodal collector drains lymph fluid into the so-called "lymphatic trunks" or the lymphatic ducts that meet in the right and the left lymphatic duct, as well as in the paired jugular lymphatic trunk. These ducts in turn meet bilaterally at the confluence of the internal jugular vein and the subclavian vein at the venous angle into the vascular system [23]. With regard to the process of lymphogenic metastatic spread, only lymphatic vessels with a diameter larger 10 μm play a role [24].

Structure of the Wall of Initial Lymph Vessels

The walls of the initial lymph vessels consist of endothelial cells that are surrounded by an incomplete and interrupted basal membrane. The endothelium measures a mere 0.1–0.2 μm. Only in the area of the cell bodies can higher volumes be observed (▶ Fig. 1.4).

The endothelial cell ends overlap like roof-tiles. They can be arranged without any contact (▶ Fig. 1.5 a) or they can be related via interendothelial junctions (▶ Fig. 1.5 b) that work as valves. Adjoining plasma membranes are mainly closed by adherent maculae and occasionally also by occluding maculae. In some cases, the overlapping cell ends may work as interlocked complex of interdigitations.

Endothelial Cells. In the endothelium of the initial lymph vessels of the upper aerodigestive tract, different ultrastructural characteristics can be observed, including:

- mitochondria
  (mainly in the perinuclear cytoplasm)
- vesicles
- poly- and monoribosomes
- centrioles
- Golgi-apparatus

Figure 1.4

Light microscopy of an initial lymph vessel

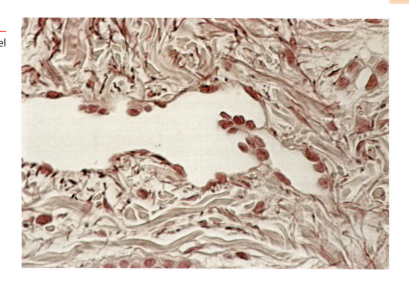

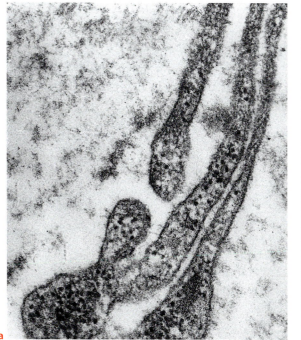

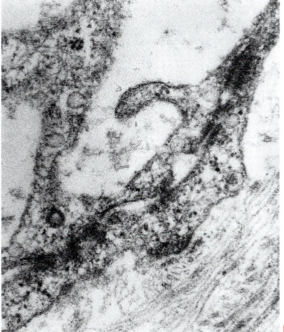

Figure 1.5 a, b

Transmission electron microscopic image of endothelial cells with interendothelial openings of initial lymph vessels. They can be arranged side by side (a) or connected via interlocked interendothelial junctions (b)

- lysosomes
- bundled microfilaments (about 4–6 nm with actinoid significance [25])

In the perinuclear cytoplasm, an endoplasmic reticulum can be observed; it is often more clearly developed in the upper aerodigestive tract than in other regions of the body [26]. This clearly developed endoplasmic reticulum of the head and neck indicates:

- intense protein synthesis
- high intracellular transport
- a membranous depot in the lymphatic endothelia

The membranous depot of the endoplasmic reticulum is obvious in view of the numerous vesicles believed to have a basically transportation function [26].

Weibel-Palade's granules [27] cannot always be detected near the initial lymph vessels in the upper aerodigestive tract. Nor are these granules seen in the lymph vessels of the milt [28], palatine tonsil [29], appendix [30] or skin [26]. The supposed lack of Weibel-Palade's granules in these lymph vessels is an important criterion in their distinction from blood capillaries, where the granules can be easily detected in the endothelium.

The lumen of the initial lymph vessels of the upper aerodigestive tract usually contains a milky or turbid material of middle electron density. Compared with interstitial fluid, the lymph fluid contains about three times more protein. This fact can be explained by the pressure exerted by the liquid exerted in the initial lymph vessels. The protein content sinks during the filling phase and increases during drainage.

Interendothelial Openings. Different examinations have revealed that the interendothelial openings near the initial lymphatic system occur mainly in the initial lymphatic capillaries and rarely in the precollectors. These interdigitations permit larger and thus more effective intercellular canals to develop for exchange between the interstitium and the lymphatic lumen without interrupting the continuous endothelial coating [31, 32]. Functionally, the idea is similar to the opening mechanism that occurs near the open foramen ovale in the atrial system of the heart, with the primary and secondary septa corresponding to the endothelial processes of the initial lymph vessels.

Subendothelial Fiber Felt. In contrast to blood capillaries, the initial lymph vessels are systematically surrounded by an elastic fibrous network, the so-called subendothelial fiber felt. Additionally, bundles of collagen fibers can be occasionally observed. These are situated adjacent to the endothelium of initial lymph vessels and sometimes seem to emanate into the abluminal cellular membrane. Due to the missing pericytes near the lymph vessels, the various forces exerting pressure on the initial lymph vessels are led along the vascular walls via the perivascular elastic fiber apparatus. This interaction has major importance for the regulation of the inflow and outflow of fluid, as well as for lymphogenic cellular migration [33].

Lymphatic Valves. In contrast to the initial lymphatic sinus, the precollectors, collectors and lymphatic trunks all possess vascular valves. The distance between the valves is about three- to ten times the size of the vascular diameter.

Different types of lymphatic valves include:
- bicuspid valves
- tricuspid valves
- quadricuspid valves
- valves with only one velum

The lymphatic valves avoid a reflux of the lymph fluid. Thus, the flowing direction of the initial lymph vessels to the collectors depends on the difference between the hydrostatic and colloid-osmotic pressure of both segments. The lymphatic flow is influenced by intrinsic and extrinsic forces. Intrinsic forces result from contractions of the actinoid filaments.

Extrinsic forces include:
- contractions of the surrounding muscles
- arterial pulsation
- respiratory movement
- tissue massage

Structure of the Wall of Lymph Collectors

Histomorphologically, the lymph collectors have three layers:

- The intima consists of endothelial cells, flimsy collagen fibers and single muscle cells.
- The media contains bundles of smooth muscle cells in corkscrew-like windings that are surrounded by collagen fibers.
- The adventitia consists of longitudinal bundles of connective tissue, elastic fiber networks and single smooth muscle cells.

The lymph collectors are surrounded by a continuous basal membrane like the successive lymphatic trunks.

Histochemistry of the Wall of Lymph Vessels

Reports on findings concerning the histochemical behavior of the lymphatic walls are very scarce in comparison to those concerning blood capillaries and walls of blood vessels. Descriptions of lymphatic histochemistry vary significantly due to differences in reported species, pathologic changes and methodological errors.

According to our own findings, the lymphatic vessels of the upper aerodigestive tract are characterized by a high activity of the enzymes adenylate and guanyl cyclase, 5'-nucleotidase and ATPase. We found most other enzymatic reactions to be negative or only slightly positive at the initial lymph vessels [34]. The first three enzymes mentioned have a special position in view of the fact that their histochemical activity at the lymph vessels is clearly higher than at the walls of blood capillaries or blood vessels. These findings confirm current reports concerning the lymphatic vessels of other organs in humans and other species for 5'-nucleotidase [28, 35–37], adenylate cyclase [38, 39] and guanylate cyclase [38, 39]. The different enzymatic activity of initial lymph vessels and blood capillaries is especially important for the histochemical differentiation of both vascular types.

Another point of interest is the functional significance of endothelial enzymatic activity in the lymphatic and vascular system. The necessary biochemical analyses of this enzymatic activity exist only for the endothelium of blood vessels. For the endothelium of the initial lymph vessels, no comparable analysis is available; hence, the discussion must rely on histochemical findings. The limited histochemical activity of 5'-nucleotidase, adenylate- and guanylate cyclase at the endothelium of the blood capillaries and blood vessels does not mean that those enzymes are missing. All of these enzymes can be detected biochemically in the endothelium of blood vessels. The histochemical findings rely on a comparison of lead or cerium fallout [40] that allows conclusions to be drawn regarding the extent of enzymatic activity.

In regard to 5'-nucleotidase, a distinction must be made between cytoplasmic (cyto 5'-nucleotidase) and ecto 5'-nucleotidase, which is related to the plasma membrane. The histochemically detectable high activity of 5'-nucleotidase in lymphatic endothelia and the comparatively low activity in blood capillaries, as in the majority of the blood vessel system, cannot be explained sufficiently at present. The lymphatic endothelia could have an increased trans-membranous absorption rate of nucleosides in comparison to the endothelia of blood capillaries. Kato [35] assumed that ecto 5'-nucleotidase plays an important role in the regulation of the blood flow and that this is dependent on the metabolic situation of the tissue. In this context, he suspected a lymphogenic regulation of the absorption rate of the tissue fluid based on 5'-nucleotidase activity. Besides nucleotide dephosphorylation, the stimulating effect of ecto 5'-nucleotidase on lymphocytes described by Andree and co-workers [41] could play a role in the endothelium of the initial lymph vessels.

Adenylate cyclase can be detected histochemically at the lymphatic endothelium where adenosine triphosphate is converted into cyclic adenosine monophosphate and pyrophosphate. Cyclic AMP is the second messenger substance in the chain of many peptide hormones; furthermore, it activates different enzymatic systems. Beta-catecholamine receptors are associated with a membranous adenylate cyclase that can elicit e.g. lipolysis and vasodilatation. In this context, the observations of Darózy [26] must be mentioned, where cyclic AMP leads to relaxation of mesenteric lymph vessels. Guanylate cyclase catalyses the conversion of guanosine triphosphate into cyclic guanosine monophosphate (cyclic GMP), detectable in the endothelium of lymph vessels.

Regarding the occurrence of factor VIII associated antigen in the lymphatic walls, reports diverge. Whereas some groups have observed rarely if at all the von Willebrand factor [33, 42–44], Svenholm [45] and Beckstead [46] confirmed clearly positive reactions in the endothelia of lymphatic vessels. Our evaluations have shown without doubt factor VIII-associated antigen in the lymph collectors and the lymphatic trunks, as already communicated by Mørck Hultberg and Svanholm [47]. In the endothelia of the initial lymph vessels, von Willebrand factor was present only in very low concentrations and sometimes it could not be detected at all histochemically. Regarding the origin of the factor VIII associated antigen in lymph vessels, it was assumed that the lymphatic endothelium produces the von Willebrand factor only in very low quantities [46]. In contrast to this, Kramer and co-workers [33] drew the conclusion in their communications on Kaposi sarcoma that the detection of the factor VIII associated antigen in the lymph vessels is possibly due to its release into the tissue and subsequent absorption into the lymph vessels.

Among the current histochemical investigations of lymph vessels, very little attention has been paid to the glyco-histochemical reaction of the lymphatic walls. In this context, UEA I-lectin has been examined extensively. While Suzuki et al. [44] detected no or at best only a very low reaction, other authors [46–48] consistently found the reaction to be positive. This corresponds to the UEA I-binding behavior of the initial lymph vessels of the upper aerodigestive tract. Furthermore, clearly positive lectin binding reactions in the initial lymph vessels of this region have been demonstrated for the lectins PNA, DBA and GS I.

In contrast to the glyco-histochemical reaction of lymphatic vessels, the composition of the discontinuous basal membrane of the initial lymph vessels (as well as the structural concretion called subendothelial fiber felt [49] in cases where there was a missing basal membrane) has been studied intensively. The

basal membrane of the initial lymph vessels of the upper aerodigestive tract contains only low concentrations of laminin, collagen type IV and fibronectin, compared with the continuous basal membrane of blood capillaries [50]. This confirms already communicated findings [51–53]. In pathologically transformed tissue, the basal membrane of the lymphatic vessel can be developed more strongly and thus have a higher concentration of the substances mentioned. As a result, the basal membrane of lymph angiomas is clearly thickened [44].

In conclusion, it may be said that histochemical findings allow a differentiation between lymphatic vessels and blood capillaries. The combined application of different histochemical techniques is critical in order to make this assessment. The histochemical differentiation of vascular types allows a reliable description of an organ-related lymphatic system, and it also provides the ability to differentiate whether tumor cell accumulations are situated in lymph vessels, blood capillaries or artificial tissue clefts.

1.1.1.4 Distribution

The lymphatic system of the mucosa of the aerodigestive tract consists of:

- a narrow-meshed, superficial vascular system
- a wide-meshed, deeply situated vascular system

The lymph vessels of the superficial network are flimsy in comparison to the deeply situated network. The superior vascular plexus is extraordinarily narrow-meshed. It is separated from the epithelium by a blood capillary network. These observations were made by Teichmann [54, 55] and can be confirmed for many parts of the aerodigestive tract. However, the technique used to identify the various structures involved cannot be generally applied due to the fact that there are initial lymph vessels that directly adjoin the epithelium.

Besides lymphatic capillaries, precollectors can occasionally be found in the superficial lymphatic network. In the deeper layer, lymphatic valves are observed more frequently than in the superficial lymphatic plexus. This is typical for the precollectors that can be discerned from the lymph collectors via the structure of the wall. Generally, the walls of the precollectors become stronger and stronger from the subepithelial to the submucous layer. This is a morphological indication for lymphatic transport into deeper layers.

Skin

Scalp

The lymph vessels of the scalp that anastomose with each other are situated in the subcutaneous layer. The midline is trespassed. Such contralateral connections exist only via the dense cutaneous capillary network.

On the scalp, there is a frontal, a parietal and an occipital territory. These do not strictly correspond to the areas supplied by the blood vessels (frontal, temporal, superficial posterior auricular and occipital artery).

Frontal Territory. Two to three lymph collectors drain around the orbicularis oculi muscle to the preauricular lymph nodes, and occasionally to the infraauricular or the deeply situated parotid lymph nodes. In addition, from two to five posterior collectors directly reach the preauricular lymph nodes.

Parietal Territory. The lymph vessels of this part drain around the parietal tuber and concentrate behind the ear in two to five lymph collectors. Part of the lymph collectors end in the preauricular lymph nodes. The major part drains into either the internal jugular lymph nodes or the infraauricular lymph nodes.

Occipital Territory. The lymph collectors of this drainage region can be divided into a medial group and a lateral group. The medial group ends in the superficial occipital lymph nodes, while the lateral group ends in the cranial portion of the deep lateral cervical lymph nodes.

Facial Region

The lymph vessels of the chin and the nose drain skin, muscles, perichondrium and the periosteum of this region. In contrast, the lymph vessels of the lip, the cheek and the eyelids also transport lymph fluid of the mucosa.

Eyelid. The drainage of the eyelids is accomplished partly by cutaneous and partly by conjunctival lymph vessels. The skin collectors and mucosal collectors are closely related in the area of the Meibomian glands. This connection is created by communicating branches that pass the tarsal plate. The lymphatic valves of the communicating branches of the tarsal plate direct the lymphatic flow of the deep cutaneous into the conjunctival lymphatic system.

Approximately six to seven collectors drain the lymph fluid from the skin of the upper lid and the lateral two thirds of the lower lid. They also transport the lymph fluid from the corresponding parts of the palpebral conjunctiva and the conjunctiva bulbi. The lymph collectors accompany the transverse facial artery and end in the preauricular lymph nodes. From the lower lid, lymph vessels may drain to the infraauricular, and, to some extent, into the preauricular lymph nodes.

The lymph fluid of the skin and the conjunctiva of the medial third of the lower lid drain alongside the facial vessels into the submandibular lymph nodes. Now and then, a medial course of the collector can be observed in the middle third of the upper lid. This is why drainage is possible into the parotid lymph nodes, as well as into the submandibularly localized lymph nodes.

Cheek. From the infraorbital region, meandering lymph collectors drain into the subcutaneous layer. Here, they run alongside the facial vessels into the submandibular lymph nodes. The skin area of the chin drains into the submental lymph nodes, while dorsal skin drains into the infraauricular lymph nodes.

Nose. The five to eight lymphatic collectors of the nose drain alongside the facial vessels and into submandibular lymph nodes. The root of the nose can be drained via a collector along the upper lid to the parotid lymph nodes. Next to the edge of the nasal ala, lymph collectors appear from the nasal vestibulum between the cartilaginous parts, and merge with the lymph vessels of the skin.

Upper Lip. The lymph vessels of the skin follow the facial vessels and drain into submandibular lymph nodes. Occasionally, a lymph collector diverging to the infraauricular or submental lymph nodes can be detected. The collectors of the skin cross the midline and thus can drain into the contralateral submandibular nodes.

Lower Lip. The skin and the mucosa of the lower lip have a superficial and deeply situated drainage region. At least two skin and two mucosal collectors transport the lymph fluid from this area. The collectors of the middle third of the lip drain into the submental lymph nodes, whereas those of the lateral third drain alongside the facial vessels and end in the submandibular lymph nodes. The drainage regions merge and cannot be clearly delineated.

Chin. The lymph collectors of the lateral chin region end in the submandibular lymph nodes. The lymph fluid from the middle chin region is transported into submental lymph nodes. This lymphatic drainage is effectuated via numerous anastomoses and crossings bilaterally into the submental, submandibular and parotid lymph nodes.

Auricle. The lobule, antitragus and lower part of the concha drain into the infraauricular lymph nodes. Lymph fluid from the skin near the tragus, the anterior part of the concha, the helix and the fossa triangularis flow into the preauricular and the deep parotid lymph nodes. The lymph vessels of the posterior part of the helix and concha, as well as the antihelix, drain into the retroauricular, infraauricular lymph nodes and into the internal jugular lymph nodes. Finally, the lymph fluid of the skin of the whole auricle is transported directly or indirectly into the internal jugular lymph nodes (level II).

Skin of the Neck

Neck Region. The lymph fluid of the posterior neck region is drained mostly without interposition of a superficial occipital lymph node directly into the accessory chain. The lymph collectors that originate from the caudal region penetrate the trapezius muscle and end in the subtrapezoid cervical lymph nodes.

Lateral Neck Region. The delineation of the lateral cervical region is made by the anterior edge of the trapezius and the sternocleidomastoid muscle and the clavicle. The lymph fluid is drained into the accessory chain, the internal jugular chain and the supraclavicular chain.

Submental and Submandibular Region. The lymph collectors in these regions drain into the submental, submandibular and infraauricular lymph nodes. There is no direct lymphatic drainage of the skin into the submandibular lymph nodes because this lymph node group is located below the platysma.

Prelaryngeal Region. The lymph fluid of the prelaryngeal skin area drains into the anterior jugular lymph nodes and into the internal jugular lymph nodes.

Nasal Cavity and Paranasal Sinuses

Nasal Cavity
The olfactory and the respiratory lymphatic systems appear to be separate.

Olfactory Region. The lymph vessels of this region are closely related to the perineural sheath of the olfactory nerves, and they overlay the blood capillaries. The lymph vessels closely communicate with the subarachnoidal space. They interdigitate along the olfactory nerves, penetrating the lamina cribrosa, and thus they may cause meningeal infections.

Respiratory Region. The lymph collectors of the lateral nasal wall drain into the nasopharynx. Near the nasopharyngeal folds they form the plexus pretubaris. The 1–2 lymph collectors originating from the sphenoethmoidal recess and the supreme nasal meatus drain via the fornix of the pharynx into the lateral retropharyngeal lymph nodes.

The plexus pretubaris is situated between the levator muscle and the tensor palatini muscle. The efferent lymph collectors drain into the subdigastric lymph nodes, whereas other lymph nodes drain to the lateral retropharyngeal lymph nodes.

The lymph collectors originating from the upper part of the nasal septum drain, together with the blood vessels of the superior nasal wall, alongside the pharyngeal roof into the lateral retropharyngeal lymph nodes. The lymph collectors near the middle and inferior part of the septum drain in caudal direction to the floor of the nose and converge in the plexus pretubaris.

Paranasal Sinuses

The lymphatic system of the paranasal sinuses is significantly more flimsy in healthy tissue than the one of the nasal cavity. Compared to other regions of the aerodigestive tract, the mucosa of the paranasal sinuses contains fewer lymphatic vessels. The mucosa of the sphenoidal and the frontal sinus contains only few lymph vessels, compared with the mucosa of the ethmoidal sinuses and the maxillary sinus. The main lymphatic drainage of the paranasal sinuses occurs via the infundibulum, where the lymph vessels of the paranasal sinuses anastomose with those of the nasal cavity (▶ Fig. 1.6). In addition, lymphatic drainage is possible via transosseous lymph vessels from the maxillary sinus into the nasopharynx. The lymphatic network of the nasal cavity and the paranasal sinuses, together with the piriform sinus, pass without interruption into the most dense nasopharynx in the head and neck region [34].

At this point it should be mentioned that, in patients with squamous cell carcinomas, management of the neck without clinically evident lymph node involvement of the maxillary sinus remains controversial. This is because of the low density of lymphatics [56].

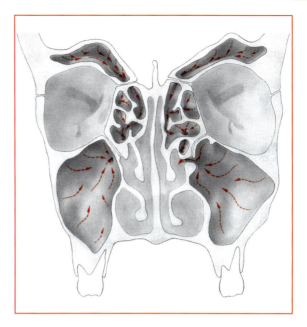

Figure 1.6

Lymphatic drainage of the paranasal sinuses in frontal section. The lymph fluid is mainly drained centripetally to the respective ostia

Nasopharynx

In the posterior wall of the nasopharynx, the lymphatic density varies regionally. High concentrations can be observed at the posterior wall at the transition to the lateral wall and near the eustachian tubal openings. Near the nasopharyngeal roof, the posterior wall and the anterior wall, numerous lymph vessels occur that cross the midline. The physiologic lymphatic drainage of the nasopharynx occurs first in dorso-lateral direction and then in dorso-lateral-caudal direction [34]. Additionally, there is a drainage parallel to the posterior midline [57] that transports the lymph fluid from the roof and the nasopharyngeal posterior wall via 8–12 collectors. The collectors penetrate the pharyngeal fascia at the level of the skull base and drain between the pharyngeal wall and the long muscle of the head. Most of the collectors drain into the retropharyngeal lymph nodes; the others drain into the deep cervical lymph nodes (level II).

Oral Cavity and Pharynx

Oral Cavity

The mucosa of the oral cavity is pervaded by an un-interrupted lymphatic system that can be divided into a superficial and a deep vascular network. The mucosa of the upper and lower lips contain numerous lymph vessels communicating at the corners of the mouth. Their density decreases at the midline of the upper and lower lips without interrupting the continuity (▶ Fig. 1.7 a). The lymphatic drainage (▶ Fig. 1.7 b) is directed mainly in medio-lateral direction in the middle part of the upper lip. The lymph fluid drains from the lateral part of the upper lip via buccal collectors. The lymph fluid originating from the medial part of the lower lip is drained in a manner similar to the lymph fluid from the vestibular gingiva to lymph collectors, i. e., in submental direction at the level of the second incisor (▶ Fig. 1.7 c). The lymph fluid of the lateral mucosa of the lower lip is transported to the collectors (▶ Fig. 1.7 d) situated at the level of the second premolar and the second molar in the submandibular fossa. These collectors also drain the lymph fluid of the lateral vestibular gingiva of the mandible [58].

The lymphatic networks of the mucosa of the lip continue regularly in the dense lymphatic system of the buccal mucosa. About 8–10 collectors absorb the buccal lymph to drain it through the buccinator muscle in the direction of the facial artery and vein, mainly to the submandibular fossa (▶ Fig. 1.7 e). The lymphatic network of the buccal mucosa continues to the alveolar ridge without interruption. The gingiva of the upper and lower jaw are pervaded by dense superficial and deep lymph vessels that cross the midline in the inner as well as the outer sulcus. In the periosteum of the upper and lower jaw, lymph vessels can be observed sporadically over very short distances. These are detected by means of interstitial dye lymphography. The lymphatic drainage of the palatine gingiva of the upper jaw occurs via the lymphatic system of the hard and soft palate. The mucosa of the hard and soft palate is pervaded by a dense superficial and deeply situated lymphatic network. In the midline of the hard palate only a few crossing lymph vessels can be detected. A significant crossing

of the midline is evident in the deep part of the soft palate, including the uvula. At the anterior and posterior palatine arch, lymph collectors are directed alongside the palatoglossal muscle and the palatopharyngeal muscle.

The lymph fluid of the lingual mandibular gingiva is drained via the lymphatic system of the floor of the mouth, where numerous lymph vessels can be detected that cross the midline in the superficial, as well as the deep, network. The lymphatic density of the floor of the mouth is higher than that of the upper and lower lip, the gingiva and the buccal mucosa. The lymphatic drainage of the floor of the mouth occurs first and primarily in dorsal direction alongside the mandibular axis and continues to the collectors draining to the submandibular fossa. Single collectors drain from the anterior part of the floor of the mouth in caudal direction to the submental area, and from the posterior floor of the mouth alongside the medial surface of the angle of the mandible to the oropharynx.

The tongue is pervaded by a dense lymphatic network. Without interruption the superficial lymphatic plexus becomes only slightly denser from the tip of the tongue to the floor of the tongue. In the deeply situated network, a clear ventral-dorsal increase in number and wall thickness of the precollectors, compared with the superficial lymphatic plexus, can be observed. The lymphatic density of the mucosa is higher than that of the muscles. The lingual lymphatic flow reveals regional differences (▶ Fig. 1.7 f). From the ventral undersurface of the tongue, the lymphatic transport occurs mainly in medial direction, and from there in dorsal direction via at least two main collectors. Together with the lymph fluid of the floor of the mouth, a small part of the lymph flows to the submandibular region. The lymph fluid from the mucosa of the dorsum of the tongue is drained mainly in lateral direction and from there to the submandibular region via marginal collectors and in the area of the floor of the tongue in cranio-jugular direction. The lymph fluid of the mucosa localized around the median line flows in vertical direction in the area of the middle third of the tongue via 5–7 collectors situated between the genioglossal muscles. From the posterior part of the tongue, the lymph fluid is drained via collectors drawing through the pharyngeal wall, together with the dorsal lingual veins. Most of these collectors run to the cranio-jugular area. The collectors of the left and right parts of the tongue communicate via precollectors that cross the midline. Crossings of the midline can be observed from the lingual surface to the mylohyoid muscle.

Although it carries a low incidence, a direct lymphatic route or pathway between the oral region and preglandular submandibular node has to be supposed [59]. Furthermore, lymph nodes located in the superficial floor of the mouth associated with the sublingual gland above the lingual nerve may drain a ventral tongue or floor of the mouth carcinoma [60].

The palatine tonsils reveal the highest lymphatic density below the squamous epithelium and in their lateral areas adjacent to the tonsillar fossa. Septal lymph vessels can also be detected, as well as lymph vessels, in the interfollicular and subreticular lymphatic tissue. Our examinations did not reveal lymph vessels in the germinal centers. Penetration of lymph vessels can be observed only where blood vessels penetrate in the capsule formed by the fascia of the upper pharyngeal constrictor muscle. The lingual tonsil and the pharyngeal tonsil reveal a similar distribution of lymph vessels.

Pharynx

The lymphatic networks of the oral cavity communicate unhindered with those of the nasopharynx, the oropharynx and the hypopharynx. The total pharyngeal mucosa is pervaded by a dense lymphatic system that reveals its highest density near the nasopharynx and the piriform sinuses. In the region of the nasopharynx, an especially dense concentration of lymph vessels can be observed at the transition of the lateral to the posterior wall, and in the area of the eustachian tubal ostium. Lymph vessels crossing the midline of the nasopharynx are numerous; they can be detected at the roof and at the posterior and anterior walls. The lymphatic drainage of the nasopharynx occurs from the roof of the nasopharynx; first in dorsal direction, then in dorso-lateral-caudal direction. From the section adjacent to the midline and the posterior wall, the lymph fluid flows via collectors

parallel to the midline. The lymph fluid of the anterior wall of the nasopharynx drains to the lateral wall, where it is transported mainly in caudal direction. The lymph fluid drained caudally is partly transported via horizontal collectors into deeper areas. The lymphatic flow directed via collectors from the posterior wall flows mainly in the direction of the retropharyngeal and accessory lymph nodes. From other regions of the nasopharynx, the flow is to the jugular lymph nodes.

Together with the lymph fluid of the glottic and supraglottic space, the lymph of the cranial hypopharyngeal area flows mainly in dorso-ventral direction, and from the retrolaryngeal mucosa in medio-lateral direction, to collectors that penetrate the lateral part of the thyrohyoid area adjacent to the superior laryngeal artery. The lymph fluid of the caudal hypopharyngeal area is drained via collectors penetrating the cricothyroid membrane. Another drainage pathway occurs in cranio-caudal direction at the posterior wall of the hypopharynx, along the midline which is crossed by numerous lymph vessels.

Larynx and Trachea

Most reports on the lymphatic system of the upper aerodigestive tract refer to the larynx. It is therefore surprising that the findings concerning the lymphatic distribution in the larynx vary more than in other areas of the aerodigestive tract. The density of lymph vessels of the laryngeal region – as well as the question about lymphatic sheaths, or the connection of the laryngeal lymphatic system to the lymphatic system of the pharynx and trachea – are all subjects of controversy.

The earliest complex data on the lymphatic system of the larynx appeared in 1785 and was published by Mascagni [10]. An extended overview of the laryngeal lymphatic system was later provided by Teichmann [55]. The reports rendered by Most [61, 62] led to our present day understanding of the lymphatic system of the larynx. However, the compartments within the lymphatic system of the larynx and regional differences in lymphatic density remain controversial even today.

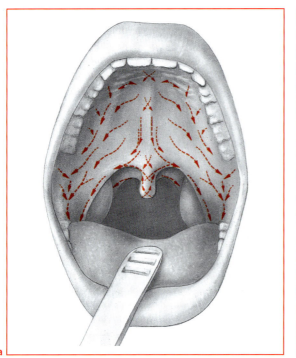

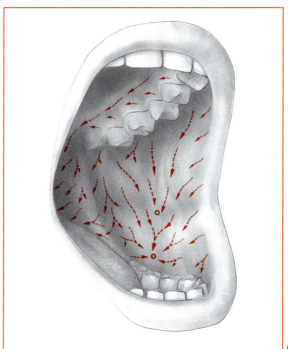

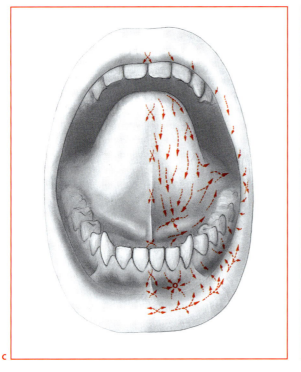

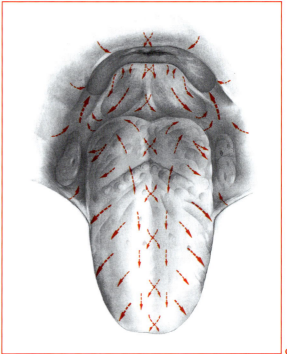

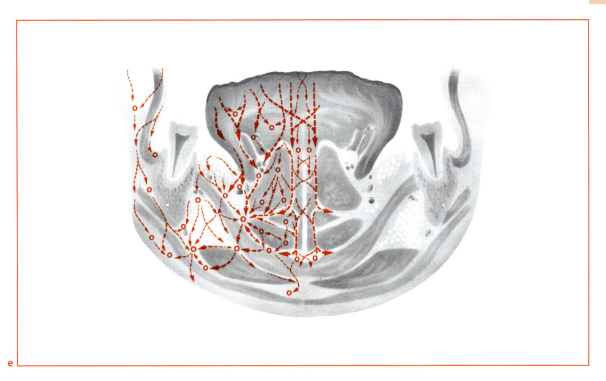

e

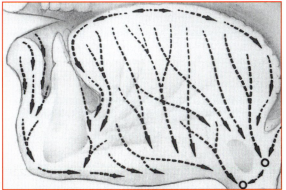

f

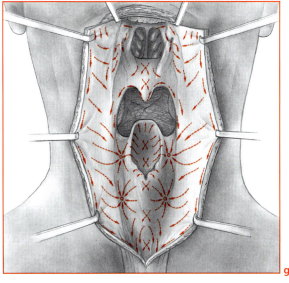

g

Figure 1.7. a–g

a–d Predominant direction of the lymphatic flow of the oral cavity; *o* collectors running deeply. e Lymphatic flow of the tongue, the floor of the mouth and the cheek. Frontal section through the medial area of the tongue and the submandibular region. *1* lingual septum, *2* buccinator muscle, *3* depressor anguli oris muscle, *4* platysma, *5* mylohyoid muscle, *6* digastric muscle, *7* hypoglossal muscle, *8* longitudinalis inferior muscle, *9* genioglossus muscle, *10* geniohyoid muscle, *11* submandibular gland, *12* uncinate process of submandibular gland, *13* sublingual gland, *14* profound lingual artery, *15* submandibular duct, *16* hypoglossal nerve, *o* sagittally arranged precollectors and collectors. f Vertical lymph flow of the tongue. Sagittal section through the tongue. Lymphatic drainage via up to seven collectors located between the genioglossal muscles, *o* collectors running horizontally. g Lymphatic drainage of the pharynx. Dorsal view of the pharynx opened in the posterior median. *1* choanal region, *2* posterior surface of the soft palate, *3* piriform sinus, *4* mucosa of the posterior laryngeal surface, *5* epiglottis, *o* sagittally draining collectors

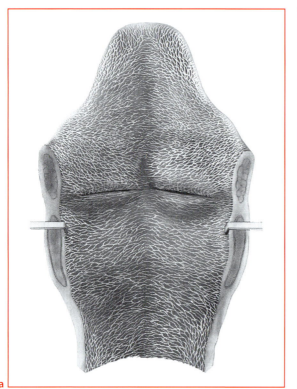

a

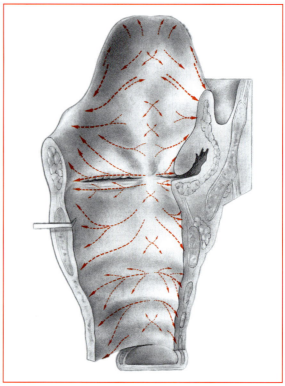

b

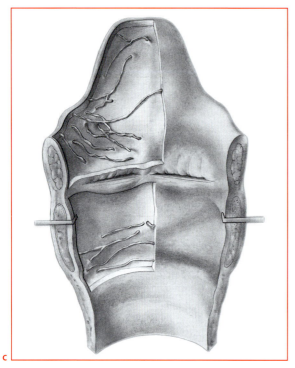

c

Figure 1.8 a–e

a Schematized description of the density of the regional lymph vessels in the laryngeal mucosa. The lymphatic network is the most dense in the supraglottic region. An exception is the area around the epiglottic petiole. Compared to the supraglottic and the subglottic region, the glottic vascular network is scarcely developed. The lymph vessels of the subglottic space are primarily oriented in a circular arrangement. b Main lymphatic drainage direction of the endolaryngeal space. Dorsal view of the larynx opened in the posterior median. c Direction and distribution of lymph collectors in the laryngeal mucosa. The lymph collectors can be detected regularly in the supraglottic and subglottic mucosa. In the area of the vocal cords, lymph collectors are present only in the deeply situated muscles. d Direction of the lymph vessels in the trachea. *Left side*: View on the mainly horizontally directed lymphatic meshes of the anterior wall of the trachea. The dorsal tracheal segment is put to the side along with the esophagus (*right side*) so that the mainly vertical lymphatic direction becomes visible at the tracheal posterior wall. e Lymphatic direction of larynx and trachea in ventral view

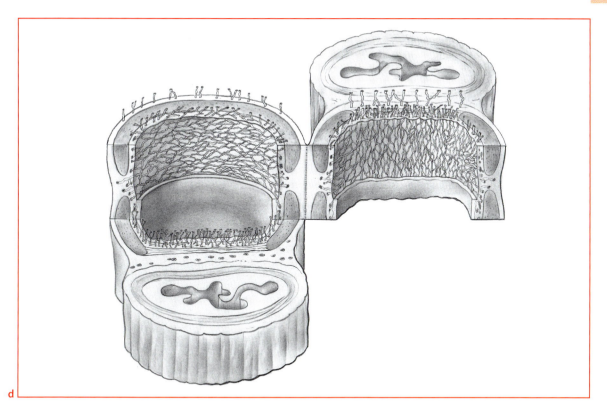

d

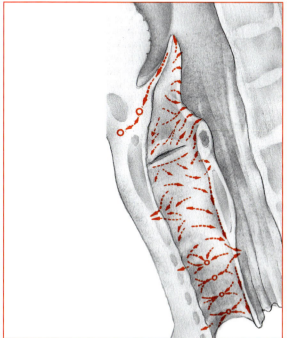

e

Mucosa, submucosa and muscles of the aerodigestive tract contain numerous initial lymph sinuses and precollectors. The number of lymph collectors is comparably lower than the number of initial lymph vessels. Differentiation between the initial lymphatic sinuses and the precollectors cannot always be made by means of light microscopy or the transmission electron microscope. This is why only the term, initial lymph vessel, is used when discussing findings. Because the initial lymph vessel includes both lymphatic parts, it is unnecessary to further complicate the discussion.

The laryngeal mucosa is pervaded by two communicating lymphatic networks, a narrow-meshed superficial one and a wide-meshed deeply situated one (▶ Fig. 1.8 a). Both vascular networks are uninterruptedly connected with those of pharynx and trachea. The lymphatic networks of the larynx are characterized by regional differences in density. There are no barriers to divide the lymphatic network of the larynx into superior and inferior, or left and right. In the superficial lymphatic network, numerous vessels crossing the midline can be observed. The submucous lymphatic network, however, rarely crosses to the contralateral side. The lymphatic density of the larynx is highest in the supraglottic area. Exceptions to this are the mucosa in the area of the epiglottic petiole and in the tissue around the thyroepiglottic ligament. The lymph fluid of the supraglottic space drains in medio-lateral direction (▶ Fig. 1.8 b) via 3–6 collectors through the lateral part of the thyrohyoid membrane. The lymph fluid of the laryngeal surface of the epiglottis drains to the lingual surface of the epiglottis. The main drainage occurs via the free epiglottic edge, although a small part of the lymph fluid flows through pore-like holes localized in the epiglottic cartilage.

The lymphatic system of the vocal fold is least developed in the anterior third. Dorsally, the lymphatic network that is mainly oriented in the direction of the vocal ligament becomes denser under the squamous epithelium. A denser zone is situated under the adjacent areas of the transitional epithelium. The entire mucosa of the vocal cords contains only a few precollectors. Collectors are missing. The vocalis muscle contains significantly more precollectors than the mucosa. The muscle tissue contains at most 2–3 lymph collectors. In the vocal ligament, lymph vessels can be observed only sporadically. The connective tissue of the tendon of the vocal cord penetrating the thyroid skeleton from the elastic noduli contains few initial lymphatic sinuses and sporadic precollectors.

The free edge of the vocal cord does not divide the lymphatic network of the larynx into subglottic and supraglottic parts. Injected dye is preferentially transported via initial lymph vessels to the arytenoid ridge that is directed primarily to the longitudinal axis of the vocal fold. The lymphatic drainage of the arytenoid region concurs with supraglottic drainage. Transportation of dye injected into the vocal cord can be observed only sporadically in the subglottic area or the Morgagni sinus. The transition of dye between the supraglottic and the subglottic areas can be observed only occasionally in the anterior two thirds of the free edge of the vocal cord at macroscopically unchanged tissue. This phenomenon is detected more often in the dorsal region of the vocal cord. The lymphatic network of the glottis continues into the subglottic network without interruption. The lymph vessels localized there are directed mainly horizontally, and the lymphatic flow is limited primarily to one side. Midline crossings, however, are always possible.

The highest density of lymph collectors can be observed in the supraglottic region in the triangle formed by the epiglottis, ventricular fold and aryepiglottic fold. Although lymph collectors are missing in the mucosa of the vocal cord, they occur in the muscles of the vocal cords. About 2cm below the glottic level, regular, mainly horizontally directed, lymph collectors can be observed in the mucosa.

The lymph fluid of the supraglottic and, in particular of the glottic, regions flows mainly to the upper and middle deep cervical lymph nodes (▶ Fig. 1.8 c). Subglottic lymph fluid leaves the endolaryngeal space in ventral direction via collectors through the conus elasticus, and in dorsal direction through the cricotracheal ligament. Lymph fluid is drained to the above-mentioned jugular lymph nodes, to the lymph nodes of the recurrent chain, to the prethyroidal and the pre- and paratracheal lymph nodes and sporadically to the prelaryngeal lymph nodes.

The laryngeal lymphatic plexus continues into the tracheal network without interruption. The lymphatic distribution of the trachea (▶ Fig. 1.8 d) is most dense in the area of the lamina propria. Continuing in subglottic direction, initial lymph vessels develop narrow meshes. The direction of the meshes is mainly transverse according to the position of the tracheal ring. The relatively dense, flimsy lymphatic network of the membranous part of the trachea goes in cranio-caudal direction (▶ Fig. 1.8 e). The efferent tracheal lymph vessels leave the organ primarily in lateral direction, between the tracheal rings, and, sporadically, in ventral direction.

The laryngeal lymphatic drainage is characterized by a high degree of variability. Descriptions of the main drainage pathways that are still valid originate from publications by Most [61, 62] and de Santi [63]. The lymph fluid drains from the supraglottic and from the main part of the glottis via 3–6 collectors at the passage of the superior laryngeal artery through the thyrohyoid membrane, along with the lymph of the cranial part of the hypopharynx. The lymph fluid from these areas is mainly transported to the deep cervical lymph nodes localized cranio- and medio-jugularly. From the subglottic area, the lymph is drained in ventral direction mainly through the conic ligament, and it is drained in dorsal direction through the cricotracheal ligament. The subglottic lymph fluid flows to the deep cervical lymph nodes, the lymph nodes of the recurrent chain, the prethyroidal lymph nodes and the pre- and paratracheal lymph nodes. The subglottic lymph also flows sporadically to the prelaryngeal lymph nodes. It should be pointed out that, in advanced cancer of the larynx, hypopharynx and cervical esophagus paratracheal lymph nodes may be involved [64].

Finally, it is important to mention that all discussions concerning direction of lymphatic drainage must be understood as preferred pathways. In individual cases, the direction and extent of the lymphatic flow can vary enormously [65, 66]. The direction is also influenced by tumors, inflammations, radiotherapy and surgery [67]. It is important to be aware of this variability whenever discussing possible directions of lymphatic drainage.

Salivary Glands

The structure of the lymphatic systems of the major salivary glands is very similar to the structures discussed above. The finger-shaped origin of the initial lymphatic system is situated intralobularly between the glandular acini. Initial lymph vessels transport lymph fluid from the glandular lobules via the interlobular plexus (localized in the interlobular connective tissue) to the subcapsular area and the hilus. In this region, valvular precollectors, as well as sporadic collectors, can be observed. It is evident that lymphatic drainage to the regional lymph nodes occurs, accompanied by blood vessels and the secretory ducts of the glands.

Parotid Gland. The lymph fluid of the parotid gland drains mainly into the deep and superficial parotid lymph nodes. Occasionally, a lymph collector may drain from the anterior inferior portion of the parotid gland, via the masseter muscle, to the submandibular lymph nodes. Drainage of the posterior part of the parotid gland into the accessory chain can also occur, but this is very rare. The efferent lymph collectors of the deep and superficial parotid lymph nodes transport the lymph fluid into the cranial portion of the internal jugular lymph nodes. Lymph nodes in the area of the Rouvière triangle are closely related to the lymph nodes of the accessory chain. This explains the frequent occurrence of secondary metastases of the parotid gland in this area.

Submandibular Gland. The lymph fluid of the anterior and superior part of the submandibular gland drains into the submandibular lymph nodes. From the posterior part of the submandibular gland, 1–2 lymph collectors drain to the subdigastric and principal lymph nodes, together with the facial artery.

Sublingual gland. The anterior part of the sublingual gland drains into the submandibular lymph nodes. The lymph fluid of the posterior part of the gland flows to the subdigastric and jugulo-omohyoid lymph nodes.

Of the cervical salivary glands, the submandibular gland has a higher density of lymph vessels than the parotid gland. The low lymphatic density of the sublingual gland may explain the low quantity of substances transported by means of lymph fluid.

1.1.2 Lymph Nodes

1.1.2.1 Embryology

During the fetal period, lymph node groups develop from the jugular and iliac lymph saccules, as well as from the peritoneal lymph saccus. Due to the invasion of neighboring mesenchymal cells, the so-called lymph sinuses evolve intranodally. Lymph nodes develop shortly before and after birth alongside the big lymph vessels from the mesenchymal reticular cells. The lymphocytes within the lymph nodes that can be detected before birth derive from the thymus and the medulla [68].

1.1.2.2 Morphology

In the human body, there are about 800 lymph nodes, 300 of which are localized in the head and neck. Their physiologic size varies from 1 to 30mm in diameter [54]. To be considered normal, the larger normal lymph nodes must be checked by differential diagnosis to rule out pathophysiologic processes.

Within the lymph node, a large number of lymph follicles are arranged within a small space so that the interstitial liquid from a body region transported through the lymph vessels into the lymph nodes can be controlled immunologically. The filtering function of the lymph node is evident in its structure of loosely meshed reticular connective tissue, as well as in the formation of preferred pathways called sinuses [68].

Lymph Node Structure. As far as function is concerned, the structure of the lymph node (▶ Fig. 1.9) can be divided into three consecutive layers (▶ Table 1.1):

- the marginal zone (with lymph follicles – mainly B-lymphocytes – and marginal sinus) which functions as a site humoral defense;
- the paracortical region (with intermediary sinus and medullar cords – mainly T-lymphocytes) which functions as a site of cellular defense; and
- the medulla (with medullary sinus and medullary cords) which functions as the main site of phagocytosis performed by lining cells and macrophages.

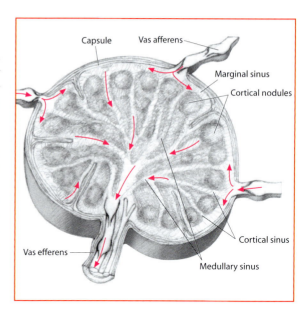

Figure 1.9

Schematized structure of a lymph node

Intranodal Lymph Flow. Lymph fluid is transported by numerous afferent vessels to the lymph node. These vessels interfuse the capsule, which consists of firm connective tissue, and drain into the marginal sinus situated directly below the capsule. Here, all the afferent lymph fluid is collected. The lymph fluid seeps from the marginal sinus through the marginal zone that harbors many lymph follicles. Via the numerous irregularly delimited marginal sinuses, the lymph fluid reaches the medulla, where the lymphat-

Table 1.1. Structure of human lymph nodes under functional aspects

Functional zones from the exterior to the interior	Cellular type	Immunologic function
Cortical zone with lymph follicles and marginal sinus	B-lymphocytes	Humoral defense
Paracortical region with intermediary sinus and medullary cords	T-lymphocytes	Cellularly induced defense
Marrow with medullary sinus and medullary cords	Macrophages and medullary sinus lining cells	Phagocytosis

ic tissue occurs in the form of a network of cords – the so-called medullary cords. Between the medullary cords, the medullary sinuses can be found. The lymph fluid flows via the medullary sinuses and terminal sinuses to the hilus at the beginning efferent vessel. In rare cases, two or three efferent vessels can be observed. Normally, however, there are more afferent than efferent vessels.

Intranodal Vascular Supply. Afferent arteries occur in the lymph nodes in the area of the hilus. They ramify in the medullary region, and, within the marginal zone, they form a dense network around the lymph follicles. Recirculation occurs via post-capillary venules and venous trunks that run parallel to the arteries.

Intranodal Immune Reaction. Antigens reaching the marginal sinus can be bound to the membrane of dendritic cells in the marginal region of the lymph follicles and elicit a defense reaction [68]. The various mechanisms localized to this region include:

- presentation of the antigen by T-helper cells and macrophages, and activation of immunocompetent lymphocytes of the mantle zone;
- conversion of activated B-lymphocytes into basophile immunoblasts that move toward the medulla;
- passage of the paracortical region with an increase or suppression of the immune reaction by T-helper cells or suppressor cells;
- invasion of differentiated plasma cells into the medulla about 5–7 days after antigen contact; and
- diffusion of humoral antibodies from the medullary sinus into the efferent lymph vessels.

1.1.2.3 Topography and Classification of Cervicofacial Lymph Nodes

History

The lymphatic drainage of the head and neck occurs via the approximately 300 lymph nodes of this region. Investigations of lymphatic drainage of the up-

per aerodigestive tract [69, 70] show that the lymph fluid is drained via relatively constant and predictable directions for the various lymph node groups. However, the lymphatic drainage directions discussed in the following section must be understood as only preferred drainage directions that have a high variability, even without prior therapeutic intervention [65, 69].

During the first four decades of the 20th century, the foundation for our current knowledge of clinically relevant anatomic structures of the cervical lymph nodes was established. Important publications include the studies by Poirer and Charpy [71], Trotter [72] and Rouvière [57, 70]. These studies elaborated a classification of the cervicofacial lymph nodes according to their topography and attributed the lymph node groups to morphologically relevant landmarks that facilitate the specific assignment for the surgeon. The anatomic principle was based upon the fact that, despite the ubiquitous lymph node distribution in the cervical soft tissue, accumulations of lymph nodes form lymph node groups at defined points [73]. The above-mentioned authors also emphasized the significance of the lymph nodes localized alongside the internal jugular vein, and they divided them into superior, intermediate and inferior jugular groups [74, 75].

The studies performed by Rouvière deserve separate mention. The final description of his results was published in 1932 [70], with the most important results being published six years later in English [57], a fact that promoted the distribution and appreciation of international literature. Rouvière was able to establish a nomenclature and topography that included information on clinical routine (▶ Table 1.2) and endured for several decades.

In the past, cervical lymph nodes were classified into chains surrounding important vascular and nervous structures of the neck. In particular, cervical lymph nodes were divided into superficial and deep chains, and each of these chains were further divided into lateral and medial chains. The superficial lateral cervical lymph nodes were located along the external jugular vein, and the superficial medial cervical lymph nodes along the anterior jugular vein. The deep lateral cervical lymph nodes were arranged in

Table 1.2. Topography of cervical lymph nodes (LN) according to Rouvière (1938)

Level	Name of LN groups	Subgroup	Characteristics
1	Occipital LN	a) superficial LN b) deep LN	1–6 LN mostly located between edge of sternocleidomastoid muscle and trapezius muscle
2	Retroauricular LN	–	1–4 LN, mostly located caudal to posterior auricular muscle
3	Parotid LN	a) extraglandular LN (a1: preauricular LN and a2: infraauricular LN) b) intraglandular LN	Up to 32 LN (mean: 20 LN)
4	Submandibular LN	a) preglandular LN b) prevascular LN c) retrovascular LN d) retroglandular LN e) intracapsular LN	4–7 LN, inconstantly located according to subgroups
5	Fascial LN	a) mandibular LN b) buccinator – LN group c) infraorbital LN group d) malar LN	Along facial vascular cord, LN above facial muscles, number variable
6	Submental LN	a) anterior LN b) middle LN (b1: medial LN and b2: lateral LN) c) posterior LN	2–8 LN, localized in adipose tissue of submental triangle
7	Sublingual LN	–	Along vessels of tongue and sublingual gland
8	Retropharyngeal LN	a) superior LN (a1: lateral LN and a2: medial LN) b) medioinferior LN	LN localized between pharynx and prevertebral fascia
9	Anterior cervical LN	a) anterior jugular LN b) juxtavisceral LN (b1: prelaryngeal LN; b2: pretracheal LN and b3: LN localized along recurrent nerve	Superior border: hyoid bone Inferior border: sternoclavicular line Dorsal border: carotid sheath
10	Lateral cervical LN	a) superficial LN b) deep LN (b1: N. XI-chain; b2: transverse chain; b3.1: anterior group, b.3.2: digastric LN, b3.3: thyroid group)	a): 1–4 LN, inconstant b): oncologically very important

Table 1.3. Comparison of the cervical lymph node classifications according to Lindberg (1972) and Robbins (2000)

Lindberg 1972			Robbins 2000		
Level	Description	Limitation	Level	Description	Limitation
1	Submental LN	Between anterior bellies of digastric muscles and hyoid bone	I A	Submental LN	Between anterior bellies of digastric muscles and hyoid bone
2	LN of subman-dibular triangle	Localized along lower edge of mandible, 3 subgroups: preglandular, prevascular and retrovascular	I B	Submandibular LN	Between anterior and posterior bellies of digas-tric muscle, stylohyoid muscle and ramus of mandible
3	Subdigastric LN	Between posterior belly of digastric muscle and hyoid bone	II	Craniojugular LN	LN localized between skull base and inferior edge of hyoid bone around internal jugular vein and along XI. nerve. Anterior (medial) limita-tion: lat. edge of sternohy-oid and stylohyoid mus-cles, posterior (lat.) limita-tion: sternocleidomastoid muscle
			II A		In front of (medial to) an imaginary line passing vertically through XI. Nerve
			II B		Behind (lat.) an imaginary line passing vertically through XI. nerve.
4	Mediojugular LN	Mostly single LN localized at carotid bifurcation directly below hyoid bone	III	Mediojugular LN	LN localized between inferior edge of cricoid cartilage around middle third of internal jugular vein. Anterior (medial) border: lat. edge of ster-nohyoid muscle, posterior border of sternocleido-mastoid muscle
5	Caudojugular LN	Localized along internal jugular vein and anterior belly of omohyoid muscle	IV	Caudojugular LN	LN localized between lower edge of cricoid cartilage and clavicle around lower third of internal jugular vein. Anterior (medial) border: lat. edge of sternohyoid muscle; posterior (lat.) border: posterior edge of sternocleidomastoid muscle

Table 1.3. (continued)

Lindberg 1972			Robbins 2000		
Level	Description	Limitation	Level	Description	Limitation
6	Cranio-posterior LN	Localized along the superior part of XI. nerve beside mastoid border of stern-ocleidomastoid muscle	V	LN of posterior triangle	LN located around the lower part of XI. nerve and transverse cervical artery including supraclavicular LN. Upper border: meeting of sternocleidomas-toid muscle and trapezius muscle. Lower border: clavicle. Anterior (medial) border: posterior edge of sternocleidomastoid muscle, posterior (lat.) border: anterior edge of trapezius muscle.
7	Medioposterior LN	Localized along XI. nerve at level of mediojugular LN	V A		Above an imaginary line passing horizontally through lower edge of cricoid cartilage
8	Caudoposterior LN	Localized along caudal part of XI. nerve	V B		Below an imaginary line passing horizontally through lower edge of cricoid cartilage
9	Supraclavicular LN	Located directly superior to clavicle between XI. nerve and internal jugular vein			
			VI	LN of anterior compartment	pre- und paratracheal LN, precricoidal (Delphian) LN, perithyroidal LN including LN along recur-rent nerve. Upper border: hyoid bone; lower border: superior edge of sternum, lateral border: common carotid arteries

three chains: the internal jugular vein, the spinal accessory nerve and the supraclavicular lymph node chains. The internal jugular and spinal accessory lymph nodes were divided into upper, middle and lower nodes. The deep medial cervical group consisted of the prelaryngeal, perithyroidal, pretracheal and paratracheal lymph nodes [76].

In 1972, Lindberg [77] described the distribution of cervicofacial metastases related to the localization of the primary tumor. In contrast to studies published earlier, Lindberg's lymph node classification was oriented directly at the preferred metastatic direction of carcinomas localized in the area of the upper aerodigestive tract. It was Lindberg who developed the concept of anatomically correlated groups of cervical lymph nodes. It was also he who categorized the lymphonodular system in the head and neck on the basis of pathophysiological mechanisms. To achieve this, Lindberg performed a retrospective examination, assessing the medical reports of 2044 patients suffering primarily from untreated squamous cell carcinomas of the head and neck. All patients had been treated at the M.D. Anderson-Hospital in Houston, USA, between 1948 and 1965. A total of 1155 patients had clinical symptoms of cervical lymphogenic metastatic spread. Lindberg described nine lymph node levels on each cervical side, as well as the parotid lymph nodes (▶ Table 1.3). His studies form the basis for our current knowledge of the direction of metastatic spread, a phenomenon which can be predicted with a certain degree of probability. This is significant when searching for occult metastases of know primary tumors, as well as when searching for unknown primary cancers involved in CUP syndrome [74, 75, 78–80].

Topography and Classification

In 1981, Shah and co-workers [81], from the Memorial Sloan-Kettering Cancer Center in New York, described a simplified version of the lymph node classification established by Lindberg. They divided seven cervical lymph node regions according to different levels. In this new classification system, cervical lymph nodes were no longer divided as cranio-jugular lymph nodes, with the cranial part of the lymph nodes arranged alongside the accessory nerve. Instead, they were integrated into level II [82].

According to Shah (1981), the lymph node groups (▶ Fig. 1.10) consisted of:

Level I: submandibular and submental lymph nodes
Level II: cranio-jugular lymph nodes
Level III: medio-jugular lymph nodes
Level IV: caudal-jugular lymph nodes
Level V: lymph nodes of the posterior triangle
Level VI: lymph nodes of the anterior compartment
Level VII: tracheo-esophageal and superior mediastinal lymph nodes

Although, following the classification performed by Shah and co-workers [81], several modifications were made – by Spiro [83] in 1985, Suen and Goepfert [84] in 1987, the American Joint Committee on Cancer (AJCC) and the International Union against Cancer

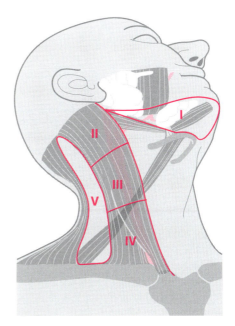

Figure 1.10

Topography of the cervical lymph nodes, according to Shah (1981) [81]

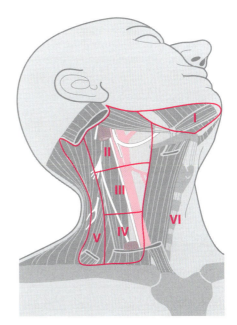

Figure 1.11

Topography of the cervical lymph nodes, according to Robbins (1991) [6]

(UICC) in 1988, followed by Medina [85] in 1989 – the basic structure has not changed significantly.

This despite the fact that head and neck surgeons at the Memorial Sloan-Kettering Cancer Center in New York elaborated a classification of the cervical lymph nodes that defines five levels representing the preferred direction of metastatic spread of carcinomas of the upper aerodigestive tract [81]. Based on this elaboration, the cervical lymph node classification of the American Academy of Otolaryngology – Head and Neck Surgery – was developed. According to this classification, the five levels discussed above are further divided by clinical and surgical assignment (▶ Fig. 1.11). In addition, a sixth level is added containing the so-called anterior compartment. The further division of the cervical lymph nodes into the levels II A and II B (described by Suen and Goepfert [84]) was initially not included in the classification.

Topography of the Cervical Lymph Node Levels
(▶ Fig. 1.12)

Level I is delimited by:
- the body of the mandible;
- the anterior belly of the contralateral digastric muscle and
- the posterior belly of the ipsilateral digastric muscle.

Level II (cranial) goes from:
- the skull base to the carotid bifurcation (surgical landmark).
- In dorsal direction, it is delimited by the posterior edge of the sternocleidomastoid muscle,
- and in ventral direction, by the lateral border of the sternocleidomastoid muscle.
- The accessory nerve divides level II into the level II A, located above the nerve (submandibular recess), and into level II B, situated caudally to the accessory nerve.

Level III (medial) is delimited by:
- the carotid bifurcation (surgical landmark) to
- the crossing of the omohyoid muscle and the internal jugular vein (surgical landmark).

Figure 1.12

Topography of the cervical lymph nodes, according to Robbins (1991). The level I (*blue*) is limited by the body of the mandible and the anterior belly of the contralateral digastric muscle, as well as the posterior belly of the ipsilateral digastric muscle. The levels of the deep jugular lymph nodes (levels II-IV) are printed in *red*. Level II (cranial) goes from the skull base to the carotid bifurcation (surgical landmark). In dorsal direction, it is limited by the posterior edge of the sternocleidomastoid muscle, and in ventral direction, by the lateral border of the sternocleidomastoid muscle. The accessory nerve divides level II into level IIa (submuscular recess), situated superior to the nerve direction, and level IIb, situated caudally to the accessory nerve. Level III (medial) is limited by the carotid bifurcation (surgical landmark) to the crossing of the omohyoid muscle and the internal jugular vein (surgical landmark). In dorsal direction, it is limited by the posterior edge of the sternocleidomastoid muscle and in ventral direction by the lateral border of the sternocleidomastoid muscle. Level IV (caudal) goes from the crossing of the omohyoid muscle and the internal jugular vein (surgical landmark) to the clavicle. In dorsal direction, it is limited by the posterior edge of the sternocleidomastoid muscle and in ventral direction by the lateral border of the sternocleidomastoid muscle. Level V (*yellow*) consists of all lymph nodes of the so-called posterior triangle. It is limited by the anterior edge of the trapezius muscle; in anterior direction, it is limited by the posterior edge of the sternocleidomastoid muscle and in caudal direction by the clavicle. Level VI (*green*) goes from the top of the hyoid bone to the sternal notch. The lateral limitation is localized bilaterally to the carotid artery (design: Gertraud M. Zotter, Berlin, Germany)

- In dorsal direction it is delimited by the posterior edge of the sternocleidomastoid muscle;
- and in ventral direction, it is delimited by the lateral border of the sternocleidomastoid muscle.

Level IV (caudal) reaches:
- from the crossing of the omohyoid muscle by the internal jugular vein (surgical landmark)
- to the clavicle.
- It is delimited, in dorsal direction, by the posterior edge of the sternocleidomastoid muscle; and
- in ventral direction, by the lateral border of the sternocleidomastoid muscle.

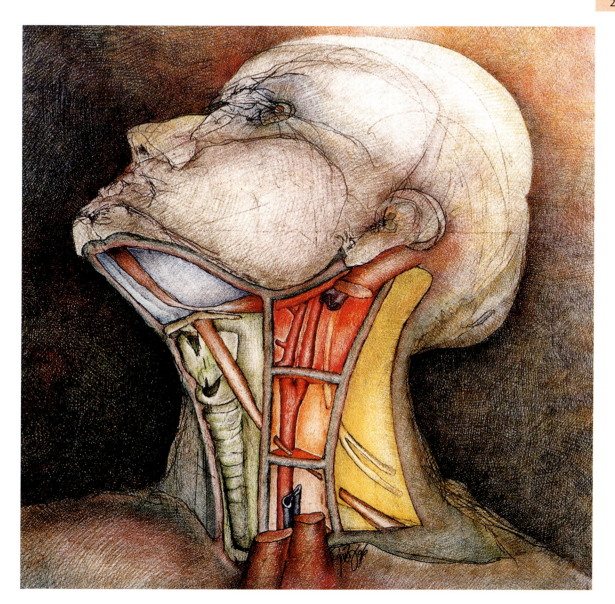

Level V includes all lymph nodes of the so-called posterior triangle. It is delimited:
- in posterior direction, by the anterior edge of the trapezius muscle;
- in anterior direction, by the posterior edge of the sternocleidomastoid muscle; and
- in caudal direction, by the clavicle.

Level VI reaches:
- from the area of the hyoid bone
- to the sternal notch.
- The lateral limitation is located bilaterally medial to the carotid artery.

Further Lymph Node Groups. The retroauricular and the suboccipital lymph noade groups, among others, are not included in the six levels. These lymph node groups are clinically relevant mainly in the context of the lymphogenic metastatic spread of malignant melanomas and squamous cell carcinomas of the back of the head [52].

The *retroauricular* lymph nodes:
- are a group of two to three lymph nodes that are manifest especially in children. In adults, these lymph nodes are mostly atrophied.

The *suboccipital* lymph nodes can be divided into three subgroups:
- three to five superficial occipital lymph nodes in the insertion area of the trapezius muscle along the inferior nuchal line;
- subfascial and deep occipital lymph nodes that are located below the superficial layer of the deep cervical fascia at the splenius capitis muscle; and finally,
- a lymph node that is often found at the so-called splenius portion of the occipital artery.

The *parotid* lymph nodes consists of about 20–30 lymph nodes located mainly lateral to the facial nerve [87]. They can be divided into:
- superficial supraaponeurotic lymph nodes (adjacent to the external jugular vein)
- superficial subaponeurotic lymph nodes
- deep intraparenchymal lymph nodes

The following areas of the head and neck are drained by the *parotid lymph nodes*:
- parotid gland
- cheek
- eye lids
- conjunctiva
- lacrimal gland
- upper lip
- retromolar triangle
- gingiva
- external acoustic meatus
- Eustachian tube

The *submandibular gland*, located in level I, does not contain lymph nodes within its capsule, in contrast to the parotid gland [88].

The *retropharyngeal lymph nodes* are of clinical relevance with respect to the metastatic direction of nasopharyngeal and oropharyngeal carcinomas.

They are divided into a *lateral* and *medial* groups.
- The lateral lymph node group is situated near the skull base, adjacent to the internal carotid artery.
- The medial group is located more caudally, adjacent to the pharyngeal muscles [34].

Modifications to the descriptions of Shah and co-workers [81] were intended to make the classification more precise and to facilitate the determination of the levels under surgical criteria [89]. Applying the classification from 1991, it became obvious that the suggested division into levels was controversial. A typical example was the ongoing discussion concerning the limits of the levels I and II.

Based on the discussions concerning the definitions of the levels and nomenclature for the neck dissection types, the Committee for Neck Dissection Classification, in the American Head and Neck Society, published a revised version (▶ Fig. 1.13 a, b) of the classification for the dissection of the neck [90]. By further defining imaging diagnosis, this published revision provided an obviously improved topographic assignment of different cervical lymph node levels [91, 92, 93]. It also contained a simplified nomenclature of selective neck dissection types, which made a distinction between lymph node groups (▶ Table 1.3) according to the following schema:

- submental and submandibular group
- a cranio-jugular group
- a medio-jugular group
- a caudo-jugular group
- a group containing the posterior triangle
- a group of the anterior compartment

Among other things, however, the classification does not include:
- retroauricular lymph nodes
- suboccipital lymph nodes

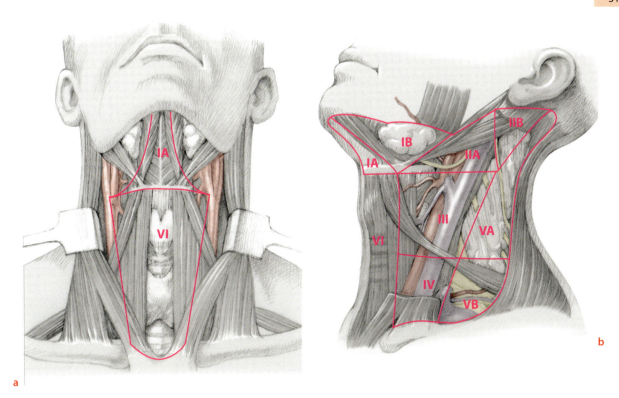

Figure 1.13 a, b

Topography of the cervical lymph node regions according to Robbins (2000) [90]

- parotid lymph nodes
- retropharyngeal lymph nodes

The inclusion of a level VII suggested by Suen and Ferlito [84, 94] will not examined in this publication [90] because the mediastinal lymph nodes are not related primarily to the cervical lymph nodes, nor are they are not involved in the classic neck dissection types.

1.1.2.4 Fascial System of the Neck

The cervical muscles form a kind of shell around the visceral organs and the neuro-vascular track. Their alignment forms the basis for the topographic classification of this region. The muscles themselves are held by three parts of the cervical fascia (▶ Fig. 1.14).

The fascial system of the neck includes the:
- superficial cervical fascia
- prevertebral cervical fascia
- pretracheal cervical fascia (deep cervical fascia)
- visceral fascia
- carotid sheath

Superficial Cervical Fascia. The superficial cervical fascia is a continuation of the body fascia – specifically, in the nuchal fascia. The superficial cervical fas-

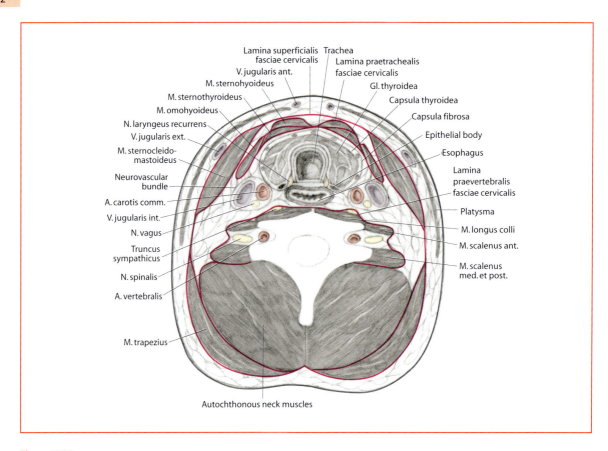

Figure 1.14

Schematized description of the fascial system of the neck using an anatomic profile

cia forms a recess for the sternocleidomastoid muscle and the trapezius muscle. It overdraws the posterior cervical triangle.

Prevertebral Cervical Fascia. The middle cervical fascia forms at the end of the upper thorax apparatus as a triangular tent between the hyoid and the clavicle. Laterally, it reaches the omohyoid muscle and bundles the infrahyoidal muscles, including the sternohyoid muscle, the sternothyroid muscle, the thyrohyoid muscle and the omohyoid muscle. The omohyoid muscle tenses the middle cervical fascia.

Prevertebral Cervical Fascia. The deep cervical fascia forms a recess for the longus colli muscle and the

longus capitis muscle, the scalene muscles, the splenius capitis and cervicis muscles, and the semispinalis cervicis muscle. Furthermore, it is the baseline of the sympathetic trunk up to the upper thoracic apparatus. The deep cervical fascia continues in the axilla, together with the brachial plexus.

The epifascial base of the platysma allows a further drawing of the body fascia in case of head movements, thus allowing a mimic not limited by movement. It divides the subcutis in the anterior cervical region into two layers.

The cervical structure of the muscles in this area is divided by three parts of the cervical fascia (▶ Table 1.4), which explains the regionally limited distribution of the subfascial processes, compared

Table 1.4. Fascial system of the neck

Cervical fascia	Muscles	Particularities
Superficial cervical fascia	Sternocleidomastoid muscle Trapezius muscle	Continuation of body fascia Continuation of fascia nuchae
Middle cervical fascia	Sternohyoid muscle Sternothyroid muscle Thyrohyoid muscle Omohyoid muscle	Tension due to omohyoid muscle
Deep cervical fascia	Longus colli and capitis muscles Anterior scalene muscle Middle scalene muscle Posterior scalene muscle Splenius capitis and cervicis muscles Semispinalis cervicis muscle	Contains sympathetic trunk

with the diffuse distribution of subcutaneous processes. The middle cervical fascia loosens in caudal direction from the superficial cervical fascia. This creates the suprasternal space. The loose connective tissue continues to the mediastinum, and, as a result, the connective tissue space allows the continuation of neck pathology into the thoracic space. Inflammatory processes (e.g. abscesses) of the spine travel along the deep cervical fascia into the posterior mediastinum or the axilla. Due to the direct location adjacent to the cervical fascia, such spinal processes may cause severe lesions.

Visceral Fascia. The so-called visceral fascia surrounds the pharynx, as well as the esophagus, in caudal direction. It also surrounds the larynx, the hyoid and the trachea with the thyroid gland.

Carotid Sheath. The internal jugular vein, the carotid artery system and the vagus nerve all run in this clearly delimited, connective tissue sheath of the neurovascular track. The intermediate tendon of the omohyoid muscle adheres to the connective tissue sheath of the neurovascular bundle and the adventitia of the jugular vein. This enables the omohyoid muscle to keep the lumen of the jugular vein open.

1.2 Physiology and Pathophysiology

The lymphatic system is a drainage system that works in parallel with the venous system. The lymph vessels drain the lymph fluid into the venous system, while the lymphatic organs, such as the spleen, tonsils, thymus and lymph nodes, serve as defense system [95].

The lymphatic system of the human body serves to:
- drain the interstitium
- filter and calculate the protein content of the lymph fluid
- impart cellular and humoral immunity

The physiologic principles necessary to perform these tasks are explained in the following section.

Diffusion

Definition: Diffusion is the accidental movement of molecules in water or gas from a region of higher concentration to a region of lower concentration.

Significance: In the context of substance exchange, the diffusion processes in the human body have an immense importance. The whole task of providing the body with oxygen and disposing of carbon dioxide is performed via diffusion processes. Likewise, the vast majority of the alimentary processes are accomplished by diffusion. Finally, catabolic products are removed by diffusion. The amount of movement occurring through the various diffusion processes in the human body is immense. For example, the amount of liquid passing the total capillary surface is about 240 liters per minute [95].

The velocity of diffusion depends on several factors, including:

- size of the particles – the larger the particles, the slower the diffusion
- difference in concentration – the higher the difference in concentration, the faster the velocity
- distance – the higher the distance, the slower the amalgamation
- total diameter – the larger the contact surfaces of both liquids, the faster the diffusion
- temperature – the lower the temperature, the slower the diffusion
- acceleration of diffusion by warming

Osmosis

Definition: Osmosis is diffusion that occurs artificially in only one direction through a semipermeable membrane.

Because the membrane is permeable for water and more or less impermeable for larger particles, osmosis leads to osmotic pressure. The part of the total osmotic pressure caused by macromolecules and/or colloids is called *colloid osmotic pressure*.

The water transport occurs passively from the region of higher concentration to the region of lower concentration. When there is sufficient permeability for water, the transport of water is practically isoosmolar, i. e., 1 l water per 290 mosmol/kg.

1.2.1 Lymph Vessels

Based on the physiologic mechanisms of diffusion and osmosis discussed above, the lymphatic vessels' primary function is to drain the interstitium and to transport substances in the venous circulation that can only be transported if dissolved in lymph fluid. The lymphatic system thus functions of a drainage system and occurs in parallel to the venous system. Sufficient filtering of the interstitium is of such decisive importance that, in the event of a local collapse of the lymphatic system, a total collapse would lead to death within 24 hours. Interstitial protein deposition leads to local edema with tissue toxicity [95].

A number of substances only soluble in lymph fluid leave the interstitium via the lymphatic system, including:

- proteins
- fats
- cells
- interstitial liquid

Proteins: About half the quantity of circulating protein is drained within 24 hours into the interstitium via the terminal capillaries and postcapillary venules. This includes not only specific protein but also foreign protein – for example: foreign serums; foreign proteins of decomposed bacteria; or cellular proteins of specific decomposed tissue. These proteins reach the lymphatic system via the initial lymphatic sinuses and precollectors, and are drained back into the blood vessels.

Fats: In the context of digestion, the nutrients are decomposed into fatty acids and glycerin. These are then reabsorbed by the intestinal epithelia and synthesized into the so-called chylomicrons (▶ Fig. 1.15). The molecular structure consists of fats in the center and proteins in the outer part. Chylomicrons are drained from the intestinal epithelia into the interstitium, where they are transported via the lymphatic vessels of the intestine, known as the chylous vessels. These meet the cisternae chyli, where an amalgamation of the fatty lymph fluid with the albuminous lymph fluid occurs.

Cells: All types of white blood cells, as well as erythrocytes, can reach the interstitium in the region of two adjacent capillary endothelia via their basal membrane. Additionally, inanimate particles, such as dust or dye, can diffuse into the interstitium by ultra-

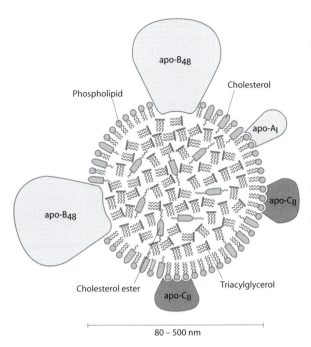

Figure 1.15

Schematized description of jejunal chylomicrons

filtration and be transported via the lymph vessels. In the same manner, the transport of pathogenic bacteria occurs via the lymph vessels.

Interstitial Liquid: This term identifies the liquid that is drained into the interstitium as a net ultrafiltration. Under physiologic conditions, it serves as a solution for the substances that can only be transported by lymph fluid. After absorption of the interstitial liquid into the lymphatic system, the liquid is called lymph fluid. The absorbed lymph fluid can leave the lymphatic vessels, as well as the lymph nodes, during transport. This system of lymphatic vessels transports more than the 2–3 liters of lymph fluid that ultimately reaches the blood circulation within 24 hours.

The formation of lymph fluid occurs in the terminal capillaries of the venous circulatory system. About 90–95 % of the interstitial fluids are generated by capillary ultrafiltration or an increased permeability in the terminal capillary. The other 5–10 % result from aerobic metabolic processes. An active organism consumes about 1000 liters of oxygen of intracellular aerobic metabolism. This leads to the production of about 150–300 ml of water [96].

The interstitial liquid and the substances dissolved in the lymph fluid flow into the lymphatic system through the initial lymphatic vessels. The loose, roof tile-like overlapping of the endothelial cell endings of the initial lymph vessels allows the inflow of free liquid and particles up to a size of 25 nm into the lymphatic system. Larger molecules and whole cells reach the initial lymph vessels via interendothelial junctions that act as valves. The apertures of the interendothelial junctions are controlled by movements of connective tissue. Specifically, this leads to a tension in the elastic fibers that are in contact with the endothelial cells of the initial lymph vessels, which, in turn, leads to openings with a diameter of 100–500 nm [97]. In the context of inflammatory processes, they may even obtain a size of 2000–3000 nm.

Around the initial lymph vessels, a negative pressure occurs under physiological conditions that stimulates the inflow of interstitial liquid and substances that can only be dissolved in lymph fluid [98]. The drainage of the interstitial area is mainly due to this mechanism. The inflow of the interstitial liquid causes an increased intraluminal pressure, which results in the closure of the interendothelial openings. Surrounding larger lymph vessels, a positive pressure can be measured between 3.9–4.5 mmHg [99, 100]. Despite the loose connections of the endothelial cell endings of the initial lymph vessels, the larger lymph vessels resist an intraluminal increase in pressure of up to 80 cm of mercury [101].

For a long time, it was assumed that the intralymphatic protein concentration was responsible for the inflow of interstitial fluid into the initial lymph vessels. Now, however, it is known that this does not play an important role [102]. Another widely discussed transportation mechanism in the lymphatic system is due the process of pinocytosis [103, 104]. Electron microscopic examinations are able to depict luminally, as well as extraluminally, directed vesicular movements in the region of the endothelial plasmatic membrane. Thus, material transport into and out of lymph vessels seems to be possible. Under physiological conditions, however, this process is of secondary importance [102].

Volume Production: The quantity of lymph produced at a certain time is highly variable. Different factors influence this process. These are mainly:

- environmental temperature
- body movement

Under physiological conditions, the organism produces lymph fluid in a quantity of about 0.003 ml/min/100 kg tissue with normal body movement [105]. Within 24 hours, about two to three liters of lymph fluid are drained via the thoracic duct or other large lymphatic trunks into the venous system [95].

The unidirectional transport of lymph fluid from the periphery into the center of the body is important [102]. Examinations with fluorescent isothiocyanate dextran are able to depict an average flow rate of 3.1 cm/min in the lymph vessels [106]. This velocity is seen especially in the post-injection phase. At the end of the filling period, a mean lymphatic velocity of 576 μm/min can be measured. This shows the high variability of the lymphatic system and its ability to adapt to situational requirements. A mean flowing velocity of 282 μm/min has been measured in animal experiments (mouse) for the lymph vessels of the skin [107].

Under physiologic conditions, the flowing velocity of the lymph fluid is influenced by intrinsic and extrinsic mechanisms.

Intrinsic mechanisms include:
- intraluminal pressure
- lymphatic pump

An increased intraluminal pressure correlates positively with the velocity of the lymphatic flow in the thoracic duct [108].

Lymphangio-Motor Function: The vasomotor contractions of single lymphatic parts are supposed to work as a lymphatic pump [102]. The contraction of the lymphatic segment below a lymphatic valve occurs immediately before the contraction of the lym-

phatic segment located above the valve [109]. These spontaneous contractions are easiest to observe in the sitting position [99]. This is how the organism performs the centrally oriented lymph transport function under physiologic resting conditions.

The pumping volume and the frequency of contractions increase when the intraluminal pressure increases to over 10 cm of water [110]. The distension leads to a higher frequency of contractions and of amplitude. The relationship between the transport velocity and the intraluminal pressure is non-linear. This is due to the pumping function of the lymph vessels, which under physiological resting conditions plays a central role in the regulation of the lymphatic flow [102].

The modulation of the vasoconstrictor activity of the lymph vessels seems to be determined mainly by the prostaglandins, thromboxane A2 and prostaglandin H2, which are synthesized in the endothelial cells of the lymph vessels [111]. The application of indomethacin, a blocker of prostaglandin receptors, avoids the perfusion-controlled change of the diameter of the lymph vessels and the vasomotor activity of the lymph vessels. The velocity of the lymphatic flow is also influenced by the undertow of the thoracic duct, which occurs as a result of negative intrathoracic pressure during inspiration [102].

The high compliance of the lymph vessels permits extrinsic mechanisms to exert an influence on velocity. [112].

Extrinsic mechanisms include:
- interstitial pressure
- movement
- temperature

Interstitial Pressure: The interstitial pressure in the area of the terminal lymph vessels influences the absorption of substances that can only be dissolved by lymph fluid into the lymphatic system. It is well known from lymphatic diagnostic procedures that the absorption of large radionuclides can be increased by application of high volumes of liquids. The increase of the interstitial pressure leads to an opening of the interendothelial apertures that allows the inflow of larger particles. It is controversial in

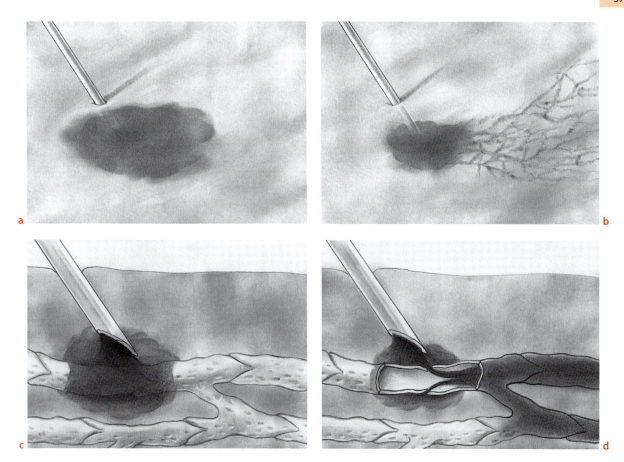

Figure 1.16 a–d

Working principle of indirect ink lymphography. The ink injected through a lymphographic canula (a) leads to an interstitial increase in pressure (b). The resulting tension of the perivascular fiber apparatus leads to an opening of the interendothelial junctions (c). This allows the ink to flow into the vascular lumen through the interendothelial apertures (d)

which manner an increased interstitial pressure leads directly to an augmented velocity of lymphatic transport [109, 113].

Movement: The absorption of substances that can only be transported into the lymphatic system when dissolved in lymph is also influenced by:

- muscular contractions
- arterial pulsations
- respiration
- movements of connective tissue

All the above mechanisms lead to contraction of the elastic collagen fibrils that reach from the surrounding connective tissue into the endothelial cells of the lymph vessels. A dilatation of the interendothelial openings occurs resulting in an increased inflow of liquid that leads to an acceleration of the lymphatic velocity due to intrinsic mechanisms (▶ Fig. 1.16 a–d). In addition, all the same mechanisms have a direct influence on the lymphangiokinetics, and, thus, also on lymphatic velocity.

Temperature: Body and environmental temperature have an influence on the physiological integrity of the organism. A clear reduction in temperature leads to a significant decrease in the absorption of substances that can only be transported when dissolved in lymph fluid and of interstitial liquid into the lymphatic system. In contrast, warming leads to an increased inflow of substances to be transported by lymph fluid and also to an increased velocity in the lymphatic flow.

Some of the mechanisms leading to pathologic changes of lymphatic production and lymphatic flow are:

- inflammation
- venous stasis
- mechanical insufficiency of the lymphatic vessels and valves
- drugs

Inflammation: Increased arterial perfusion seen in inflammatory processes seems to parallel an increase in the volume of the lymph fluid produced [102]. Higher body temperature leads to an increased inflow of substances to be transported by lymph into the lymphatic system. Both mechanisms lead to an accelerated velocity of the lymphatic flow.

Venous Stasis: Venous occlusion leads to an increased production of lymph due to the higher venous pressure. Under physiological conditions, a higher production of lymphatic fluid results in an increased velocity of lymphatic flow. Patients with chronic venous insufficiency have a reduced lymphatic transport [114]. The reduced lymphatic drainage is a possible co-factor in the development of venous ulcers.

Mechanical Insufficiency of Lymphatic Vessels and Valves: There are several types of mechanical insufficiency.. Due to intense dilatation of the lymphatic vessels, the lymphatic valves are dispersed. A functional valvular insufficiency results. Lymphedema that can be observed with filariasis is due to lymphangioparalysis. The lymphatic vessels dilate maximally and no longer pulsate. An increased permeability of the lymphatic wall leads to an unphysiolog-

ically high outflow of lymph into the perilymph-vascular tissue. This type of dysfunction is called insufficiency of the membrane.

Drugs: The vasoconstrictor activity of certain lymphatic parts can be influenced medicinally [102, 111, 115]. Contractions can be elicited by application of:

- noradrenaline
- 5-Hydroxytryptamine
- prostaglandins
- thromboxan-A2 mimetics

A *blockage* of vasoconstrictor activity can be observed with:

- phentolamine
- prostaglandin receptor blockers

Beta-blockers of the propranolol type do not influence the vasoconstrictor activity of the lymphatic vessels [115].

Changes in lymphatic production and lymphatic flow lead to an accumulation of the substances to be transported by lymph in the interstitial space. Within 24 hours, edema develops with circulatory disorders and resulting metabolic tissue injury [95]. Manual physiotherapeutic therapy for the treatment of lymph edemas is based on the influence of extrinsic forces on lymphatic transport.

1.2.2 Lymph Nodes

The defense and immune system consists of, on one hand, the thymus, spleen and lymph nodes, and on the other hand, the lymphatic tissue. The latter can be found in the region of the upper aerodigestive tract, as well as in the mucosa of the gastro-intestinal tract. Due to antigen contact with nutrients and respiratory air, the upper aerodigestive tract can be called the first defense station of the body.

The lymph nodes, located mainly in the fatty tissue and interposed in the lymphatic flow, can be described in groups or as nodular chains along the blood vessels. They represent lymphatic organs with multiple functions.

Shape: Under physiological conditions, there is a high degree of variability in the shape of lymph node groups. Inguinal lymph nodes are usually described as large and rotund. Outer iliac lymph nodes appear as longish masses, whereas inner iliac lymph nodes are small and rotund. Cervical lymph nodes are mostly oval, spindle- or kidney-shaped.

Size: The size of lymph nodes is determined primarily by their function. Another factor influencing size is constitution and age. Conspicuously large nodes generally indicate pathological changes. However, size increase can also be due to diagnostic procedures such as previous lymphography.

Number: The number of lymph nodes in the human body amounts to about eight hundred – three hundred of which are localized in the head and neck region.

Absorption Capacity of the Lymph Nodes: Filling experiments for the calculation of the dose for radionuclide therapy have revealed an average filling volume of 0.07ml per lymph node [116].

Under physiological conditions, the lymph nodes have three main functions:

- biologic filtering
- production of lymphocytes in the context of immune reactions
- calculation of the protein contents of the lymph fluid

Biologic Filtering: Basically, the lymph node is structured as wide-meshed reticular connective tissue (▶ Fig. 1.16 a–d). It works as a filter for the preferred flowing pathways, the so-called "sinuses." The reticular connective tissue contains B- and T-lymphocytes, macrophages, and reticulocytes. Lymph fluid flows from the periphery to the center, i.e., from the capsule to the hilus. The thin-walled lymph vessels that are mostly equipped with valves (vasa afferentia) transport the lymph fluid to the lymph nodes. They

intersperse the capsule and meet the marginal sinus that is located directly below the capsule and surrounds the whole lymph node. Here the total afferent lymph fluid is collected. The lymph then fluid flows over the marginal zone, which harbors numerous lymph follicles, into the marrow, where the lymphatic tissue is arranged mainly in the form of a network of medullary cords. The lymph fluid is transported via the so-called medullary sinus through the terminal sinuses to the hilus and from there to the beginning effluent lymph vessel (vas efferens).

Traveling through the ramified, narrow and wide-meshed sinuses, the lymphatic flow is slowed down. This allows the macrophages located in the sinuses, and the reticular and lining cells located adjacent to the sinuses, to perform phagocytosis, destroying corpuscular elements, bacteria, cellular debris and antigens. The phagocytosis of foreign substances from the filtered lymph fluid occurring in the marrow is an acute defense mechanism of the body. This generally happens prior to immunologic defense reactions.

Immune Reactions: The antigens reaching the marginal sinus, together with the afferent lymph vessels, elicit an immune reaction in the marginal zone that generally proceeds according to the scheme explained below.

The antigens are bound to macrophages and reticular cells at the edges of the lymph follicles. Adjacent T-helper cells and macrophages present the antigen to immunocompetent lymphocytes of the so-called mantle zone (memory cells, B-lymphocytes). The activated B-cells pass in the dark zone of the lymph follicles, proliferate and become extended basophilic immunoblasts. These immunoblasts move into the germinal center of the lymph follicles, where they differentiate into sensitized immunocytes and plasma cells.

About 5–7 days after initial antigen contact, the plasma cells move into the so-called medullary cords. In doing so, they pass the paracortical zone, where many T-lymphocytes are situated within the interdigitating reticular cells. These T-lymphocytes play an important role in the context of immune reactions. Before plasma cells emit the synthesized antibodies into the medullary sinuses, and thus into the lymph vessels, the T-helper cells or suppressor cells must either increase or decrease the immune reaction. From the medullary sinus, the synthesized antibodies reach the efferent lymph vessels and then proceed on to the circulation. This occurs about a week after antigen contact [117].

Recirculation: Generally, the afferent lymph contains about 200–2000 lymphocytes, whereas the efferent lymph contains about 17.000–150.000 lymphocytes. This indicates that a major part of the intranodally measured T-lymphocytes are not sedentary, but leave the lymph nodes from time to time in order to circulate in the bloodstream. The T-lymphocytes situated primarily in the paracortical and parafollicular zone leave the lymph nodes at regular intervals to become sedentary after about 15–20 hours in the same lymph node. This process is called recirculation [68]. The vascular network is probably the precondition for this recirculation. It allows the lymphocytes circulating in the blood to get back into the lymph follicles – specifically, into the adjacent paracortical zones. The precondition for this process is the special wall construction of the postcapillary venules (epithelioid venules). The venules reveal an almost cubic endothelium with a particularly well-structured cellular membrane that is assumed to be recognized by the circulating T-lymphocytes.

The task of the recirculating immunocompetent, and thus specifically sensitized, lymphocytes is to control the lymph according to specific antigens. In the event of specific antigen contact, the T-lymphocytes become sedentary in the respective lymph nodes and elicit a clonal proliferation and differentiation of equal, antigen-determined cells. In the lymph nodes that are not antigen simulated, the number of newly generated lymphocytes distributing the immune response in the whole body is superior in the efferent lymph [116].

Regulation of the Protein Concentration of the Lymph Fluid: Another important role of the lymph nodes is regulating protein concentration in the intercellular fluid. With higher protein concentrations in the afferent lymph, protein-free liquid is filtered into the lymph fluid, which, as a result, is diluted. With lower protein concentrations in the afferent lymph, water is resorbed from the lymph fluid in order to concentrate it. Thus, by modulating the quantity of lymph fluid, the lymph node controls the protein concentration. The dilution of the lymph leads to an increased volume of the lymph fluid draining from the lymph nodes. The resorption of water from the intranodal lymph fluid, however, leads to reduction of the volume of the draining lymph. The volume of afferent and efferent lymph is only equal when the hydrostatic and osmotic pressures are balanced [95].

Tumor draining to regional lymph nodes reveals morphologic and functional changes.

Structural Changes: Tumor draining to lymph nodes generally shows an expansion of the B- and T-lymphocytes, with consecutive enlargement of the cortical region [117]. It also reveals a significant increase in the number of macrophages in the area of the sinuses, especially in the medullary sinus. Histologically, this phenomenon is referred to as sinus histiocytosis. These structural changes are not specific to the tumor draining lymph nodes. They represent a frequently occurring phenomenon that, to date, has not been sufficiently clarified.

Functional Changes: First, reduced filtering capacity must be mentioned. As an example, reduced sequestration of carbon particles with a size of 150 nm has been described in the metastatic colonization of the lymph node [118].

In additional, the immune system is activated via tumor draining lymph nodes [119]. The antigen presentation of tumor cells by means of sinusoidal macrophages and marginal T-lymphocytes leads to an activation of B-lymphocytes. In lymph nodes stimulated by tumor cell antigens, an increased number of macrophages, neutrophil granulocytes and, in particular, natural killer cells, can be observed [117, 119].

Activated T-lymphocytes produce cytokines such as, for example, macrophage stimulating factor, tumor necrosis factor alpha, interferons and epithelial growth factors. These cytokines stimulate other T-lymphocytes, as well as natural killer cells. In the context of this process, some B-lymphocytes differentiate to become memory cells [120].

Activated B-lymphocytes produce antibodies that are directed against the surface of the presented antigens of the tumor cells. In most cases, these are non-specific antigens. As a result, the antibodies produced by the B-lymphocytes are mostly inadequate. Occasionally, however, a presentation of representative antigen structures occurs so that the antibodies can be effective in the control of the tumor cells.

Tumor-Associated Immune Suppression: In spite of local immune stimulation, a generalized, tumor-induced immune suppression occurs in the context of malignancy. This is often magnified by the necessary chemotherapy that alters B- as well as T-lymphocytes.

References

1. Maasa N (1532) Lib Introd Anat
2. Asellius G (1627) De lactibus sive lacteis venis quarto vasorum mesaraicorum genere. Apud Jo. Baptam Bidellium, Mediolani (Exemplar der Universitätsbibliothek Basel)
3. Asellius G (1640) De lactibus sive lacteis venis, quarto vasorum mesaraicorum genere, Ex Officina Johannis Maire Lugduni Batavorum (Exemplar der Universitätsbibliothek Basel)
4. Asellius G (1968) De lactibus sive lacteis venis. Faksimile der Originalausgabe von 1627. Edition Leipzig
5. Bartholinus TH (1653b) Vasa lymphatica nuper Hafniae in Animantibus inventa, et Hepatis exsequiae. G. Holst, Hafniae
6. Rudbeck O (1653) Nova exercitatio anatomica, exhibens Ductus Hepaticos Aquosos et Vasa Glandularum Serosa, nunc primum inventa, aeneisque figuris delineata. Euchar. Lauringerus, Arosiae
7. Pecquet J (1653) New Anatomical Experiments (English translation). London: O Pulleyn
8. Pecquet J (1661) Experimenta nova anatomica, quibus incognitum hactenus chyli receptaculum et ab eo per thoracem in ramos usque subclavios vasa lactea deteguntur. Janssonium, Amstelaedam
9. Glenn WWL (1981) The Lymphatic System. Some Surgical Considerations. Arch Surg 116:989–995
10. Mascagni P (1787) Vasorum lymphaticorum corporis humani historia et ichnographia. Carli, Senis
11. Ludwig C (1858) Lehrbuch der Physiologie des Menschen. Leipzig and Heidelberg, Germany, Winter
12. Kaufman MH (1999) Observations on some of the plates used to illustrate the lymphatics session of Andrew Fyfe's compendium of the anatomy of the human body, published in 1800. Clin Anat 12:27–34
13. Sappey MCP (1874) Anotomie, Physiologie, Pathologie des vaisseaux Lymphatiques consideres chez L`homme at les Vertebres, edited by A. DeLahaye and E. Lecrosnier, Paris
14. Recklinghausen FDv (1862) Die Lymphgefässe und ihre Beziehung zum Bindegewebe. Berlin, Hirschwald
15. Fohmann V (1821) Anatomische Untersuchungen über die Verbindung der Saugadern mit den Venen. Heidelberg
16. Starling E (1908) The Fluids of the Body. Chicago, Kenner
17. Field ME, Drinker CK (1931) Conditions governing the removal of protein deposited in the subcutanenous tissues of the dog. Am J Physiol 98:66–69
18. Yoffey JM, Courtice FC (1956) Lymphatics, lymph and lymphoid tissue. 2nd ed., Arnold, London
19. Cooper A (1840) The anatomy of the breast. Longman, London
20. Moore KL, Lütjen-Drecoll E (1980) Embyologie. Lehrbuch und Atlas der Entwicklungsgeschichte des Menschen. Stuttgart, Schattauer, 291–292
21. Berens von Rautenfeld D, Lüdemann W, Cornelsen H (1996) Die peripheren Lymphgefässe – eine Blackbox der anatomischen Ausbildung – der Versuch eines Kataloges von Mindestanforderungen an Medizinstudenten. In: Tiedjen K U (ed) Lymphologica, Medikon, München, 5–10
22. Dünne AA, Werner JA (2000) Functional anatomy of lymphatic vessels under the aspect of tumor invasion. Recent Results Cancer Research, 157:82–89
23. Kaplan BR, D'Angelo A, Johnson CB (1985) The carbon dioxide laser in pediatric medicine. Clin Pediatry 2:519–522
24. Hannen EJ, van der Laak JA, Manni JJ, Freihofer HP, Slootweg PJ, Koole R, de Wilde PC (2002) Computer assisted analysis of the microvasculature in metastasized and nonmetastasized squamous cell carcinomas of the tongue. Head Neck 24:643–650
25. Schipp R (1968) Feinbau filamentärer Strukturen im Endothel peripherer Lymphgefässe. Acta Anat 71:341–351
26. Daroczy J (1988) The dermal lymphatic capillaries. Springer, Berlin
27. Weibel E R, Palade G E (1964) New-cytoplasmatic components arterial endothilia. J Cell Biol 23:101–112
28. Heusermann U (1979) Morphologie der Lymphgefässe, der Nerven, der Kapsel und der Trabekel der menschlichen Milz. Habilschrift Medical Faculty, University of Kiel, Germany
29. Loose R (1987) Das Lymphgefässsystem der menschlichen Gaumenmandel. Enzymhistochemische und elektronenmikroskopische Untersuchungen zum Vorkommen und Verlauf. Medical Dissertation, University of Kiel, Germany
30. Labusch D M (1988) Das Lymphgefässsystem des menschlichen Appendix. Enzymhistochemische und elektronenmikroskopische Untersuchungen zum Vorkommen und Verlauf. Medical Dissertation, University of Kiel, Germany

31. Berens von Rautenfeld D, Castenholz A (1987) Neues zur Form und Funktion der interendothelialen Öffnungen. Verh Anat Ges 81:751–752

32. Leak L V, Burke J F (1986) Ultrastructural studies on lymphatic anchoring filaments. J Cell Biol 36:129–149

33. Burgdorf WH, Mukai K, Rosai J (1981) Immunohistochemical identification of Factor VIII-related antigen in endothelial cells of cutaneous lesions of alleged vascular nature. Am J Clin Pathol 75:167–171

34. Werner JA (1995) Untersuchungen zum Lymphgefäss der oberen Luft- und Speisewege. Shaker, Aachen

35. Kato S, Gotoh M (1990) Application of backscattered electron imaging to enzyme histochemistry of lymphatic capillaries. J Electron Microsc 39:186–190

36. Okada E (1992) Enzyme-histochemical observation of the cardiac lymphatic vessel using serial paraffin sections. In: Cluzan RV, Pecking AP, Lokiec FM (eds) Progress in lymphology-XIII, Excerpta Medica, Amsterdam

37. Weber E, Lorenzoni P, Lozzi G, Sacchi G (1994) Cytochemical differentiation between blood and lymphatic endothelium: bovine blood and lymphatic large vessels and endothelial cells in culture. J Histochem Cytochem 42:1109–1115

38. Nishida S, Ohkuma M (1990) Ultrastructural-cytochemical demonstration of adenylate cyclase activity in the human lymphatic and blood capillary. In: Nishi M, UchinoS, Yabuki S (eds) Progress in lymphology, Bd.XII, Excerpta Medica, Amsterdam 275

39. Nishida S, Ohkuma M (1990) Enzyme-histochemical differentiation of the human cutaneous lymphatic from the blood capillary-adenylate cyclase In: Nishi M, Uchino S, Yabuki S (eds) Progress in lymphology, Bd.XII, Excerpta Medica, Amsterdam 275

40. Werner JA, Schünke M (1989) Cerium-induced light-microscopic demonstration of 5'-nucleotidase activity in the lymphatic capillaries of the proximal oesophagus of the rat. Acta Histochem 85:15–21

41. Andree T, Gutensohn W, Kummer U (1987) Is ecto-5'-nucleotidase essential for stimulation of human lymphocytes? Evidence against a role of the enzyme as mitogenic lectin receptor. Immunobiology 175:214–225

42. Mukai K, Rosai J, Burgdorf WH (1980) Localization of factor VIII-related antigen in vascular endothelial cells using an immunoperoxidase method. Am J Pathol 4:272–276

43. Sehestedt M, Hou-Jensen K (1981) Factor VIII-related antigen as an endothelial cell marker in benign and malignant diseases. Virchows Arch. (A) 391:217–225

44. Suzuki Y, Hashimoto K, Crissmann J, Kanzaki T, Nishiyama S (1986) The value of group-specific lectin and endothelial associated antibodies in the diagnosis of vascular proliferations. J. Cutaneous Pathol. 13:408–419

45. Svanholm H, Nielsen K, Hauge P (1984) Factor VIII-related antigen and lymphatic collecting vessels. Virchows Arch. (A) 404:223–228

46. Beckstead JH, Wood GS, Fletcher V (1985) Evidence for the origin of Kaposi's sarcoma from lymphatic endothelium. Am J Pathol 119:294–300

47. Mörck Hultberg B, Svanholm H (1989) Immunohistochemical differentiation between lymphangiographically verified lymphatic vessels and blood vessels. Virchows Arch (A) 414:209–215

48. Ordonez NG, Brooks T, Thompson S, Batsakis JG (1987) Use of Ulex europaeus agglutinin I in the identification of lymphatic and blood vessel invasion in previously stained microscopic slides. Am J Surg Pathol 11:543–550

49. Herberhold C (1993) Manuelle Lymphdrainage im Kopf-Hals-Bereich? Laryngorhinootologie 72:580

50. Lubach D, Nissen S (1992) Immunelektronenmikroskopische Untersuchungen der Wandstrukturen initialer Lymphgefässe. In Berens v. Rautenfeld D, Weissleder H (eds) Lymphologica. Jahresband 1992. Kagerer, Bonn 1992

51. Alessandrini C, Guarna CM, Pucci AM, Crestini F, Losi M, Fruschelli M (1992) An immunohistochemical study of basement membrane componentsin human lymphatic capilaries. In: Cluzan RV, Pecking AP, Lokiec FM (eds) Progress in lymphology-XIII, Excerpta Medica, Amsterdam 51

52. Auto-Hermainen HT, Karttunen T, Apaja-Sarkkinen M, Dammert K, Ristelli L (1988) Laminin and type IV collagen in different histological stages of Kaposi's sarcoma and other vascular lesions of blood and lymphatic vessel origin. Am J Surg Pathol 12:469–476

53. Nerlich AG, Schleicher E (1991) Identification of lymph and blood capillaries by immunohistochemical staining for various basement membrane components. Histochemistry 96:449–453

54. Teichmann L (1871) Die Lymphgefässe des Kehlkopfes. In: Luschka v (ed) Der Kehlkopf des Menschen. Tübingen

55. Teichmann L (1861) Das Saugadersystem vom anatomischen Standpunkte. Engelmann, Leipzig

56. Magari S, Asano S (1978) Regeneration of the deep cervical lymphatics. Light and electron microscopic observation. Lymphology 11:57–61

57. Rouviére H (1938) Lymphatic system of the head and neck. In: Tobias MJ (translator) Anatomy of the Human Lymphatic System. Ann Arbor, Edwards Bros

58. Werner JA (1995) Untersuchungen zum Lymphgefässsystem von Mundhöhle und Rachen. Laryngorhinootologie 74:622–628

59. Abe M, Murakami G, Noguchi M, Yajima T, Kohama GI (2003) Afferent and efferent lymph-collecting vessels of the submandibular nodes with special reference to the lymphatic route passing through the mylohyoid muscle. Head Neck 25: 59–66

60. Dutton JM, Graham SM, Hoffman HT (2002) Metastatic cancer to the floor of mouth: the lingual lymph nodes. Head Neck 24: 401–405

61. Most A (1899) Über die Lymphgefässe und Lymphdrüsen des Kehlkopfes. Anat Anz 15:387–393

62. Most A (1900) Über den Lymphgefässapparat von Kehlkopf und Trachea und seine Beziehungen zur Verbreitung krankhafter Prozesse. Dtsch Z Chir 57:199–230

63. De Santi PRW (1904) The lymphatics of the larynx and their relation to malignant disease of the organ. Lancet I: 1710–1713

64. Timon CV, Toner M, Conlon BJ (2003) Paratracheal lymph node involvement in advanced cancer of the larynx, hypopharynx, and cervical esophagus. Laryngoscope 113: 1595–1599

65. Hildmann H, Kosberg RD, Tiedjen KU (1987) Lymphszintigraphische Untersuchungen der regionalen Lymphwege bei Patienten mit Kopf-Hals-Tumoren. HNO 35:31–33

66. Werner JA (1995) Morphologie und Histochemie von Lymphgefässen der oberen Luft- und Speisewege: Eine klinisch orientierte Untersuchung. Laryngorhinootologie 74:568–576

67. Buchali K, Winter H, Blesin HJ, Schürer M, Sydow K (1985) Scintigraphy of lymphatic vessels in malignant melanoma of the skin before operation (en bloc excision). Eur J Nucl Med 11:88–89

68. Rohen JW, Lütjen-Drecoll E (1990) Lymphknoten und Lymphgefässsystem. In: Rohen JW, Lütjen-Drecoll E (eds) Funktionelle Histologie. Schattauer, Stuttgart, 226–232

69. Fisch UP (1964) Cervical lymphography in cases of laryngeo-pharyngeal carcinoma. J Laryngol Otol 122:712–726

70. Rouviére H (1932) Anatomie des lymphatiques de l`homme. Masson et cie, Paris

71. Poirer P, Charpy A (1909) Traité d' anatomie humaine. ed 2, vol 2, fasc 4. Paris

72. Trotter HA (1930) The surgical anatomy of the lymphatics of the head and neck. Ann Otol Rhinol Laryngol 39:384–397

73. Snow GB (1998) Chirurgie des zervikalen Lymphsystems, Teil 1. Laryngorhinootologie 77: A93–9

74. Werner JA, Dünne AA (2001) Value of Neck dissection in patients with squamous cell carcinoma of unknown primary. Onkologie 24:16–20

75. Werner JA, Dünne AA, Lippert BM (2001) Die Neck dissection im Wandel der Zeit. Der Onkologe 7:522–532

76. Ferlito A, Robbins KT, Medina JE, Shaha AR, Som PM, Rinaldo A (2002) Is it time to eliminate confusion regarding cervical lymph node levels according to the scheme originated at the Memorial Sloan-Kettering Cancer Center? Acta Otolaryngol 122:805–807

77. Lindberg R (1972) Distribution of cervical lymph node metastasis from squamous cell carcinoma of the upper respiratory and digestive tracts. Cancer 29:1446–1449

78. Werner JA, Dünne AA, Brandt D, Ramaswamy A, Külkens C, Lippert BM, Folz BJ, Joseph K, Moll R (1999) Untersuchungen zum Stellenwert der Sentinel Lymphonodektomie bei Karzinomen des Pharynx und Larynx. Laryngorhinootologie 78:663–670

79. Werner JA, Dünne AA, Brandt D (2001) Sentinel Lymphonodektomie bei Plattenepithelkarzinomen im Kopf-Hals-Bereich. In: Schlag PM (ed) Sentinel Lymphknoten Biopsie. Ecomed, Landsberg, 129–139

80. Zimmermann I, Stern J, Frank F, Keiditsch E, Hofstetter A (1984) Interception of lymphatic drainage by Nd:YAG laser irradiation in rat urinary bladder. Lasers Surg Med 4:167–172

81. Shah JP, Strong E, Spiro RH, Vikram B (1981) Surgical grand rounds. Neck dissection: Current status and future possibilities. Clin Bull 11:25–33

82. Som PM, Curtin HD, Mancuso AA (1999) An imaging-based classification for the cervical nodes designed as an adjunct to recent clinically based nodal classifications. Arch Otolaryngol Head Neck Surg 125:388–396

83. Spiro RH (1985) The management of neck nodes in head and neck cancer: A surgeon's view. Bull NY Acad Med 61: 629–637

84. Suen JY, Goepfert H (1987) Standardization of Neck dissection nomenclature. Head Neck 10:75–77

85. Medina JE (1989) A rational classification of Neck dissections. Otolaryngol Head Neck Surg 100:169–176

86. Robbins KT, Medina JE, Wolfe GT, Levine PA, Sessions RB, Pruet CW (1991) Standardizing Neck dissection terminology. Official report of the Academy's Committee for Head and Neck Surgery and Oncology. Arch Otolaryngol Head Neck Surg 17:601–5

87. McKean ME, Lee K, McGregor IA (1985) The distribution of lymph nodes in and around the parotid gland: An anatomical study. Br J Plast Surg 38:1–5

88. Spiro JD, Spiro RH (1994) Submandibular gland tumors. In: Shockley WW, Pillsbury III HC (eds) The neck. Diagnosis and Surgery. Mosby, St. Louis, 295–306

89. Robbins KT (1999) Integrating radiological criteria into the classification of cervical lymph node disease. Arch Otolaryngol Head Neck Surg 125:385–387

90. Robbins KT, Denys D and the committee for Neck dissection classification, American Head and Neck Society (2000) The American head and neck society's revised classification for Neck dissection. In: Johnson JT, Shaha AR (eds). Proceedings of the 5th International Conference in Head and Neck Cancer. Madison, Omnipress, 365–371

91. Gregoire V, Coche E, Cosnard G, Hamoir M, Reychler H (2000) Selection and delineation of lymph node target volumes in head and neck conformal radiotherapy. Proposal for standardizing terminology and procedure based on the surgical experience. Radiother Oncol 56:135–150

92. Som PM, Curtin HD, Mancuso AA (2000) Imaging-based nodal classification for evaluation of neck metastatic adenopathy. Am J Roentgenol 174:837–844

93. Som PN, Curten HD, Mancuso AA (2000) The new imaging-based classification for describing the location of lymph nodes in the neck with particular regard to cervical lymph nodes in relation to cancer of the larynx. ORL 62:186–198

94. Ferlito A, Som PM, Rinaldo A, Mondin V (2000) Classification and terminology of Neck dissections. ORL 62:212–216

95. E. Földi, M. Földi (1991) Physiologie und Pathophysiologie des Lymphsystems. In: M. Földi, S. Kubik (eds) Lehrbuch der Lymphologie. 2. Auflage, Stuttgart, Fischer, 185–228

96. Shields JW (1992) Lymph, lymph glands, and homeostasis. Lymphology, 25:147–153

97. Leak LV (1971) Studies on the permeability of lymphatic capillaries. J Cell Biol 50:300–323

98. Allen L (1938) Volume and pressure changes in terminal lymphatics. Am J Physiol 123:3–4

99. Franzeck UK, Fischer M, Costanzo U, Herrig I, Bollinger A (1996) Effect of postural changes on human lymphatic capillary pressure of the skin. J Physiol 494:595–600

100. Spiegel M, Vesti B, Shore A (1992) Pressure of lymphatic capillaries in human skin. Am J Physiol 262:H1208-H1210

101. Delamere G, Poirier P, Cuneo B (1903) The lymphatics. In: Charpy PP (ed) Treatise of human anatomy. Westminster, Archibald Constable and Co. Ltd.

102. Uren RF, Thompson JF, Howmann-Giles RB (1999) Lymphatics. In: Uren RF, Thompson JF, Howmann-Giles RB (eds) Lymphatic drainage of the skin and breast. Singapur, Harwood, 1–20

103. Gangon WF (1979) In: Gangon WF (ed) Review of Medical Physiology. Gulec SA, Moffat FL; Carroll RG (1997) The expanding clinical role for intraoperative gamma probes. In: Freeman LM (ed) Nuclear Medicine Annual 1997, Philadelphia, Lippincott

104. Yoffey JM, Moffat FL, Carroll RG (1997) Lymphatics, Lymph and the Lymphomyeloid Complex. London, Academic Press

105. Jacobsson S, Kjellmer L (1964) Flow and protein content of lymph in resting and exercising skeletal muscle. Acta Physiol Scand 60:278–285

106. Crandell LA, Barker SB, Graham DG (1996) Ultrastructural study of the dermal microvasculature in patients undergoing tetrograde intravenous pressure infusions. Dermatology 192:103–109

107. Berk DA, Swartz MA, Leu AJ, Jain RK (1996) Transport in lymphatic capillaries. II. Microscopic velocity measurement with fluorescence photobleaching. Am J Physiol 270: 330–337

108. Inagki M, Onizuka M, Ishikawa S, Yamamoto T, Mitsui T (2000) Thoracic duct lymph flow and its driving pressure in anesthetized sheep. Lymphology 33:4–11

109. Swartz MA, Berk DA, Jain RK (1996) Transport in lymphatic capillaries. I. Macroscopic measurements using residence time distribution theory. Am J Physiol 270: 324–329

110. McHale NG, Roddie IC (1976) The effect of transmural pressure on pumping activity in isolated bovine lymphatic vessels. J Physiol 261:255–269

111. Koller A, Mizuno R, Kaley G (1999) Flow reduces the amplitude and increases the frequency of lymphatic vasomotion: role of endothelial prostanoids. J Physiol 277:1683–1689

112. Deng X, Marinov G, Marois Y, Guidoin R (1999) Mechanical characteristics of the canine thoracic duct: what are the driving forces of the lymph flow? Biotheology 36:319–399

113. Fischer M, Franzeck UK, Herring I (1996) Flow velocity of single lymphatic capillaries in human skin, Am J Physiol 270:358–363

114. Mortimer PS (1995) Evaluation of lymphatic function: abnormal lymph drainage in venous disease. Int Angiol 14: 32–35

115. Sjoberg T, Steen S (1991) Contractile properties of lymphatics from the human lower leg. Lymphology 24:16–21

116. Kubik S (1974) Anatomische Voraussetzungen zur endolymphatischen Radionuklidtherapie. Die Med Welt 23:3–19

117. Carr I (1983) Lymphatic metastasis. Cancer Metast Rev 2: 307–317

118. Liotta L, Stetler-Stevenson WG (1989) Principles of molecular cell biology of cancer: Cancer metastasis. In: DeVita V, Hellmann S, Rosenberg S (eds) Cancer. Principles and Practice of Oncology. Philadelphia, Lippincott, 98–112

119. Roitt I, Brostoff J, Male D (1989) Immunology. St. Louis, Mosby

120. Hoon, DSB, Korn, E.L., Cochran, A.J (1987) Variations in functional immunocompetence of individual tumor-draining lymph nodes in humans. Cancer Res 47:1740–1744

Lymphogenic Metastatic Spread

The direction and extent of lymphatic drainage and related lymphogenic metastatic spread are influenced among other things by:

- tumor growth
- accompanying inflammations
- surgical measures
- and radiotherapy

The significance of these factors is also critically important in the metastatic process in contralateral cervical lymph nodes for which Ossof and Sisson [1] consider three mechanisms as being responsible.

- The first pathway of metastatic spread occurs via afferent lymph vessels crossing to the contralateral side. This is especially true when ipsilateral lymph vessels are interrupted [2].
- The second pathway of contralateral metastatic spread occurs in areas that are not divided by a midline.
- The third pathway of metastatic spread occurs via retrograde metastatic spread along crossing, efferent lymph vessels; this is observed in cases of extended regional lymph node involvement.

Another example of altered lymphatic drainage direction and related lymph node metastases in unusual locations is the development of metastases at the base of a myocutaneous pedicle of a flap placed after previous extirpation of a carcinoma of the oral cavity or the pharynx. In such cases, lymphogenic metastatic spread can occur through the myocutaneous flap in levels where usually no metastases develop [3].

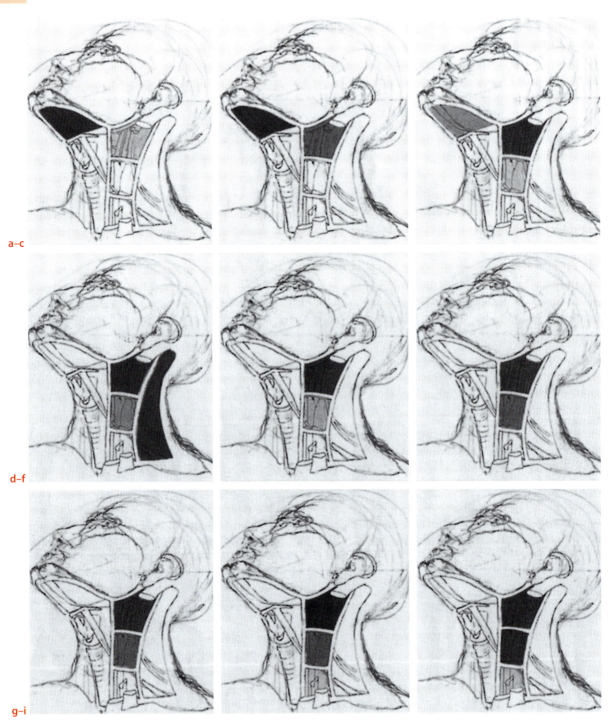

a–c

d–f

g–i

Table 2.1. Metastatic frequency of squamous cell carcinomas of the head and neck

Location of primary tumor	Occult metastatic spread (%)	Metastatic rate (%)	Bilateral metastatic spread (%)
Nasopharynx	28–50	48–90	25–50
Lower lip	3–10	7–37	10–25
Gingiva	17–22	18–52	9–15
Buccoalveolar complex	7–25	9–43	7–13
Floor of mouth	10–31	30–65	8–12
Oral tongue	20–36	34–75	10–15
Retromolar triangle	10–30	32–45	6–12
Soft palate	22–30	30–68	20–32
Tonsil	25–32	58–76	7–22
Base of tongue	22–38	50–85	20–50
Piriform sinus	30–50	52–87	8–15
Supraglottis	16–43	31–70	20–32
Glottis	0.5–12	0.5–39	7–16

Figure 2.1a–i

Schematized description of the main metastatic direction of squamous cell carcinomas of the upper aerodigestive tract. These figures show the initial lymphogenic metastatic pattern of carcinomas in different locations, elaborated by means of an intensive review of the literature; they do not describe the entire metastatic frequency: **a** lower lip; **b** floor of mouth; **c** anterior two thirds of tongue; **d** nasopharynx; **e** palatine tonsil; **f** base of tongue; g supraglottis; **h** glottis; **i** piriform sinus. The probability of initially affected regions increases with the degree of blackening (see [43a])

Examinations of the direction and frequency of lymphogenic metastatic spread are often flawed due to a number of possible sources of error. A significant number of the manuscripts on this topic give insufficient information on their methods. Statements can be variable if the description of location of the metastases is based only on palpation, or only on imaging studies, or, again, only on histological evaluation of the neck dissection (ND) specimen. Likewise, the exact localization of the primary tumor must be accurately defined.

If the preferred direction of lymphogenic metastatic spread is examined in light of the location of the primary tumor, it is useful to examine the untreated sonographic N0 neck, which is then treated with unilateral or bilateral neck dissection with exactly defined dissected lymph node neck levels. Selective neck dissection will give less information on this question than RND or modified RND. This is a critical point to consider when analyzing the often quoted paper by Byers et al. [4], who identified metastatic direction partly on the basis of selective ND.

Examinations fulfilling all mentioned requirements are very rare, a fact that makes clear the already known problem of retrospective analyses. However, the compilation of a large statistical series as performed e.g., by Ganzer [5], who evaluated more than 7000 cases in the literature, can lead to conclusions in regard to certain regularities.

The results taken from the literature and established in our own patient population are summarized in ▶ Table 2.1 and in ▶ Fig. 2.1. In the following discussion, we will not provide another listing of these results; instead, we will focus on the different tumor locations.

2.1 Squamous Cell Carcinomas

2.1.1 Nasal Cavity and Paranasal Sinuses

Carcinomas of the nasal cavity and the paranasal sinuses occur in about 5 % of all malignancies of the head and neck [6, 7]. They metastasize mainly in:

- lymph nodes of level I
- parotid and retropharyngeal lymph nodes
- lymph nodes of level II

With a frequency of 60 %, squamous cell carcinomas form the largest group of sinunasal carcinomas, followed by anaplastic carcinomas, which occur in about 10 % of the cases. This second group is characterized by significantly earlier lymphogenic metastatic spread [8].

The lymphogenic metastatic spread of squamous cell carcinomas of the nasal cavity is about 10 % [9, 10]. It is higher [6] in cases of infiltration of:

- the columella
- the floor of the nose
- the upper lip

Ganzer [5] explains the obvious discrepancy reported in the medical literature of values ranging from 13–89 % for carcinomas of the nasal cavity and the paranasal sinuses. On the one hand, small tumors lead only rarely to regional spread, due to the sparsely developed lymphatic network in this region. On the other hand, carcinomas of the nasal cavity are usually diagnosed only at an advanced stage, when they have already transgressed the borders of their point of origin.

2.1.2 Lip and Oral Cavity

Ninety-five percent of lip cancers involve the lower lip, which usually has a low lymphogenic metastatic frequency. In the upper lip, however, 50 % of all carcinomas develop lymph node metastases in the further course of the disease. Because of this, the presence of occult metastases must be considered when establishing a therapeutic strategy [11].

Ranking second after the carcinomas of the lip, squamous cell carcinomas of the anterior two thirds of the mobile tongue are the most frequently occurring carcinomas of the oral cavity. 75 % of all carcinomas of the tongue develop in this area.

- The lymph fluid of the oral cavity flows mainly in its anterior part to the lymph nodes of level I.
- The lymph fluid from the upper lip additionally drains to parotid lymph nodes.
- The lymph fluid also flows from the lateral tongue and the posterior floor of the mouth into level II.

A tumor that occurs mainly in the oral cavity or, less often, in the larynx [12], rarely metastasizes, according to some authors [13]. Others report that it metastasis does not occur at all [14]. A selective ND does not seem to be appropriate for this tumor entity.

One aspect which has possibly been neglected too much is the metastatic spread of carcinomas of the tongue into lingual lymph nodes [15], which can be divided into lateral and median groups [16]. Ozeki et al. [15] were able to detect three cases of metastases of carcinomas of the tongue in the lingual lymph nodes (one metastasis occurred in the median and two in the lateral group). The possibility of metastatic spread into lingual lymph nodes has led the authors to seriously consider the advisability of en-bloc resection in certain cases. This is because the lingual lymph nodes located above the omohyoid muscle are not dissected in the context of classic neck dissection.

With respect to the dissection of metastatically affected level I lymph nodes, the question as to whether the platysma is to be included in the dissection preparation must be considered [17]. Median submandibular lymph nodes, which frequently have a paramandibular versus submandibular location, are closely related to the platysma. Furthermore, superficial cervical lymph nodes are sometimes situated between the fibers of the platysma. The treating surgeon must be conscious of these problems.

2.1.3 Nasopharynx

The physiological lymphatic drainage of the naso- or epipharynx occurs from the roof of the nose, first in dorso-lateral direction, and then in dorso-latero-caudal direction [18]. Furthermore, there is a lymphatic drainage parallel to the posterior midline, as noted by Rouvière [16]. He stated that the lymph fluid drains from the roof of the nose and the nasopharyngeal posterior wall via 8–12 collectors parallel to the posterior midline. The collectors drain to the retropharyngeal lymph nodes, as well as to lymph nodes of levels II and V. Thus, nasopharyngeal carcinomas metastasize mainly into the lymph nodes of levels II and V.

Lymphoepithelial carcinomas of the nasopharynx have an extraordinarily early and nearly regular involvement of the regional lymph nodes [19]. In many cases, cervical lymph node metastases are the first symptom of a lymphoepithelial carcinoma of the nasopharynx (so-called Schmincke–Regaud tumor).

2.1.4 Oropharynx

The lymphatic drainage of the palatine tonsil and the base of the tongue mainly occurs directly to the lymph nodes of level II [20]. Sporadically, collectors drain to the retropharyngeal lymph nodes and to the lymph nodes of level III.

A notable feature of lymphogenic metastatic spread of oropharyngeal carcinomas is the often detected, but occasionally occult, primary tumor in cases of cystic cervical lymph node metastases that are regressively transformed. These are frequently described as branchiogenic carcinomas (carcinomas in a lateral cervical cyst). In the context of such a diagnosis, an intensive search of the primary tumor must occur (see Chap. 9). In our own patient population, we regularly perform laser surgical resection of the lingual tonsil, which often leads to the diagnosis of a microscopically small carcinoma on the base of tongue with cystically degenerated cervical lymph node metastasis, rather than branchiogenic carcinoma (see Chap. 9.9).

2.1.5 Hypopharynx and Cervical Esophagus

From the hypopharynx, the lymphatic fluid flows mostly via collectors into the lymph nodes of levels II and III. A direct relationship to level I has not been detected. Drainage via collectors into level IV occurs frequently.

The lymphatic drainage of the posterior wall of the pharynx occurs normally first into the retropharyngeal lymph nodes, where the lymph fluid is drained via lymph collectors to the lymph nodes of the levels II and III. As a result, the metastatic spread of a carcinoma of the posterior wall of the pharynx into retropharyngeal lymph nodes amounts to over 40 % [21].

2.1.6 Larynx and Trachea

The descriptions, still valid today, concerning lymphatic drainage of the larynx (▶ Fig. 2.2) originated mainly from examinations by Most and De Santi [22, 23, 24].

The lymph fluid of the supraglottic, and generally also the glottic region, drains to the lymph nodes of levels II and III, along with lymph fluid from the cranial part of the hypopharynx.

From the subglottic space, lymph fluid is drained in ventral direction through the conus elasticus and in dorsal direction through the cricotracheal ligament. The subglottic lymph fluid flows to:

- the lymph nodes of level III, and
- the lymph nodes of level VI.

The prelaryngeal lymph node (the so-called Delphian lymph node) is located on the fascia above the thyroid isthmus, and it lies between the cricoid and the thyroid cartilage [25]. Usually there is only one lymph node, but there may be as many as three, especially in cases where the pyramidal lobe of the thyroid is present. The Delphian node is a midline node and may be seen anywhere in the lower half of the thyroid cartilage itself. Other midline nodes located anterior to the trachea are known as sub-Delphian nodes. The presence of a prelaryngeal lymph node is related to

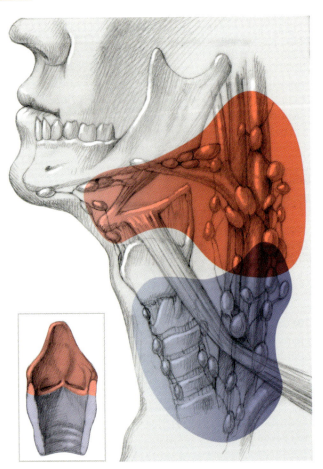

Figure 2.2

Main lymphogenic drainage direction from the supraglottic and glottic space (*red*) – as well as the subglottic region (*blue*) – especially into the deep jugular lymph nodes

the age of the patient. While this lymph node can be detected regularly in children up to the age of 10, only about half of examined adults between the ages of 40 and 75 still have this lymph node.

The *Delphian lymph node* gets lymph fluid from the level of the:

- petiolus;
- the anterior commissure; and the
- subglottis.

The metastatic direction of *laryngeal carcinomas* corresponds in most cases to the described lymphatic drainage of levels II and III.

Regarding the metastatic potential of laryngeal carcinomas, we want to point out that extralaryngeal cancer growths lead to metastasis considerably more often than endolaryngeal carcinomas [26, 27]. In this context, it is also interesting to note that the lymphatic vessels are directed mainly at the pharyngeal clefts according to the embryological development. In cases of tumor invasion in adjacent parapharyngeal spaces, e.g., penetration of a laryngeal carcinoma in ventral direction, lymph node metastases must be expected in atypical levels.

2.1.7 Skin

Squamous cell carcinomas of the skin account for about 20% of malignant cutaneous neoplasms. The majority of these tumors occur in the skin of the head. Carcinomas of skin exposed to sun lead to the development of lymph node metastases in about 5% of the cases.

Squamous cell carcinomas of the facial skin metastasize frequently in the lymph nodes situated in the area of the parotid gland [28]. Squamous cell carcinomas localized in the area of the back of the head mainly metastasize into levels II and V.

Squamous cell carcinomas of the auricle have lymph node metastases in up to 11% of the cases [16]. Metastases of carcinomas of the auricle accumulate in the preauricular parotid lymph nodes (especially when the primary tumor is situated in the ventral part of the auricle), and they also accumulate in the

Table 2.2. Metastatic frequency and survival rate of malignant melanoma patients correlated to the manifestation site

Type of melanoma	Ratio (%)	5-year survival rate (%)
Malignant melanoma of skin	91.2	80.8
Choroid melanoma	5.2	74.6
Melanoma of unknown primary	2.2	29.1
Mucosal melanoma	1.3	25.0

lymph nodes of level II. Initial metastatic spread to occipital lymph nodes is observed only rarely.

2.2 Malignant Melanoma

Malignant melanomas can occur on the skin, in the area of the eye or in the mucosa. According to an extensive analysis made by Chang [29], the survival rate correlates directly with the manifestation site (▶ Table 2.2). Furthermore, different metastatic directions must be considered, depending on the type of melanoma (▶ Figs. 2.3, 2.4). The metastatic frequency of malignant melanomas of the mucosa of the upper aerodigestive tract amounts to about 20– 25 % [30, 31]. Melanomas of the mucosa metastasize in cervical, as well as in axial, inguinal and mediastinal lymph nodes. In comparison, 90 % of melanomas of the choroids metastasize into the liver, whereas pulmonary filiae are observed in only about 20 % of cases, and lymph node involvement in only 6 % of the cases. The lymphogenic metastatic frequency of malignant melanomas of the skin with a greater tumor thickness (>4.0 mm) is between 19 % and 32 %. In malignant melanomas with intermediate tumor thickness (1.5–3.99 mm), the incidence of lymph node metastases is about 7 % [32]. Based on extensive evaluations concerning the so-called sentinel node concept (see Chap. 7.6), extensive knowledge exists on the main metastatic direction of melanomas localized in the area of the skin [33]. Melanomas in the area in front of an imaginary coronal, preauricular line, running from the vertex to the anterior cervical soft parts, metastasize mainly into the parotid gland and into levels I–III (▶ Fig. 2.4). Melanomas situated

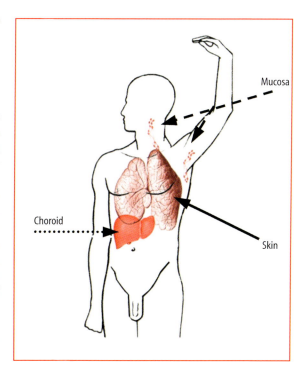

Figure 2.3

Main metastatic direction of malignant melanomas in relation to the location of the primary tumor. Melanomas of the mucosa metastasize into cervical, axial, inguinal or mediastinal lymph nodes. In contrast, melanomas of the choroid metastasize primarily into the liver, whereas melanomas of the skin metastasize mainly into the lung

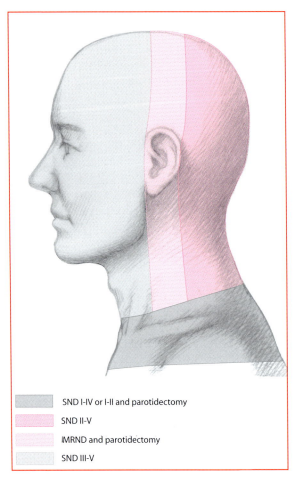

SND I-IV or I-II and parotidectomy

SND II-V

IMRND and parotidectomy

SND III-V

Figure 2.4

Lymphogenic metastatic spread of malignant melanomas from the head and neck; the location determines the indication of selective dissection of cervical lymph node levels (according to Pathak et al. [33])

between a coronal line running pre- and postauricularly metastasize into the parotid gland, as well as into levels I-V. Melanomas situated behind an imaginary coronal postauricular line metastasize mainly into levels II-V, as well as into occipitally located lymph nodes. In individual cases, however, patients can develop lymph node metastases in level I.

2.3 Merkel Cell Carcinoma

The Merkel cell belongs to the so-called APUD system (amine precursor uptake and decarboxylation system). It transmits tactile sensations from the dermal neural endings. Carcinoma of Merkel cells is a rare but very aggressive endocrine tumor entity of the skin, which was first described by Toker [34] in 1972. About 50 % of Merkel cell carcinomas manifest in the head and neck region, mainly in areas exposed to the sun [35, 36]. The red-violet and nodular tumor is located subcutaneously and shows a mean manifestation age of 79 years. The five-year-survival rate is about 60 %. Histopathologically, a distinction is made between the trabecular, or intermediary, type, and the parvicellular type. Merkel cell carcinomas tend to develop early lymphogenic metastatic spread into the regional cervical lymph nodes, which always precedes distant metastatic spread. In about 50–100 % of the cases, histologically detected micrometastases are present, despite a clinically inconspicuous cervical lymph node status [37].

2.4 Carcinomas of the Salivary Glands

Carcinomas of the salivary glands account for about 7 % of all malignant epithelial head and neck tumors, with an incidence of about 1 case per 100,000 inhabitants per year [21]. Spiro [38] reported on tumors of the salivary glands in 2807 patients, the largest series to date of this type of investigation. It became obvious in this series that the highest frequency of lymphogenic metastatic spread occurred when the primary tumor was localized in the submandibular gland, whereas there was no difference in the frequency of lymphogenic metastatic spread when the primary tumor was localized in smaller salivary glands or in the parotid gland. For both primary parotid malignancies and metastatic squamous cell carcinomas, the presence of pathological nodes has a negative influence on survival [39].

The frequency of regional lymph node metastases of carcinomas of the salivary glands is between 20–72 % [5, 40]. Their incidence is directly related to the histological type of the neoplasm (▶ Tables 2.3, 2.4).

Table 2.3. Occult metastatic spread of carcinomas of the parotid gland

	Occult metastases (%)
Acinic cell carcinoma	10
Adenoid cystic carcinoma	10
Carcinoma in a pleomorphic adenoma	21
Adenocarcinoma	35
Mucoepidermoid carcinoma (intermediate grade differentiation)	25
Mucoepidermoid carcinoma (high-grade differentiation)	44
Squamous cell carcinoma	40

Table 2.4. Lymphogenic metastatic spread of the various types of carcinoma of the salivary gland

Tumor entity	Lymphogenic metastatic spread (%)
Acinic cell carcinoma	8–19
Mucoepidermoid carcinoma (high-grade differentiation)	60
Adenoid cystic carcinoma (parotid gland)	10
Adenoid cystic carcinoma (submandibular gland)	34
Polymorphic low-grade adenocarcinoma	10
Epithelial myoepithelial carcinoma	17–25
Basal cell adenocarcinoma	10
Papillary cystadenocarcinoma	30
Oncocytic carcinoma	40–60
Carcinoma of salivary duct	60–80
Myoepithelial carcinoma	10–20
Carcinoma in a pleomorphic adenoma	55
Squamous cell carcinoma	20–58
Undifferentiated carcinoma	40–50
Carcinoma in a cystadeno lymphomatosum	30

Regarding the lymphogenic metastatic spread of carcinomas of the salivary glands, Ganzer [30] noted the importance of differentiating between genuine metastatic involvement, versus direct tumor extension. This is especially important with respect to *adenoid-cystic carcinoma*, where often an infiltration of the lymph nodes by the tumor can be observed. Genuine lymphogenic metastases occur only rarely. However, when they do develop, the prognosis becomes even poorer. In regard to adenoid-cystic carcinomas, it must also be mentioned that they tend to metastasize hematogenously with rates up to 40 % [41].

Finally, the exceptional case of squamous cell carcinoma of the parotid gland must be considered. In contrast to the vast majority of carcinomas (discussed above), this diagnosis requires that an intra- or periglandular lymph node metastasis be ruled out as the origin of the carcinoma. This explains the significantly varying data concerning metastatic frequency, as well as the high rate (up to 70 %) of occult metastases in squamous cell carcinomas of the parotid gland.

Lymph node metastases of *primary parotid carcinomas* are found initially mainly in the parotid lymph nodes and in level II. Carcinomas of the *submandibular gland* metastasize lymphogenously in the same direction as squamous cell carcinomas occurring in this site.

2.5 Carcinomas of the Thyroid Gland

The lymph fluid of the thyroid gland is transported below the fibrous capsule, along the draining veins of the thyroid gland and into the deep superficial cervical lymph nodes. From there, it is transported into the submandibular lymph nodes and into the jugulodigastric lymph nodes situated dorsally to the digastric muscle, as well as into the deep inferior cervical lymph nodes that are localized dorsally to the internal jugular vein and ventrally to the anterior scalene muscle and branchial plexus fibers.

In considering the lymphogenic metastatic potential of carcinomas of the thyroid gland, it is very important to understand that the lymphatic drainage regions of both thyroid lobes are not strictly separat-

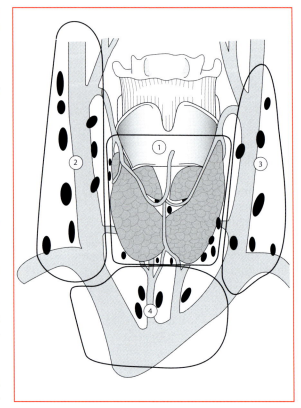

Figure 2.5

In the context of thyroid gland surgery, the described division of the cervical lymph nodes into compartments is widespread. A distinction is made between the central compartment (K1), the right (K2) and the left (K3) cervico-lateral compartments and the mediastinal compartment (K4)

ed. In fact, there is a widely ramified network of lymphatic interconnections by which the prelaryngeal and pretracheal lymph nodes communicate. Furthermore, connections are known to the retropharyngeal lymph nodes and to lymph nodes located in the area of the superior mediastinum [1, 42].

Surgical Division of Lymph Nodes. Compared with the division of the cervical lymph nodes into 6 levels by the North-American Head and Neck Surgeons, the classification made by general surgeons is oriented with respect to the course of the head and neck vessels, and the single lymph node regions are divided into compartments (▶ Fig. 2.5). Accordingly, a differentiation is made between a central compartment (K1), a right compartment (K2), a left (K3) cervico-lateral compartment and a mediastinal compartment (K4) [43].

Central Compartment. The central compartment (K1) includes the lymph node groups located bilateral and medial to the neuro-vascular sheath from the hyoid bone to the left brachio-cephalic vein and the right subclavian vein, respectively. Within the central compartment (K1), a distinction is made between a left central compartment (K1b) and a right central compartment (K1a). The border between the left and the right compartment is the trachea.

Cervico-Lateral Compartment. Here, a distinction is made between the right cervico-lateral compartment (K2) and the left cervico-lateral compartment (K3), which extend laterally from the neuro-vascular sheath to the anterior edge of the trapezius muscle.

Mediastinal Compartment This compartment includes the lymph node groups located inferior to the left brachio-cephalic vein and the right subclavian vein.

In up to 40 % of the cases, metastasis is the first symptom of a malignancy of the thyroid gland. Carcinomas of the thyroid gland show different metastatic patterns depending on the tumor entity.

- The metastatic frequency of *papillary* carcinomas of the thyroid gland amounts to about 50 %. In the literature, the values vary between 25 and 84 %. According to an evaluation by Frazell and Foote [44], in about 61 % of the cases, occult metastases must be expected with papillary thyroid carcinoma.
- For *follicular* carcinoma of the thyroid gland, the metastatic frequency has been described as 2–15 %.
- For the *undifferentiated* (*anaplastic*) carcinoma, the rate is 30 %.
- Finally, for *medullar* carcinoma of the thyroid gland, the rate of metastatic spread is about 70 % [37].

References

1. Ossof RH, Sission GA (1981) Lymphatics of the floor of the mouth and neck: anatomical studies related to contralateral drainage pathways. Laryngoscope 91:1847–1850
2. Larson DL, Lewis SR, Rapperport AS, Coers CR, Blocker TG (1965) Lymphatics of the mouth and neck. Am J Surg 110: 625–630
3. Werner JA (1995) Untersuchungen zum Lymphgefäßsystem der oberen Luft- und Speisewege. Shaker, Aachen
4. Byers RM, Wolf PF, Ballantyne AJ (1988) Rationale for elective modified neck dissection. Head Neck 10:160–167
5. Ganzer U (1992) Das Metastasierungsverhalten von Kopf-Halskarzinomen. In: Vinzenz K, Waclawiczek HW (eds) Chirurgische Therapie von Kopf-Hals-Karzinomen. Springer, Wien, 129–134
6. Barnes EL (1985) Surgical pathology of the head and neck. Vol 1. Dekker, New York
7. von Ilberg C, Kleinmann H, Arnold W (1976) Das Schmincke-Karzinom des Nasopharynx. Laryngorhinootologie 55:420–428
8. Ganzer U, Donath K, Schmelzle R (1992) Geschwhlste der inneren Nase, der Nasennebenhöhlen, des Ober- und Unterkiefers. In: Naumann HH, Helms J, Herberhold C, Kastenbauer E (eds) Oto-Rhino-Laryngologie in Klinik und Praxis. Bd 2. Thieme, Stuttgart, 312–359
9. Stern SJ, Hanna E (1996) Cancer of the nasal cavity and paranasal sinuses. In: Myers EN, Suen JY (eds) Cancer of the head and neck. 3rd ed. Saunders, Philadelphia, 205–233
10. Wustrow J, Rudert H, Diercks M, Beigel A (1989) Plattenepithelkarzinome und undifferenzierte Karzinome der inneren Nase und der Nasennebenhöhlen. Strahlenther Onkol 165:468–473
11. Rudert H (1983) Tumoren des Oropharynx. In: Naumann HH, Helms J, Herberhold C, Kastenbauer E (eds) Oto-Rhino-Laryngologie in Klinik und Praxis. Bd 4/2. Thieme, Stuttgart, 10.1–10.115
12. Glanz H, Kleinsasser O (1978) Verrukköse Akanthose (verruköses Karzinom) des Larynx. Laryngorhinootologie 57: 835–843
13. Schrader M, Laberke HG, Jahnke K (1987) Lymphknotenmetastasen beim verrukösen Karzinom (Ackermann-Tumor). HNO 35:27–30
14. Lee RJ (1988) Verrucous carcinoma of the larynx. Otolaryngol Head Neck Surg 98:593–595
15. Ozeki S, Tashiro H, Okamoto M, Matsushima T (1985) Metastasis to the lingual lymph node in carcinoma of the tongue. J Max Fac Surg 13:277–281
16. Rouviére H (1932) Anatomie des lymphatiques de l`homme. Masson et cie, Paris
17. Lentrodt J (1992) Indikation und Technik der radikalen Neck dissection. In: Vinzenz K, Waclawiczek HW (eds) Chirurgische Therapie von Kopf-Hals-Karzinomen. Springer, Wien, 135–141

18. Jung H (1974) Intravitale Lymphabflussuntersuchungen vom Nasenrachendach beim Menschen. Laryngorhinootologie 53:769–773

19. Thiel HJ, Rettinger G (1986) Der heutige Stand der Erkennung und Behandlung maligner Nasen- und Nasennebenhöhlen-Tumoren. 1. Teil: Pathologie, Diagnostik und Stadieneinteilung der Nasen- und Nebenhöhlentumoren. HNO 34:91–95

20. Rudert H (1992) Maligne Tumoren der Lippen, der Mundhöhle und des Oropharynx. In: Naumann HH, Helms J, Herberhold C, Kastenbauer E (eds) Oto-Rhino-Laryngologie in Klinik und Praxis. Bd 2. Thieme, Stuttgart, 648–668

21. Nicolson GL (1994) Tumor microenvironment: Paracrine and autocrine growth mechanisms and metastatis to specific sites. In: Meyer JL (ed) The lymphatic system and cancer. Vol 28. Front Radiat Ther Oncol. Karger, Basel,11–24

22. Most A (1899) Über die Lymphgefässe und Lymphdrüsen des Kehlkopfes. Anat Anz 15:387–393

23. Most A (1900) Ueber den Lymphgefässapparat von Kehlkopf und Trachea und seine Beziehungen zur Verbreitung krankhafter Prozesse. Dtsch Z Chir 57:199–230

24. Most A (1901) Über den Lymphapparat von Nase und Rachen. Arch Anat Physiol 75–94

25. Ferlito A, Shaha AR, Rinaldo A (2002) Prognostic value of Delphian lymph node metastasis from laryngeal and hypopharyngeal cancer. Acta Otolaryngol 122:456–457

26. Shah JP, Tollefsen HR (1974) Epidermoid carcinoma of the supraglottic larynx. Am J Surg 128:494–499

27. von Ilberg C, Arnold W (1972) Halslymphknotenbeteiligung beim Larynxkarzinom. Laryngorhinootologie 51:258–282

28. O'Brien CJ, Malka VB, Mijailovic M (1993) Evaluation of 242 consecutive parotidectomies performed for benign and malignant disease. Aust NZ J Surg 63:870–877

29. Chang AE, Karnell LH, Menck HR (1998) The National Cancer Data Base report on cutaneous and noncutaneous melanoma: a summary of 84,836 cases from the past decade. The American College of Surgeons Commission on Cancer and the American Cancer Society. Cancer 83:1664–1678

30. Einhorn LE, Burgess M, Vallejos C, Bodey GP, Gutterman J, Mavligit G, Hersh EM, Luce JK, Frei III E, Freireich EJ, Gottlieb JA (1974) Prognostic correlations and response to treatment in advanced metastatic melanoma. Cancer Res 34:1995–2004

31. Shah JP, Huvos AG, Strong EW (1977) Mucosal melanomas of the head and neck. Am J Surg 134:531–535

32. Hansson J, Ringborg U, Lagerlof B, Afzelius LE, Augustsson I, Blomquist E, Boeryd B, Carlin E, Edstrom S, Eldh J, et al. (1994) Elective lymph node dissection in stage I cutaneous malignant melanoma of the head and neck. A report from the Swedish Melanoma Study Group. Melanoma Res 4:407–411

33. Pathak I, O'Brien C, Peterson-Schaeffer K, McNeil EB, McMahon J, Quinn MJ, Thompson JF, McCarthy WH (2001) Do nodal metastases from cutaneous melanoma of the head and neck follow a clinically predictable pattern? Head Neck 23:785–790

34. Toker C (1972) Trabecular carcinoma of the skin. Arch Dermatol 105:107

35. Heenan PJ, Cole JM, Spagnolo DV (1990) Primary cutaneous neuroendocrine carcinoma (merkel cell tumor): an adnexal epithelial neoplasm. Am J Dermatopathol 12:7–16

36. Petrasch S (1998) Management hämatologischer Systemerkrankungen und seltener Tumorentitäten bei Manifestation im Mund-Kiefer-Gesichtsbereich. Mund Kiefer Gesichts Chir 2:172–180

37. Röher, HD (1997) Die Schilddrüse. In: Siewert, JR (ed) Chirurgie, 6. Auflage Berlin, Springer

38. Spiro RH (1986) Salivary neoplasms: Overview of a 35 year experience with 2,807 patients. Head Neck Surg 8:177–184

39. Bron LP, Traynor SJ, McNeil EB, O'Brien CJ (2003) Primary and metastatic cancer of the parotid: comparison of clinical behavior in 232 cases. Laryngoscope 113:1070–1075

40. Spiro RH, Huvos AG, Strong EW (1975) Cancer of the parotid gland: A clinicopathologic study of 288 primary cases. Am J Surg 130:452–459

41. Conley J, Dingmann DL (1974) Adenoid cystic carcinoma in the head and neck (cylindroma). Arch Otolaryngol Head Neck Surg 100:81–90

42. Lanz, T. von, Wachsmuth, W. (1955) Die Schilddrüse. In: Lanz, T. von, Wachsmuth, W. (eds) Praktische Anatomie, Band I/2. Berlin, Springer

43. Dralle, H, Damm, I; Scheumann, G.F, Kotzerke, J, Kupsch, E, Geerlings, H, Pichlmayer, R (1994): Compartment-oriented microdisection of ritgenel lymph nodes in medullary thyroid carcinoma. Surg Today 24:112–121

44. Frazell EL, Foote FW (1955) Papillary thyroid carcinoma. Pathological findings in cases with and without clinical evidence of cervical node involvement. Cancer 8:1165–1166

The Pathology of Lymphogenic Metastatic Spread

R. Moll, A. Ramaswamy

The pathologic examination of cervical lymph nodes aims first at diagnosing a malignant tumor and classifying it histopathologically. This chapter will focus mainly on the cyto- and histopathology of lymph node metastases of squamous cell carcinomas of the mucosa of the mouth, the pharynx and the larynx. For these conditions, the performance of an exact histopathologic staging is very important, both to therapy and to the determination of the patient's prognosis. Another extremely important item is the detection of micrometastases and a determination their prognostic significance. A differentiation must be made between conventional squamous cell carcinomas and special variants that are distinct from a histopathological and/or clinical point of view. Non-squamous malignant tumors within or outside the head and neck region can also develop cervical lymph node metastases. Often the pathologist is asked about the type of primary tumor. Benign tumors and tumor-like lesions of cervical lymph nodes are rare and will only be discussed briefly in this chapter. Additionally, reactive changes and inflammatory diseases of the cervical lymph nodes will be dealt with in view of their significance for differential diagnosis.

3.1 Examination Methods

The least invasive pathologic examination method is fine needle aspiration (FNA) cytology, which has become a highly important diagnostic tool (see also chapters 3.2.2 and 4). By means of a fine needle, the suspect lymph node is punctured –ultrasound directed as needed – and the aspirated cellular material is appropriately smeared on microscope slides. It is recommended that half of the specimens be left unfixed, while the other half be fixed immediately with a commercial alcohol-based fixative spray. The specimens are then sent to the pathologist who stains the unfixed, air-dried specimens according to the method described by May-Grünwald-Giemsa, with hematoxylin and eosin (H&E). The specimens initially fixed with alcohol should be stained according to the method described by Papanicolaou, with H&E and PAS. Both methods are considered to be helpful and complementary [1].

Generally, a histologic examination of completely removed lymph nodes is necessary to make a definitive pathologic diagnosis of cervical lymph node disease. Diagnosis by core biopsy or partial excision is unusual. The exact procedure for both the physician, as well as the pathologist, depends on the clinical question. When the physician suspects a malignant lymphoma (or if FNA cannot definitively diagnose the tumor), excisional biopsy of the lymph node must be performed. The sampling of unfixed frozen lymph node tissue, which was previously necessary in order to achieve an exact diagnosis of lymphoma, is no longer required, due to improved immunohistochemical and molecular biologic techniques, which use formalin–fixed and paraffin–embedded tissue. The complete lymph node specimen should be fixed immediately after resection in buffered 10 % formalin (corresponding to a formaldehyde concentration of 4 %) and taken to pathology. After fixation (normally, 18 to 24 hours – any longer fixation can impair the imunohistochemical and molecular biologic examinations), the lymph node is cut macroscopically in the pathology lab and samples are dehydrated and embedded in paraffin. About 4 µm thick paraffin sections are then routinely stained with H&E. Additional stains needed in cases of malignant lymphomas are PAS and Giemsa. Occasionally, Gomori stains are used.

Immunohistochemical examinations are added in cases of lymphoma, as well as in cases of cancers where routine staining does not allow an exact diagnosis. Additionally, molecular biologic tests can be required in cases of malignant lymphoma. The diagnosis of infectious pathogens is the domain of microbiologic examinations; however, staining techniques

can detect some microorganisms. For example, mycobacteria can be seen with Ziehl-Neelsen or auramine-rhodamine staining. They can also be seen using procedures in molecular biologically, by means of PCR techniques. A significant precondition for a specific pathologic examination is the exact transfer of patient and clinical data from the surgeon to the pathologist. This is facilitated when the pathologist comes to the operating room for frozen section analyses (or when the surgeon goes to pathology), and when the surgeon appropriately orients specimens.

An important area in the surgical pathology of cervical lymph nodes relates to neck dissection specimens. Here, it is not only the diagnosis of the tumor type, but, equally importantly, the exact histopathologic staging that stands at the forefront. First, the neck dissection specimen must be separated into the defined lymph node levels, which need to be analyzed and reported on separately. Ideally, the neck dissection specimen should remain intact and be oriented at the time of surgery with colored needles on cork or polystyrene. The needles should mark the limits of the levels. The specimen is then put into sufficient volume of a fixative (4% formalin). The surgeon should record on an appropriate form this orientation, as well as the clinical history [2].

The pathologic investigation of the fixed specimen begins with a careful visual inspection. If enlarged lymph nodes are visible on the surface of the specimen, it is recommended that the resection margin be marked with dye in order to later determine histologically whether there is extracapsular tumor growth [3, 4]. During sectioning, lymph nodes contained in the fatty tissue of each single level are identified by means of fine laminar sectioning. The use of narrow sectioning, together with careful palpation, is sufficient to detect all lymph nodes (from 2–3 mm) contained in the specimen. Today, complex techniques for rendering the fat tissue transparent, and thus for better identifying lymph nodes [5, 6], are generally not used. Basically, all suspected lymph node structures, even if unclear, should be embedded because metastases can also occur in small lymph nodes. A sufficient edge of perinodal fatty/connective tissue should remain on all lymph nodes, including those that macroscopically are free of tumors, in order to determine microscopic extracapsular spread [7]. The macroscopic documentation includes, for every level, the number of detected lymph nodes, the maximal diameter (i.e., the diameter of the largest lymph node) and the macroscopic suspicion of metastatic involvement. The macroscopic finding of extracapsular tumor extension in particular should be documented, as it is one of the most significant prognostic parameters [8]. The number of examined lymph nodes that can be considered as a certain measure for the quality of the surgery, as well as the pathological examination, depends largely on individual variation. From a potential anatomical total of about 300 cervical lymph nodes [9, 10], an average of 20 to 30 nodes can be found in a neck dissection specimen [11]. In a series of 154 consecutive patients, Woolgar [7] achieved an average of 45 lymph nodes in cases of radical neck dissection, and 21–36 lymph nodes in cases of modified radical neck dissection.

The manner in which lymph nodes are put into cassettes for paraffin embedding depends on their size. Lymph nodes that are smaller than 5 mm in diameter are put in completely without being cut. Larger lymph nodes follow a simple, routinely performed scheme to embed a plate corresponding to the highest diameter, so that the number of the histological lymph node sections is equal to the number of macroscopically prepared lymph nodes [11]. When the focus is placed on the detection of micrometastases, a more extended embedding of larger lymph nodes according to the following scheme is useful. Middle-sized lymph nodes are halved in their longitudinal axis at the level of the highest perimeter, and both halves are put into the cassettes. Lymph nodes larger than 9mm are divided into several parallel sections of 3–4 mm, and they are completely embedded [12]. Care must be taken to ensure that the label for each specimen ensures the definitive counting of lymph nodes for the histological section, especially when there are a large number of sections. The number of lymph nodes detected by histology is decisive, although a false positive number of nodes can be recorded from macroscopic sectioning where dense local connective tissue or vascular sheaths simulate nodes.

After embedding in paraffin, a 4 μm histological section is made from each paraffin block (with complete sectioning of all contained lymph nodes). This is then stained with H & E. Most authors consider one section from each block to be sufficient [7, 11, 12]. However, this procedure (which was investigated by Shingaki et al. [13]) can leave some micrometastases undetected. Shingaki et al. examined 716 cervical lymph nodes that were considered to be tumor-free in the routinely performed diagnosis. Using numerous 5μm serial sections, they discovered that only two of the examined lymph nodes (0.3%) contained mcrometastases (up to a size of 0.5mm) in the marginal sinus. These authors concluded that complex serial sections have no significant diagnostic importance for the detection of lymph node metastases. Another investigator (Woolgar [14]) arrived at a similar conclusion. In a Japanese study, however, 4.2% of seemingly tumor-free lymph nodes had micrometastases detected by means of semiserial sections, which led to a higher PN stage in 12.3% of the patients [15]. These authors recommended an examination of lymph nodes in paraffin blocks by step sectioning at 1mm intervals in order to ensure detection of most micrometastases (see Chap. 3.2.4). The current standard remains nonetheless to create one histological section specimen per paraffin block. Each block corresponds to an interval of 3–4mm between the histologically examined levels, due to how larger lymph nodes are sectioned (see above). To complete the examination, immunohistochemical procedures performed with a cytokeratin antibody can be used to identify small tumor cell groups. Generally speaking, with of squamous cell carcinomas, immunohistochemical procedures do not lead to higher diagnostic precision, when compared with conventional H&E staining [16, 17]. As a result, immunohistochemical examinations are not generally recommended for routine use, even though some studies describe an improved rate of detection of micrometastases in head and neck [18,19] or esophageal carcinomas [20]. With sentinel lymph nodes, however, a more extended histological examination should be performed.

In reporting the microscopic findings, the number of tumor-negative and tumor-positive lymph nodes should be specified for each anatomic region. Morphological parameters of the tumor tissue, such as degree of differentiation or necrosis, must also be recorded. It is important to describe carefully any extracapsular tumor growth (see Chap. 3.2.5). Here, also, the tissue reaction from extracapsular tumor extension, as well as observed vascular invasion, should be documented [11]. Finally, the summary of the findings in the pathological diagnosis must include the definitive pN stage according to TNM classification [21].

3.2 Squamous Cell Carcinomas of the Head and Neck

The origin of cervical lymph node metastases is most often an epithelial primary tumor in the head and neck. One of the tasks of the pathologist is to classify the tumor histologically. The standards used in this classification are documented by the World Health Organization (WHO), and distributed worldwide [22–24]. The spectrum of histological tumor types is very different in the various anatomic regions and organs of the head and neck. ▶ Table 3.1 describes the malignant epithelial tumors included in the WHO definitions [22–24] that may lead to cervical lymph node metastases (with varying frequency) for the most important locations of the head and neck.

In the following discussion, conventional squamous cell carcinomas that occur most often and in nearly all primary locations (▶ Table 3.1) will be described, together with their pathological characteristics. Subsequently, the distinctive variations in squamous cell carcinomas will be addressed. Other tumors will be discussed later in this chapter (Sects. 3.2.3, 3.3, 3.4, 3.5).

3.2.1 Conventional Squamous Cell Carcinoma

Metastases to cervical lymph nodes develop most frequently from squamous cell carcinomas of the head and neck. Sites include the mucosa of the oral cavity, the pharynx, the larynx and the lip. Carcinomas of the cervical esophagus must also be included because, according to the UICC, cervical lymph nodes

are also part of the regional lymph node distribution area [21]. On rare occasion, squamous cell carcinomas occurring in the scalp, facial skin, paranasal sinuses and salivary glands metastasize regionally into the cervical lymph nodes (▶ Table 3.1).

The basis for development of lymph node metastases from squamous cell carcinoma is primary site invasion that breaks into the lymph vessels. Tumor cells are transported to regional lymph nodes. While most of the tumor cells die in this process, due to factors of the microenvironment and the immune response, some cells grow and proliferate, mostly in the subcapsular sinus of the lymph node. Macrometastases develop via the stage of micrometastasis, together with angiogenesis and induction of a mesenchymal stroma [25]. This metastatic focus can further develop locally or spread extranodally. Alternatively, it may metastasize further to new lymphogenic sites along the anatomic lymph node chain, or it may spread hematogenously.

The topographic pattern of the cervical lymph node spread depends on the anatomy of the lymphatic drainage and thus on the location of the primary cancer (described in Chap. 2). Carcinomas of the oral cavity metastasize first into levels I and II, and later into level III, whereas tumors of the pharynx and the larynx spread first into levels II and III [26, 27]. Carcinomas localized at the midline may metastasize bilaterally [27], which is related to a significantly poorer prognosis, compared with unilateral metastatic spread [28]. The assumption that the topographic pattern mentioned really reflects the spatial and timely process of lymphogenic metastatic spread is based on the fact that micrometastases demonstrate these patterns [14, 15]. In certain cases, the location alone of the primary cancer also influences the frequency of lymphogenic metastatic spread. For example, squamous cell carcinomas of the lower lip, the alveolar process and the vocal cords metastasize significantly less frequently than squamous cell carcinomas in other head and neck locations [2, 27].

The lymphogenic metastatic spread of squamous cell carcinomas of the head and neck is correlated with certain morphological characteristics of the primary tumor, e.g., tumor size or the extent of the tumor at the primary site. Two features in particular

Table 3.1. Histological classification of malignant epithelial tumors of the head and neck[a] with lymphogenic metastatic potential (according to WHO: International Histological Classification of Tumours [22–24])

Tumor type	ICD-O-/SNOMED-key[b]	Oral mucosa	Nose, paranasal sinuses	Nasopharynx	Larynx, Hypopharynx, Trachea	Salivary glands
Squamous cell carcinoma	8070/3	x	x	x	x	x
Basaloid squamous cell carcinoma	8094/3	x	–	–	x	–
Adenoid squamous cell carcinoma	8075/3	x	–	–	x	–
Spindle cell carcinoma	8074/3	x	x	–	x	–
Adenosquamous carcinoma	8560/3	x	x	–	x	–
Undifferentiated carcinoma	8020/3	x	–	–	–	x
Undifferentiated lymphoepithelial carcinoma	8082/3, 8020/3[c]	–	x	x	x	x[d]
Sinonasal columnar (transitional) cell carcinoma	8121/3	–	x	–	–	–
Giant cell carcinoma	8031/3	–	–	–	x	–
Adenocarcinoma	8140/3	–	x	x	x	x
Papillary adenocarcinoma	8260/3	–	x	x	–	–
Adenocarcinoma of the intestinal type	8144/3	–	x	–	–	–
Mucinous adenocarcinoma	8480/3	–	x	–	–	x
Acinar cell carcinoma	8550/3	–	x	–	x	x
Mucoepidermoid carcinoma	8430/3	–	x	x	x	x
Adenoid-cystic carcinoma	8200/3	–	x	x	x	x
Polymorphous low-grade adenocarcinoma	–	–	x	x	–	x
Papillary cystadenocarcinoma	8450/3	–	–	–	–	x
Carcinoma in a pleomorphic adenoma	8941/3	–	x	–	x	x
Malignant myoepithelioma	8982/3	–	x	–	–	x
Epithelial-myoepithelial carcinoma	8562/3	–	x	–	x	x
Clear cell carcinoma	8310/3	–	x	–	x	–
Salivary duct carcinoma	8500/3	–	–	–	x	x
Basal cell adenocarcinoma	8147/3	–	–	–	–	x
Sebaceous gland carcinoma	8410/3	–	–	–	–	x
Oncocytic carcinoma	8290/3	–	–	–	–	x
Atypical carcinoid tumor	8246/3	–	x	–	x	–
Small cell (neuroendocrine) carcinoma	8041/3	–	x	–	x	x

x = presence; – = absence
a Not including skin, eye, ear, oropharynx, tonsils and thyroid gland
b According to ICD-O (International Classification of Diseases for Oncology) and SNOMED (Systematized Nomenclature of Medicine)
c Undifferentiated nasopharyngeal carcinoma
d Especially occurring in Inuit and Chinese [23]

seem to be responsible for the risk of developing lymph node metastases. These include the diameter of the tumor [29] and the invasion depth, i.e., the distance between the (virtual) level of the basal layer of the normal mucosa and the level of the deepest tumor infiltration [16, 30]. In a series of 128 patients, those with tumors infiltrating deeper than 4mm showed a statistically significantly higher positive nodal status than those with less deeply infiltrating tumors [16]. The extent of the vertical tumor is not considered in the Pt classification of the UICC or the AJCC. Only the largest extent (in terms of the horizontal diameter) is included [21], which, by itself, is less relevant in predicting lymph node metastases.

Important histopathologic factors for lymphogenic metastatic frequency are the histological degree of malignancy (excluding nuclear polymorphism), the detection of tumor cells in lymph vessels (lymphangiosis carcinomatosa) and perineural invasion [2, 29]. All of these findings correlate with a high invasive potential.

The histopathological appearance of metastases from squamous cell carcinomas generally corresponds to that of the primary tumor, although, occasionally, a varying degree of differentiation or malignancy can be observed between the primary site and metastasis. Generally, histological classification is not a problem for metastases from conventional squamous cell carcinomas, where aggregations of atypical squamous cells with or without keratinization are observed. Difficulties arise only in cases of tumors with a low degree of differentiation (see below).

The most important morphological indicator as far as conventional squamous cell carcinomas are concerned is the grading, i.e., the determination of the degree of differentiation (or the degree of malignancy). The parameters defining the degree of differentiation include, on the one hand, general criteria for differentiation and, on the other hand, cytologic and histological criteria for malignancy. The general differentiation parameters for squamous cells include signs of tissue maturity, such as a diversification from peripheral basal cells to larger squamous cells migrating in central direction, the formation of intercellular bridges (analogous to the prickle cell layer) and keratinization, which occurs in the form of

single cell keratinization or so-called keratin pearls. The keratinization of a squamous cell carcinoma represents mostly a focal terminal differentiation of squamous cells that can be sustained in cases of malignant keratinocytes, and it is related to an excessive synthesis of keratin proteins (squamous epithelial-type cytokeratins of the maturity subgroup) [31]. The keratin pearls that develop centrally in tumor cell aggregations generally correspond to a parakeratosis (still visible pyknotic cell nuclei) or, considerably less often, to orthokeratosis. In some lymph node metastases, the keratinization even results in extended keratin-laden masses that can also calcify. The tendency towards keratinization depends only to a small degree on the keratinized or unkeratinized character of the normal original epithelium. For example, carcinomas of the lip are often well differentiated and highly keratinizing [32], whereas the unkeratinized squamous cells of the floor of the mouth, the oropharynx or the hypopharynx can develop keratinizing squamous cell carcinomas. With respect to these last tumor types, the biologic alteration of the subtype of squamous differentiation, a fact that is also reflected in the expression pattern of the cytokeratins [31], should be stressed.

While the above parameters of differentiation decrease in the course of the spectrum from well-differentiated to less-differentiated squamous cell carcinomas, the cytological and histological criteria of malignancy increase. The cytological parameters of malignancy include the enlargement, pleomorphism and hyperchromasia of the cell nuclei, an increased nuclear-cytoplasmatic ratio and increased (and partly atypical) mitoses. These morphological findings reflect disturbances in the genetic material of the tumor cells. The most important histological criterion for malignancy is the pattern of infiltration at the invasion site. A high dissociating growth shows a higher degree of malignancy. Accordingly, squamous cell carcinomas are divided into the degrees G1, G2, G3 and (when necessary – see below) also G4. Well differentiated (G1) squamous cell carcinomas (▶ Fig. 3.1) show characteristic differentiation patterns, such as a cytological differentiation in basal cells and maturing squamous cells, well developed intercellular bridges and a clear keratinization, while nuclear

Figure 3.1

Cervical lymph node metastasis of a well differentiated squamous cell carcinoma (G1) with atypical squamous cell aggregations with only low-grade nuclear pleomorphism and central keratinization in the surrounding intact lymphatic tissue. H&E

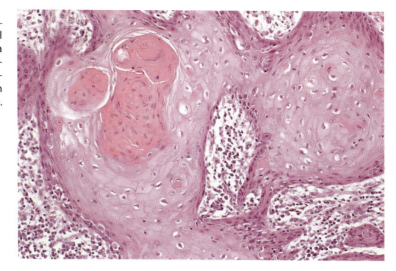

Figure 3.2

Moderately differentiated metastasis of squamous cell carcinoma (G2) in a lymph node with squamous cells showing middle-grade nuclear pleomorphism and partial central keratinization with a smaller area of necrosis. H&E

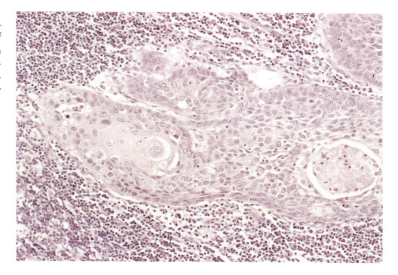

pleomorphism as a criterion of malignancy is minimal. Moderately differentiated (G2) squamous cell carcinomas (▶ Fig. 3.2) are characterized by less developed intercellular bridges and a low degree of keratinization, but moderate nuclear pleomorphism. Poorly differentiated (G3) squamous cell carcinomas (▶ Fig. 3.3) have rare or even missing intercellular bridges and keratinization, but they have highly developed cytological criteria of malignancy, such as severe nuclear pleomorphism.

With respect to the above-mentioned parameters, the WHO defines [22] the manner in which to elaborate on the degree of differentiation during the routinely performed pathological evaluation. This grading is based in principle on an old concept developed by Broders [33], who considered the percentage of differentiated cells in the tumor as decisive. While in many cases grading can be established in a satisfactory way, occasionally significant difficulties can arise concerning the exact determination of the degree of

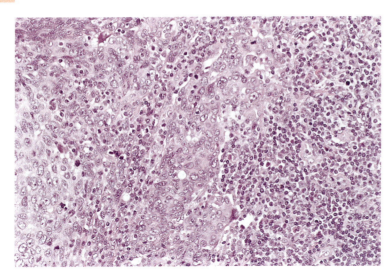

Figure 3.3

Lymph node metastasis of a non-keratinized, poorly differentiated squamous cell carcinoma (G3) with solid epithelial cell aggregations with clear nuclear irregularities without light microscopic detection of intercellular bridges or keratinization. H&E

differentiation. The problem is that the parameters of differentiation and malignancy represent a more or less continuous spectrum and are not defined quantitatively. For this reason, the grading is rather subjective, and the consensus of different examiners (the "interobserver agreement") is low [22]. Furthermore, single parameters can be dissociated – e.g., keratinization with formation of keratin pearls can be observed in cytologically very atypical tumors with a high degree of nuclear pleomorphism, while, vice versa, keratinization can be missing in carcinomas with a relatively bland nuclear appearance (corresponding to G2). Another problem results from the histological heterogeneity often observed in squamous cell carcinomas. If the parameters of differentiation and malignancy vary regionally within the macroscopically homogeneous tumor nodule, then, according to accepted convention, the least differentiated part of a malignancy is decisive for the assignment of the grade [22]. It remains the decision of the examiner whether to consider very circumscribed, poorly differentiated areas. Generally, a tumor must be classified as poorly differentiated when at least 30 % of the tumor area corresponds to the degree of differentiation.

In view of these problems, a number of efforts have been made to modify the grading procedure – e.g., by adding completing parameters, such as the

invasion pattern and the peritumoral lymphoplasmacellular infiltration, which shows a local (however insufficient), immune response [34]. Another interesting approach is selective tumor front grading [35]. This determines the degree of differentiation only at the tumor front, i. e., in the area of the deepest invasion. This zone seems to be especially representative for the invasive characteristics of the tumor and, thus, particularly relevant for the prognosis. In other types of cancer, such as breast cancer, for example, the definition of the grading is much clearer, due to the semi-quantitative and quantitative nature of the criteria [36, 37]. In the future, it might be possible to better determine the malignant potential of individual squamous cell carcinomas using molecularly defined parameters (see discussion below). When comparing primary tumors and associated lymph node metastases, often an identical degree of differentiation can be determined. However, variations in one or the other direction can also occur.

The grading G4 – undifferentiated – is not used by all authors. It represents squamous cell carcinomas with significant portions that are undifferentiated, yet which nonetheless exhibit to a high degree the cytological criteria of malignancy. There are also *completely* undifferentiated carcinomas for which the squamous origin can only be deduced immunohistochemically from the expression of primary squamous-epithelial cytokeratins, such as CK_5 and CK_{14} [31, 38]. Together with the absence or scarcity of simple-epithelial cytokeratin CK_7, immunohistochemistry can differentiate a metastasis from an adenocarcinoma, which is generally characterized by missing squamous-epithelial cytokeratins and strong expression of simple-epithelial cytokeratins – primarily CK_7. Such immunohistochemical examinations are primarily indicated when metastases from an unknown primary cancer occur (see Chap. 9), making an exact histogenetic classification of the tumor type particularly relevant.

In the area of the sinonasal mucosa, the nasopharynx and, also, the tonsil, carcinomas can occur that are morphologically similar to transitional cell carcinomas of the bladder, but without urothelial superficial cells. These tumors, which also show a transitional cell-like morphology in lymph node metastases, are currently attributed to non-keratinizing squamous cell carcinomas [39].

Under the electron microscope, squamous cell carcinomas of the head and neck reveal the ultrastructural criteria of squamous cells that diverge in their quality, as well as in their quantity, from the regular structures of healthy cells [32, 40]. Beside the atypical features of the cell nuclei associated with malignancy, disturbances appear in the tonofilaments, with formation of whorls and clumps, as well as alterations in the plasma membrane. Additionally, alterations can be found in the desmosomes. These include a reduction in number, as well as a change in appearance, with abnormal, partially shortened forms and internalized intracytoplasmatic desmosomes dominating. The basal membrane zone also varies in relation to that of healthy squamous epithelium, showing laminations and abnormal openings, all the way up to the complete absence of the basal membrane.

Beyond the mere morphological examinations of conventional histopathology, immunohistochemical and molecular-biologic markers may provide an even better biologic characterization of squamous cell carcinomas. Although extensive research in this area is currently being done, these markers are not yet included in the diagnostic routine. Among the candidates for potentially relevant biological markers of squamous cell carcinomas that can influence lymphogenic metastatic spread, a distinction can be made between markers associated with the level of differentiation and markers associated with the extent of malignancy. The markers associated with the level of differentiation include the cytokeratins, in addition to the epithelium-specific proteins of the cytoskeleton, with their highly diverse expression pattern [31, 38]. Here, the mostly stable cytokeratin markers for squamous cells, CK_5, CK_6 and CK_{14}, must be mentioned. These markers remain even in poorly differentiated and metastatic squamous cell carcinomas, and, thus, they serve as basic markers of squamous cell type, even in cases of undifferentiated morphology and unknown primary tumor. In contrast, CK_7 – which is characteristic of simple-epithelial cells and only rarely expressed ($\blacktriangleright$ Figs. 3.4, 3.5) – is typically found in adenocarcinomas (see Chap. 3.2.3.4). Other cytokeratin components typical for simple epithelia, especially CK_8, CK_{18} and CK_{19}, are potentially interesting because they increase with a higher degree of malignancy [31, 41, 42]. Whether this fact has prognostic relevance remains to be clarified. Systematic studies of the pattern of expression of cytokeratins in lymph node metastases currently do not exist.

Components of cellular adhesion may also be interesting markers for squamous cell carcinomas. It has been demonstrated that the cell-cell adhesion molecule E-cadherin, localized in certain non-desmosomal adhesive structures, occurs less often in squamous cell carcinomas with lymph node metastases [43, 45]. A reduction of E-cadherin in squamous cell carcinomas is also associated with poor differentiation [44, 46] and invasive growth [45, 46]. One of the studies [43] showed for the first time a statistically significant correlation between reduced E-cadherin and reduced survival rate. In addition, desmosomal cell connections and their protein components (which can be detected immunohistochemically) are reduced in cases of poorly differentiated squamous cell carcinomas, especially in carcinomas with lymph node metastases [45]. The metastatic potential of squamous cell carcinomas of the head and neck thus seems to be associated with a reduction in several cellular adhesive mechanisms.

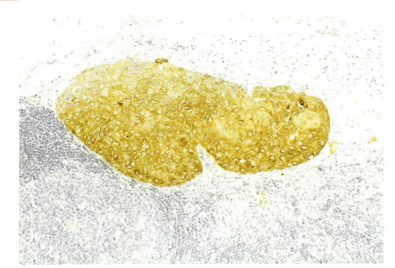

Figure 3.4

Micrometastasis of a squamous cell carcinoma in the marginal sinus of a cervical lymph node. Immunohistochemically, strongly positive reaction against the stratified epithelium-type cytokeratin CK_5

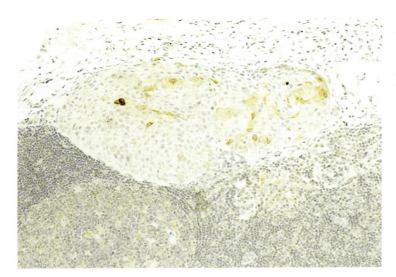

Figure 3.5

The same micrometastasis with immunohistochemically scarce expression of the simple epithelium-type cytokeratin CK_7 in about 10% of the carcinoma cells

In comparison to the parameters associated with the level of differentiation, cellular and molecular-biologic markers associated with the extent of malignancy must be mentioned (literature in the references of [32]). Among these, proteolytic enzymes (e.g., matrix metalloproteinases) and extracellular matrix components (integrins, laminin, tenascin, fibronectin, collagens, especially collagen IV and VII as components of the basal membrane) are correlated with growth behavior and tumor invasiveness. The immunohistochemical demonstration of such markers in squamous cell carcinomas, or in the peritumorous mesenchyme, can provide more information about the biologic behavior of the tumor. Among the markers that are associated with the extent of malignancy, those that are directly or indirectly related to cellular growth are of particular importance. These include oncogenes, tumor suppressor genes and regulators of the cell cycle. Among the oncogenes, the epidermal growth factor receptor (EGF-R) has been

Figure 3.6

Immunohistochemically positive reaction in about 2% of the tumor cell nuclei of this micrometastasis for p53 as sign of a pathological accumulation and possibly the functional loss of this tumor suppressor protein

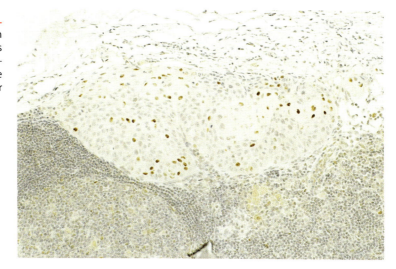

examined the most extensively. Recent studies reveal that EGF-R is an important oncogene product for these tumors, and that it is related to proliferative behavior. For other oncogenes, the relationship is still unclear. Among tumor suppressor genes, p53 in particular (▶ Fig. 3.6) has been examined extensively in squamous cell carcinomas, but the significance of p53 gene mutations [32, 43] is not fully understood at this point. Furthermore, regulators of the cell cycle, such as the cyclins D, A and B, are known to play an important role in squamous cell carcinomas (literature in references of [32]). Additional studies are required, however, to determine the precise clinical relevance of these molecular markers.

3.2.2 Cytologic Diagnosis

A minimally invasive diagnostic procedure, fine needle aspiration cytology of cervical lymph nodes, generally allows a reliable diagnosis of metastasis of squamous cell carcinomas, at least at the stage of macrometastasis [1]. In FNA specimens, atypical squamous cells with hyperchromatic nuclei having a coarser chromatin pattern and irregular nuclear contour can be detected cytologically (▶ Fig. 3.7). The character of squamous cells is revealed in a relatively broad eosinophilic cytoplasm. Dyskeratotic cells with dense acidophilic cytoplasm and small hyperchromatic, round to oval, partly deformed cell nuclei are diagnostically very helpful. Further criteria are enlarged, prominent nucleoli and a "dirty" background with cellular debris. Differential diagnostic problems can arise in the case of poorly differentiated metastases of squamous cell carcinomas when compared with other malignant tumors, or in cases of well-differentiated metastases of squamous cell carcinomas (when compared with benign tumor-like lesions, such as lateral cervical cysts).

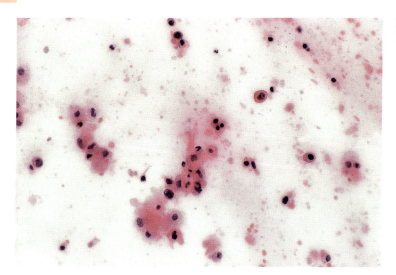

Figure 3.7

Cytologically positive cervical lymph node specimen with atypical squamous cells with middle-grade enlarged chromatin-dense irregular cell nuclei and eosinophilic cytoplasm. "Dirty" background with cellular debris and blood. H&E

3.2.3 Variants of Squamous Cell Carcinomas of the Head and Neck

A series of particular morphologic variants must be differentiated from the conventional type of squamous cell carcinoma (▶ Table 3.1). These variants, the most important of which will be discussed in the following sections, can also be observed in lymph node metastases.

3.2.3.1 Basaloid Squamous Cell Carcinoma

The basaloid squamous cell carcinomas [22, 34] regularly contain portions of conventional squamous cell carcinoma which are often very circumscribed. The real basaloid parts superficially show certain histological similarities to basal cell carcinoma of the skin. The malignant cells are similar to basal cells and have a narrow cytoplasm. Also, they can develop a palisading pattern in the periphery of the tumor cell aggregations. Keratinization is missing in the basaloid tumor component. Numerous mitoses, single cell necrosis and central necrotic accumulations can be observed: all indicators of rapid tumor cell growth. The tumor cells grow partly in larger solid aggregations and partly into more narrow cellular strands. Extracellularly, a hyaline stroma or mucinous mater-

ial, causing a cribriform pattern, often occurs. This leads to the differential diagnosis of adenoid-cystic carcinoma of the salivary glands – which can also affect lymph nodes, but in which the degree of cellular and nuclear pleomorphism is much lower. The basaloid squamous cell carcinoma occurs mainly in the area of the hypopharynx, the base of tongue, and the supraglottic larynx. It is histologically a special type that corresponds biologically and clinically to a poorly differentiated conventional squamous cell carcinoma and often leads to the development of cervical lymph node metastases.

3.2.3.2 Adenoid Squamous Cell Carcinoma

This uncommon variant does not reveal a genuine glandular differentiation, although pseudoglandular structures occur due to degenerative acantholysis of the tumor cells in the center of tumor cell aggregations. These structures can even develop pseudocysts [22, 32, 39]. The primary tumors are often localized in the area of the light-exposed skin and the lower lip. The prognosis seems to be rather good.

3.2.3.3 Undifferentiated (Lymphoepithelial) Carcinoma (Schmincke Tumor)

Undifferentiated lymphoepithelial carcinoma [22, 39, 47] is an independent clinical-pathological entity that must be correctly diagnosed as such. This type of tumor typically develops in the nasopharynx; however, it can also occur in the area of the tonsils. The age distribution of patients is remarkably broad. Even children can develop this cancer. Most of the cases are associated with the Epstein–Barr virus (EBV). Undifferentiated lymphoepithelial carcinomas typically lead very early to the development of lymph node metastases, which can be the initial clinical sign, while the primary cancer remains occult.

Histopathologically, the undifferentiated lymphoepithelial carcinoma consists of undifferentiated tumor cells, with large, round vesicular nuclei, having prominent nucleoli and a high mitosis index. Cellular boundaries are hardly visible, which simulates a syncytial cell aggregation. An abundant, diffuse lymphoplasmacellular infiltration is very typical and spreads between the tumor cells; this in turn leads to a drifting and a strong dispersion of the malignant cells. Frequently, the epithelial character gets morphologically lost, and the tumor cells resemble immunoblasts or Hodgkin cells. Because of this, malignant large cell lymphomas, as well as Hodgkin lymphomas, must be part of the histological differential diagnosis of an undifferentiated lymphoepithelial carcinoma. In cases of a high lymphatic component, the tumor can be difficult to distinguish from local lymphatic tissue. For these difficult cases, immunohistochemical staining for the detection of cytokeratin is recommended. This procedure clearly stains the epithelial tumor cells of the lymphoepithelial carcinoma, while malignant lymphomas remain negative. Another relevant differential diagnosis is the discernment of conventional non-keratinizing squamous cell carcinoma. In lymph node metastases of undifferentiated lymphoepithelial carcinoma, the lymphoplasmacellular infiltration is often present, but it can be missing.

3.2.3.4 Adenosquamous Carcinoma

The uncommon adenosquamous carcinomas are primarily highly malignant tumors. Histologically, they exhibit a biphasic structure [32, 39]. Often the squamous component dominates, frequently keratinizing, while the glandular component, along with the glandular lumina and/or intracellular mucus, is poorly developed. The primary tumors may arise from the superficial epithelium of the mucosa, from small seromucous glands or from salivary glands. The most important histological differential diagnosis is the high-grade mucoepidermoid carcinoma of the salivary glands. This carcinoma consists of distinct cell types and can be easily differentiated.

3.2.3.5 Spindle Cell Carcinoma

This biphasic special form of head and neck carcinoma is characterized by the presence of a predominant spindle cell component and a less prominent component of squamous cell carcinoma. Spindle cell carcinomas develop mainly in the larynx and, macroscopically, frequently have an exophytic-polypoid structure. The characteristic malignant spindle cell component is morphologically similar to a malignant mesenchymal tumor (sarcoma). The epithelial origin is generally reflected in at least focal cytokeratin expression [32, 39]. The spindle cell component can be absolutely undifferentiated, and it can consist of irregular pleomorphic spindle cells, divided by a fibrous matrix that resembles an undifferentiated sarcoma. The spindle tumor cells can also be arranged in loose fascicles. In other cases, they form storiform patterns that are reminiscent of a malignant fibrous histiocytoma. Alternatively, however, they can develop osteoid or chondroid structures and resemble osteosarcoma or chondrosarcoma. However, squamous cellular differentiation can always be identified, thereby allowing the diagnosis to be made. The histological differential diagnosis includes squamous cell carcinomas with increased stroma proliferation, several true sarcomas (including rhabdomyosarcoma) and the spindle cell variant of malignant melanoma [39]. Etiologically, cigarette smoke is the most com-

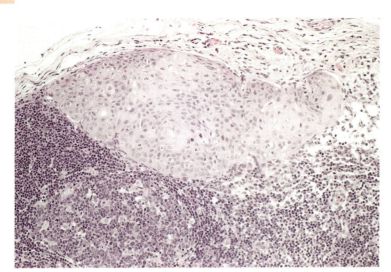

Figure 3.8

Micrometastasis of a squamous cell carcinoma presenting as an atypical squamous cell aggregation with a size of less than 1 mm in the marginal sinus of the cervical lymph node. H&E

mon significant carcinogen related to the development of these carcinomas, as it is also of conventional squamous cell carcinomas. Some patients develop this tumor after prior radiotherapy [32, 39]. The lymph node metastases of these carcinomas can reveal squamous cell differentiation, as well as a sarcoma-like spindle cell, or even, biphasic growth [39].

3.2.4 Micrometastases of Squamous Cell Carcinomas

The process of lymphogenic metastatic spread of a squamous cell carcinoma begins with invasion of the lymphatic vessels by a subpopulation of tumor cells. This can manifest in the surroundings of the primary tumor as the morphological image of lymphangiosis carcinomatosa. The tumor cells are then transported with the lymph fluid via afferent lymphatic vessels to the draining regional lymph nodes and appear there as tumor cell emboli, which become histologically visible in the subcapsular sinus and/or occasionally in a capsular lymphatic vessel [48]. If the tumor cells survive within the lymph node and are not destroyed by the immunologic defense system, these cells start to proliferate and to develop larger tumor cell aggregations. At this point, the situation is called micrometastasis, although not in the case of

single intrasinusoidal tumor cells or miniscule tumor cell emboli. Micrometastasis as the earliest stage of lymph node metastasis (▶ Fig. 3.8) is histologically defined as a metastatic focus originating from a lymph node sinus which is less than 3mm in diameter in all histologic section levels and which alters only minimally the lymph node architecture [12, 14, 15]. Micrometastases are mostly free of mesenchymal stroma, as angiogenesis has not occurred in this stage. Approximately 66–75 % of all micrometastases are located in the area of the subcapsular sinus, where lymphatic fluid flows into the lymph node. Only 25–33 % of the micrometastases are located in the area of the medullary sinus [12, 14, 15]. In rare cases, micrometastases develop from capsular or juxtacapsular lymphatic vessels and then break through the capsule or the wall of the afferent lymphatic vessel, which, in turn, may lead to an early primary extracapsular growth of the tumor [48].

Hamakawa et al. [15] reported in an extensive study with semiserial sections that all except one of twenty-nine detected micrometastatic foci of oral squamous cell carcinomas found in twenty-three cervical lymph nodes had a size of at least 0.3 mm (0.3–3 mm diameter, mean: 1.36 mm). Thus, the comparably large and compact micrometastases from head and neck carcinomas are different from micrometastases from breast carcinomas, which are

< 0.2 mm [49]. Squamous cell carcinomas seem to have greater cellular adhesion, possibly due to the relatively high number of desmosomes, while breast cancer tends to develop greater dispersion, with the ability to manifest multiple micrometastatic foci in one lymph node.

Generally, lymph nodes with micrometastases are of normal size [14] or only slightly larger than tumor-free lymph nodes [15]. However, small lymph nodes with a diameter of less than 5mm may contain micrometastases [50]. In activated lymph nodes with sinus histiocytosis and/or follicular hyperplasia, Hamakawa et al. [15] found micrometastases only rarely. Most micrometastases manifest alone, while sometimes two or three micrometastatic focuses can be detected in one lymph node [15].

While additional micrometastases in macrometastatically positive neck dissection specimens do not play an important role in tumor staging, some cases are interesting in light of the possible prognostic significance where only micrometastases are detected. As to the histological procedure (see Chap. 3.1), the sensitivity of the histopathological detection of micrometastases is generally improved by a more extensive examination procedure, such as the inspection of multiple serial sections, although this increases the detection rate only marginally [13]. Data in the literature concerning the incidence of micrometastases in neck dissection specimens varies significantly. Exact conventional histopathological examination has shown that 10% [51] to 20% [14] of all N+ specimens have only micrometastases. A significantly higher rate of 53% was found when the analysis was limited to patients with clinical N0 status [52]. The majority of patients showing micrometastases had only one lymph node affected by micrometastatic spread [14]. An extensive examination revealed micrometastases in 0.3% [13], 0.8% [16] or 4.2% [15] of the lymph nodes, even though conventional histological examination led to the result of tumor-free lymph nodes in 50–100% of cases. The two last-mentioned studies resulted in a higher pN stage in 10–12% of the patients.

How the presence of micrometastases in lymph nodes influences patient prognosis has been demonstrated for some tumor entities (e.g., breast cancer) [53], but this has not yet been clarified for head and neck cancers. Hamakawa et al. [15] observed a correlation; however, their data were collected from a very small patient population. In contrast, Woolgar [7, 14] did not observe any significant difference between patients with micrometastases, versus those without any metastases at all in the lymph nodes. Their data, however, must be considered only preliminary, given that the study was retrospective and had only a short follow-up period. In comparison to other tumor entities [53], only very few investigations on micrometastases from head and neck cancers have been performed [15]. In order to truly estimate the prognostic significance of micrometastases in cases of squamous cell carcinomas of the head and neck, controlled prospective studies are needed. From a diagnostic histopathology perspective, standard examination performed with one histological section specimen per paraffin block should be sufficient (see Chap. 3.1). This is because micrometastases of squamous cell carcinomas are relatively large [15]. However, careful macroscopic serial section of larger lymph nodes in 3–4 mm slices, together with the preparation of even the smallest lymph nodes, should be done.

Micrometastases should be delineated from isolated carcinoma cells, which have drifted into the lymph nodes sinus. This is because it is only in the case of metastasis that the tumor cells proliferate, or at least start to develop a multicellular tumor cell aggregation, at the site to which they have drifted. The detection of isolated disseminated tumor cells requires immunohistochemical examinations of serial sections or molecular-biologic analyses. Such methods give indications of occult tumor cells in lymph nodes, which cannot be detected by conventional histological examination. In one study, the lymph nodes of patients suffering from oral squamous cell carcinomas that were considered to be tumor-free in conventional H&E microscopy were discovered to harbor micrometastases and/or tiny tumor cell aggregations in 7% of the patients when cytokeratin immunohistochemistry was added to the evaluation. The influence on the prognosis was not obvious [18]. However, a recent multivariate analysis showed an independent prognostic relevance for cervical and other micrometastases of squamous cell carcinomas of the esophagus when detected by use of cytokeratins [20].

In some studies, the reverse-transcriptase-polymerase chain reaction (RT-PCR) was used to detect miniscule quantities of tumor-specific mRNA in lymph node specimens. Relatively reliable tumor-specific markers, including certain cytokeratins and other differentiation antigens characteristic of squamous epithelia, were chosen. In 37% of the lymph nodes that were considered tumor-free, tumor-specific mRNA, and thus the expression of the cytokeratin CK_5 (which is typical for squamous cell carcinoma cells), was evident [54]. Using a similar approach, Hamakawa et al. [17] detected the mRNA for CK_{13} in 14% of the histologically tumor-free cervical lymph nodes of patients suffering from an oral squamous cell carcinoma. CK_{13} is a marker also typical for squamous cell carcinomas, but it is expressed less often [31]. This group also found 19% RT-PCR positive lymph nodes when they applied the squamous cell carcinoma antigen (SCCA), a differentiation antigen, as an mRNA marker [55]. A much higher reliability for the identification of tumor cell specificity is assured by using tumor-specific gene mutations. By means of this strategy, Brennan et al. [56] could detect nucleic acid chains with tumor-specific p53 mutations occurring in primary head and neck squamous cell carcinomas in 21% of histopathologically tumor-free lymph nodes. It was clear that these chains originated from otherwise undetected, probably very sparse, tumor cells located in the lymph nodes. The biological and prognostic relevance of all these findings has not yet been clarified sufficiently.

3.2.5 Extracapsular Extension of Lymph Node Metastases

Extracapsular tumor growth mostly occurs in an advanced stage of the lymphogenic metastatic spread. While, initially, the metastatic tumor mainly does not penetrate the lymph node capsule, later, an invasion of the capsular connective tissue occurs, leading to a complete break through and/or rupture of the capsule. However, initially, extracapsular tumor extension can only be detected microscopically. In addition to direct break through of intranodal tumor tissue, Toker [48] postulated another potential mechanism, in which the stasis of afferent lymph vessels, due to metastatic involvement of the lymph node, favors the adhesion of secondary, newly identified tumor cell emboli in ectatic capsular and juxtacapsular lymph vessels. This could lead directly to extranodal tumor growth. In rare cases, small peripherally situated metastases can spread early extracapsularly, especially when tumor cell emboli have settled primarily in intra- or juxtacapsular lymph vessels [48] (see Chap. 3.2.5).

Further tumor growth makes the extracapsular tumor cell aggregations macroscopically visible during sectioning of the specimen: this is the case with macroscopic extracapsular tumor extension. Such extension can lead to the fusion of adjacent metastatic lymph nodes. The extending extranodal tumor formations can then invade other tissues, such as the submandibular gland, the wall of the internal jugular vein, skeletal muscles or the skin [7]. In larger series, the frequency of extracapsular tumor extension is estimated to be 74–85% of tumor-positive neck dissection specimens [8, 57]. As expected, extracapsular tumor extension correlates with the size of the metastatic lymph node and is typically found in cases of nodal metastases larger than 3 cm [3]. However, it must be kept in mind that about 20% of all lymph node metastases with proven extracapsular extension are smaller than 1cm in diameter [3, 9, 58].

The clinical implication of extracapsular tumor extension is its prognostic significance [7, 9, 59]. Multivariate analyses have revealed that only macroscopic extracapsular tumor extension is an independent prognostic parameter. In contrast, microscopic extracapsular tumor growth seems to be less significant [8, 57]. If these results can be confirmed in further studies, it will be important from an histopathological point of view to define a clear delineation between microscopic and macroscopic extracapsular spread, such as, for example, the invasion depth into the perinodal tissue in millimeters. Currently, such a generally acknowledged definition is missing. The findings mentioned indicate the importance for very precise macroscopic and microscopic documentation of extracapsular tumor spread [3]. Macroscopic extracapsular extension can be confused with non-tumorous, perinodal fibrosis, which can be caused by local inflammation or prior radiotherapy. The histological description of extracapsular tumor growth should take into consideration these tissue reactions, as well as vascular invasions [11]. Regarding the approach for precise histological documentation of extracapsular tumor growth, a detailed histopathological evaluation scheme was presented recently and verified with regard to its prognostic relevance [32, 60, 61]. This scheme considers seven histomorphological types of lymph node metastases, namely:

- type I: island-like metastasis without contact with the capsule
- type II: direct contact of the metastasis with the capsule
- type III: infiltration of the capsule
- type IV: desmoplasia of the lymph node with an intact capsule
- type V: desmoplasia of the lymph node with destruction of the continuity of the capsular laminae
- type VI: capsular rupture with infiltration into perinodal fatty tissue
- type VII: breakthrough of the capsule and infiltration into cervical soft tissue

When used in correlation with the number of metastatic lymph nodes, this histopathological subclassification was found to be a useful prognostic indicator of tumor-associated survival rate.

3.2.6 Cystic Cervical Lymph Node Metastases

True cystic cervical lymph node metastases represent a special clinical pathologic entity. Here, we are talking mainly about solitary cystic tumors of a size of up to 10cm, often located subdigastrically, which still show lymph node architecture at the margins, with mostly an intact capsule. These nodes consist of a cystic epithelial tumor, with a conspicuously papillary structure of the cyst wall [62]. Histologically (▶ Fig. 3.9), the cyst wall consists of a more or less atypical non-keratinizing, or transitional cell-like, squamous epithelium [62, 63]. In some cases, the epithelium can be permeated by lymphocytes, similar to the situation with a lymphoepithelial carcinoma. Remarkably, some parts of the epithelial lining of the cysts can appear bland, and thus be confused with non-neoplastic squamous epithelium. As a result, in isolated cases, the delineation of a benign lateral cervical cyst (branchial cleft cyst) can be difficult to determine. This is one reason for the long-standing

Figure 3.9

Cystic cervical lymph node metastasis with lining by narrow, mostly mature, squamous cells, and (below) lymphatic tissue in the cyst wall. H&E

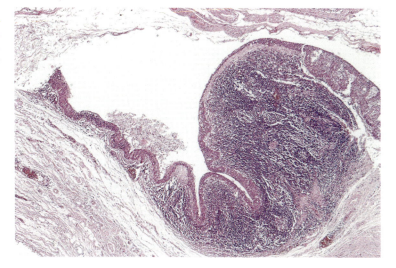

controversy concerning whether such tumors arise primarily in the neck region from a branchiogenic cyst through carcinomatous transformation, and, therefore, should be considered as primary branchiogenic carcinoma. However, numerous studies have shown that in these cases, nearly always the specially configured cervical lymph node metastasis is from a primary squamous cell cancer or lymphoepithelial carcinoma, which are typically located in the area of Waldeyer's ring. Such cystic cervical lymph node metastases probably indicate a primary cancer in the palatine tonsil or, less frequently, in either the tonsillar tissue of the base of the tongue or the nasopharynx [47, 62–66]. Often the papillary cystic metastases manifest earlier than the initially occult primary tumor. The prognosis is better than it is in cases of conventional metastasizing squamous cell carcinoma [64]. Differentiation must be made between genuine cystic metastases and a pseudocyst originating from central necrosis in metastases of conventional squamous cell carcinomas where the primary cancer is localized outside of Waldeyer's ring.

3.2.7 Changes of Cervical Lymph Node Metastases After Radiation and Chemotherapy

Preoperative irradiation or neoadjuvant chemotherapy lead to morphological alterations of metastatic tumor tissue, which may reflect the desirable effect of tumor regression. This, however, is dependent on the individual therapeutic response. Cytologically, a relatively early alteration after irradiation is the increase of abnormal nuclear types, such as micronuclei, double or multiple nuclei or nuclear buds. These are already evident in the initial stage of radiotherapy and depend on the radiation dose [67]. Electron-microscopic alterations can be found in the cell nucleus (swelling, inclusions, fragmentation), as well as in the cytoplasm, where edema and/or clumping of tonofibrils is seen [40]. Radiosensitive tumors manifest tumor regression initially by increased apoptosis [32]. After degeneration of larger tumor components by the so-called keratin granulomas, viable tumor cells can disappear altogether [57, 68]. After chemotherapy, similar alterations can be detected: increased

apoptosis is induced, and multiple ultrastructural alterations of the cell nuclei and the cytoplasm become visible [40]. In some cases after chemotherapy, an exaggerated differentiation with hyperkeratinization and the development of extended keratin masses results, which leads to granulomatous inflammatory reactions with multinucleated giant cells, which in turn leads to the formation of keratin granulomas [40, 69]. It would be of clinical interest if biopsy of the primary tumor could provide an indicator for the sensitivity of radiochemotherapy. In this context, the definition of apoptosis-associated parameters, such as p53, or chemotherapy-resistance associated parameters, such as p-glycoprotein, could be interesting [32, 69].

In summary of the pathology of cervical lymph node metastases of squamous cell carcinomas, it can be said that an important task of the pathologist is to determine the correct classification (► Table 3.1), especially of the clinically relevant subtypes of squamous cell cancer. These include undifferentiated lymphoepithelial carcinoma and spindle cell carcinoma. With regard to the staging of the cervical lymph node metastases, micrometastases and their detection play an important role. Extensive examination with serial sections is not a recommended diagnostic routine; however, it is useful in special situations, such as investigations of sentinel lymph nodes. The prognostic relevance of micrometastases has not yet been conclusively clarified and requires future prospective studies. Regarding macrometastases, capsular rupture with extracapsular tumor spread is of high prognostic relevance and should be described precisely in the histopathologic documentation. The results of histological lymph node staging are usually summarized in the pN stage of the TNM system [21].

In this pN classification for head and neck carcinomas, some of the important pathological parameters mentioned above are not specifically considered, including micrometastases (in contrast to the situation for breast cancer) and extracapsular tumor extension. Recommendations for including extranodal growth patterns in the pN stage for head and neck carcinomas have been presented. In general, however, the current N classification scheme of the TNM system [21] is of clinical prognostic relevance [70], even though a prognostic difference between N2 metastases and N3 metastases has not yet been found.

3.3 Metastases of Salivary Gland Tumors and Thyroid Gland Carcinomas

Cervical lymph node metastases can sometimes develop from a primary tumor of the major and minor salivary glands (parotid gland, submandibular gland and sublingual gland, as well as from the minor salivary glands of the oral cavity, the pharynx and the larynx) [71].

Among the multitude of salivary gland tumors (▶ Table 3.1), adenoid cystic carcinoma must be first mentioned [72]. Histomorphologically, this type of carcinoma is characterized by local perineural infiltration and thus a high recurrence rate. It manifests lymphogenic metastatic spread only late. In cases of metastases to cervical lymph nodes, histologically, an infiltration of the lymphatic tissue by atypical glandular (cribriform or tubular) cell aggregations with PAS positive basal membranes can be detected. This corresponds to the histomorphological appearance of the primary tumor (see Chap. 3.2.3 for information on differential diagnosis).

Metastases to cervical lymph nodes from undifferentiated salivary gland carcinomas are less common. These include polymorphic, low-grade adenocarcinomas or mucoepidermoid carcinomas (see Chap. 3.2.3) [71], and they occur primarily in the major salivary glands (in particular, in the parotid gland). Occasionally, they arise within a preexisting pleomorphic adenoma [72, 73]. Mucoepidermoid carcinomas are malignant epithelial tumors, consisting of various differentiated components, such as mucinous, ciliated, clear-cell or squamous cell complexes. They often show cystic growth, due to the development of mucus, which can also be found in the lymph node metastases. With regard to low-grade mucoepidermoid carcinoma, only rarely (in fewer than 5% of the cases) is lymphogenic metastatic spread observed, while in cases of high-grade mucoepidermoid carcinoma, lymphogenic metastatic spread is seen up to 80% of the time [71]. More than 50% of all mucoepidermoid carcinomas are histologically high-grade

tumors. Assignment of lymph node metastases to this tumor type, compared with an undifferentiated carcinoma or a poorly differentiated adenocarcinoma, can be difficult. In such cases, knowledge of the primary tumor is helpful.

Lymphogenic spread of benign pleomorphic adenomas is described in the literature in isolated cases of patients, often those with a history of multiple local recurrences [74–76] even after decades of latency. Histomorphologically, these lymphogenic metastases show a benign morphology corresponding to the primary tumor, with mature myxoid, or chondroid stroma, and myoepithelial cell complexes without nuclear pleomorphism. Intranodal salivary gland adenomas, such as the cystadenolymphoma (the so-called Warthin tumor), which can develop on the basis of salivary gland heterotopia in lymph nodes [71], must not be confused with lymph node metastases. Such heterotopias are commonly found adjacent to the major salivary glands. Other tissue heterotopias, such as thyroid tissue or nevus cells, occur in cervical lymph nodes and must not be confused with metastases from thyroid carcinomas or malignant melanomas.

Cervical lymph node metastases may lead to the diagnosis of primary thyroid carcinomas (often of the papillary type), which can be discerned by the typical morphology of papillary or follicular growth patterns. In cases of doubt, the diagnosis may be ensured by means of the immunohistochemical proof of thyroglobulin. Metastases of medullary carcinomas are diagnosed by the immunohistochemical detection of calcitonin, in addition to other neuroendocrine markers.

3.4 Uncommon Cervical Lymph Node Metastases

In the histopathologic analysis of cervical lymph node metastases, the above-mentioned squamous cell carcinomas of the head and neck and their variants must be differentiated from other malignant tumors that can also develop cervical lymph node metastases. Occasionally, cervical lymph node metastases are detected from an unknown primary cancer (the so-called occult carcinoma) or from carcinomas outside the head and neck region. In these cases, the histomorphology and the application of immunohistochemical testing may lead to the diagnosis of the tumor entity and facilitate the detection of the primary tumor. In lymphogenic metastases of undifferentiated tumors, examination of the tissue using immunohistochemical methodology is essential. This is true of any neoplasm that cannot be clearly identified by histomorphology. It is also important to realize that the lung is the most frequent site of a primary tumor outside the head and neck region when unclear cervical lymph node metastases are found. However, there are numerous other possibilities.

In addition to squamous cell carcinomas that develop outside the head and neck region in the lung (squamous cell carcinoma is the most frequent type of lung cancer), squamous cell carcinomas also frequently develop in the intrathoracic esophagus. Histologically, metastases from these origins cannot be clearly separated from metastases of squamous cell carcinomas of the head and neck. However, the cytokeratin analysis may suggest a primary squamous cell carcinoma of the lung, rather than a carcinoma of the mouth or the pharynx. This differentiation is aided by the high expression of simple-epithelial cytokeratins – in particular, CK_8, CK_{18} and CK_{19} [19, 31, 77, 78].

Adenocarcinomas and small cell neuroendocrine carcinomas (see below) can appear in the thoracic esophagus, as well as in the lung, and can metastasize into the cervical lymph nodes as part of their distant metastatic spread. In the event of a cervical metastasis from an adenocarcinoma, the possibility of the location of the primary tumor in the head and neck must be taken into consideration (see ▶ Table 3.1). Head and neck primary sites include the salivary glands, and the nasal or paranasal mucosa (particularly sinonasal adenocarcinoma of the intestinal type). More frequently, however, the primary tumor is located outside the head and neck. In addition to the lung and the thoracic esophagus, the breast, stomach, colon and rectum, as well as the ovaries and the prostate gland, must be considered as sites to which primary adenocarcinomas can distantly metastasize into cervical lymph nodes. Frequently,

the primary tumor is initially unknown in such cases (see Chap. 9) and is then sometimes detected in the further course of clinical examinations. When not found it is classified as CUP syndrome (cancer of unknown primary).

In the head and neck region, the most frequently unknown primary tumor sites are the nasopharynx, the base of tongue and the tonsil. Outside the head and neck, the lung is the most common site [2, 66, 79]. When exact histomorphology is coupled with immunohistochemical analyses, possible conclusions can be drawn concerning the primary tumor in metastatic adenocarcinoma. In this regard, intermediate filaments, especially cytokeratins [31, 38], can serve as immunohistochemical markers (see below). An increasing number of organ-specific markers are also available. The simultaneous expression of the apocrine marker, Gross-Cystic-Disease-Fluid-Protein-15 (GCDFP-15), and the estrogen-receptor is highly specific for breast cancer. Adenocarcinomas of the lung often express the thyroidal transcription factor 1 (TTF-1). As far as the role of the cytokeratins is concerned, pulmonary adenocarcinomas are highly positive for CK_7, while CK_{20} is mostly missing. The abundant expression of the simple-epithelial cytokeratin, CK_7, allows a differentiation of these tumors from the metastases of squamous cell carcinomas (▶ Fig. 3.5). Colorectal adenocarcinomas and their metastases are characterized by a typical cytokeratin pattern distinct from the pulmonary phenotype, with expression of CK_{20}, and the lack of CK_7 [31]. Adenocarcinomas of the ovaries express the cell surface antigen CA_{125}. Adenocarcinomas of the prostate can be diagnosed immunohistochemically by antibodies against the prostate-specific antigen (PSA) or prostatic acid phosphatase (PAP). Renal cell carcinomas, which metastasize rather frequently in cervical lymph nodes [80], are characterized immunohistochemically by a coexpression of cytokeratins and vimentin [22, 31, 38], and they may be positive for CD10. The detection of a primary adenocarcinoma through immunohistochemical means, as well as through clinical examinations, can be relevant for the choice of a specific therapy, although it is often palliative in nature in these patients.

Cervical lymph node metastases from a small cell neuroendocrine carcinoma can be identified immunohistologically via their expression of the epithelial markers (cytokeratins) and the neuroendocrine markers N-CAM (CD56), as well by means of synaptophysin. This diagnosis refers to the lung as the probable primary tumor site; however, such tumors can also occur in many other organs (▶ Table 3.1). Among these sites the skin, especially of the head, is where Merkel cell carcinomas occur as primary cutaneous neuroendocrine carcinomas in elderly patients. These cancers metastasize into the cervical lymph nodes, and they also express neuroendocrine markers, but due to their specific CK_{20} expression, they can be distinguished clearly from small cell lung carcinomas [81].

Finally, the possibility of metastatic melanoma must be considered in all cases of diagnostically unclear situations. When metastases of malignant melanoma are discerned, the primary tumor should be searched for in the sun-exposed skin of the head and neck, in the eye (although its occurrence here is rare), and in the mucosa of the head and neck, especially the sinonasal region. About 15% of all malignant melanomas occur in the head and neck region, with 1% of all melanomas arising in the nasal and paranasal sinuses. At the time of first diagnosis, 40% of all sinonasal melanoma patients suffer from advanced tumor with metastases. The prognosis is generally poor, with a mean survival after diagnosis of 2–3 years [39].

Mucosal melanomas can be characterized histologically by a small, blue round, spindle or epitheloid cell, or by pleomorphic differentiation, which is atypical for skin melanomas. These features can also be found in the metastases. Additionally, amelanotic melanomas occur in this area and can be problematic due to their lack of melanin pigment. Thus, morphologically, metastases from malignant melanomas can resemble the metastases of squamous cell carcinomas, spindle cell carcinomas or sarcomas. The typical marker expression of malignant melanomas includes the detection of the S100 protein, the HMB-45-antigen and vimentin, coupled with missing or only low expression of cytokeratins.

With malignant melanoma, the lymphogenic metastatic spread leads first to the development of micrometastases in an inactive, non-vascularized stage. Later, macrometastases develop. These are vascularized and have a significantly higher proliferation rate than micrometastases [82].

3.5 Non-Neoplastic Reactive Lymph Node Alterations

Enlarged lymph nodes are caused not only by metastases, but also by a series of non-neoplastic reactive lymph node alterations. Very often, reactive benign lymph node enlargement occurs in patients suffering from head and neck cancer and leads to a clinically false positive estimation of tumor extent. Histological examination of the lymph nodes generally shows a reactive follicular hyperplasia [83], with lymph nodes achieving a diameter of more than 2cm. The hyperplasia can be caused by ulceration and bacterial inflammation in the area of the primary tumor and/or it can be due to the inflow of tumor antigens into the cervical lymph nodes. Such immunological stimulation of the cervical lymph nodes in cancer patients can be associated with a better prognosis, while patients with lymphocytic depletion in cervical lymph nodes, and corresponding reduced immune response, seem to have a poorer prognosis [3, 84]. On occasion, a granulomatous inflammatory reaction of the sarcoidosis type (the so-called sarcoid-like lesion) can be observed in the lymph nodes of cancer patients [83, 85].

Besides such lymph node alterations indirectly influenced by tumors, there are a number of well-known benign lymph node enlargements that are not associated with tumors. Although a systematic description is outside the realm of this text, a few important lymph node diseases should be mentioned. These are associated with enlarged lymph nodes and, as a result, must always be distinguished from cervical lymph node metastases (see above) or malignant lymphoma. In this context, granulomatous inflammations, such as cervical lymph node tuberculosis, are very important [3]. Cervical lymph node tuberculosis often leads to caseating of the epitheloid cell granulomas, which contain giant cells. Different methods can be used to identify the mycobacteria. In case of sarcoidosis, fibrosis instead of caseation of the granulomas occurs. Uncommon diseases, such as Mediterranean fever, can lead to granulomatous inflammations in the lymph nodes. Granulomatous reactions in the drainage pathways of carcinomas have already been mentioned. More often than such specific inflammations, non-specific inflammatory lymph node enlargements (non-specific lymphadenitis) occur in cases of bacterial or viral infections in the head and neck. Significant enlargement and induration of cervical lymph nodes can also be caused by amyloidosis in very rare cases [86, 87]. In the cases described above, histological examination of the lymph nodes is needed to establish a correct diagnosis.

Acknowledgements. We want to thank Dr. Ulrich Feek for the electron-microscopic photos, and Mrs. Magdalena Jung for her careful writing.

References

1. Orell SR, Sterrett GF, Walters MN-I, Whitaker D (1999) Punktionszytologie: Handbuch und Atlas. Kapitel 4: Kopf und Hals, Speicheldrüsen. Thieme, Stuttgart, 33–59
2. Werner JA (1997) Aktueller Stand der Versorgung des Lymphabflusses maligner Kopf-Hals-Tumoren. Eur Arch Otorhinolaryng (Suppl I), Springer, Berlin, 47–85
3. Carter RL (1993) The pathologist's appraisal of neck dissections. Eur Arch Otorhinolaryngol 250:429–431
4. Slootweg PJ, de Groot JAM (1999) Surgical pathological anatomy of head and neck specimens: a manual for the dissection of surgical specimens from the upper aerodigestive tract. Chapter 7: Neck dissections. Springer, Berlin, 111–119
5. De La Pava S, Pickrein JW (1966) On lymph node clearing as applied to head and neck tumours. In: Ruttiman A (ed) Progress in Lymphology. Proceedings of the International Symposium on Lymphology, Zurich, Switzerland, Thieme, Stuttgart, 290–292
6. Schmitz-Moormann P, Thomas C, Pohl C, Söhl R (1982)Patho-anatomical demonstration of lymph node metastases in a surgical specimen. Pathol Res Pract 174: 403–411
7. Woolgar JA (1997) Detailed topography of cervical lymph-node metastases from oral squamous cell carcinoma. Int J Oral Maxillofac Surg 26:3–9
8. de Carvalho MB (1998) Quantitative analysis of the extent of extracapsular invasion and its prognostic significance: a prospective study of 170 cases of carcinoma of the larynx and hypopharynx. Head Neck 20:16–21
9. Snyderman NL, Johnson JT, Schramm VL, Myers EN, Bedetti CD, Thearle P (1985) Extracapsular spread of carcinoma in cervical lymph nodes: impact upon survival in patients with carcinoma of the supraglottic larynx. Cancer 56:1597–1599
10. Werner JA (1995) Untersuchungen zum Lymphgefäßsystem der oberen Luft- und Speisewege. Shaker, Aachen
11. Devaney SL, Ferlito A, Rinaldo A, Devaney KO (2000) The pathology of Neck dissection in cancer of the larynx. ORL J Otorhinolaryngol Relat Spec 62:204–211
12. van den Brekel MWM, van der Waal I, Meijer CJLM, Freeman JL, Castelijns JA, Snow GB (1996) The incidence of micrometastases in Neck dissection specimens obtained from elective Neck dissections. Laryngoscope 106:987–991
13. Shingaki S, Ohtake K, Nomura T, Nakajima T (1991) The value of single versus multiple sections for detection of lymph node metastasis. J Oral Maxillofac Surg 49:461–463
14. Woolgar JA (1999) Micrometastasis in oral/oropharyngeal squamous cell carcinoma: incidence, histopathological features and clinical implications. Br J Oral Maxillofac Surg 1999;37:181–186
15. Hamakawa H, Takemura K, Sumida T, Kayahara H, Tanioka H, Sogawa K (2000) Histological study on pN upgrading of oral cancer. Virchows Arch 437:116–121
16. Ambrosch P, Kron M, Fischer G, Brinck U (1995) Micrometastases in carcinoma of the upper aerodigestive tract: detection, risk of metastasizing, and prognostic value of depth of invasion. Head Neck 17:473–479
17. Hamakawa H, Fukuzumi M, Bao Y, Sumida T, Kayahara H, Onishi A, Sogawa K (2000) Keratin mRNA for detecting micrometastasis in cervical lymph nodes of oral cancer. Cancer Lett 160:115–123
18. Enepekides DJ, Sultanem K, Nguyen C, Shenouda G, Black MJ, Rochon L (1999) Occult cervical metastases: immunoperoxidase analysis of the pathologically negative neck. Otolaryngol Head Neck Surg 120:713–717
19. Hamakawa H, Bao Y, Takarada M, Fukuzumi M, Tanioka H (1998) Cytokeratin expression in squamous cell carcinoma of the lung and oral cavity: an immunohistochemical study with possible clinical relevance. Oral Surg Oral Med Oral Pathol Oral Radiol Endod 85:438–443
20. Komukai S, Nishimaki T, Watanabe H, Ajioka Y, Suzuki T, Hatakeyama K (2000) Significance of immunohistochemically demonstrated micrometastases to lymph nodes in esophageal cancer with histologically negative nodes. Surgery 127:40–46
21. Sobin LH, Wittekind C (2000) TNM classification of malignant tumours. 6th ed. Wiley, New York
22. Pindborg JJ, Reichart PA, Smith CJ, van der Waal I (1997) International histological classification of tumours / World Health Organization: Histological typing of cancer and

precancer of the oral mucosa. 2nd ed. Springer, Berlin 1–87

23. Seifert G (1991) International histological classification of tumours / World Health Organization: Histological typing of salivary gland tumours. 2nd ed. Springer, Berlin 1–113

24. Shanmugaratnam K (1991) International histological classification of tumours / World Health Organization: Histological typing of tumours of the upper respiratory tract and ear. 2nd ed. Springer, Berlin 1–201

25. Tarin D (1996) Metastasis: secondary proliferation in distant organs. In: Pusztai L, Lewis CE, Yap E (eds). Cell proliferation in cancer. Regulatory mechanisms of neoplastic cell growth. Oxford University Press, Oxford, 316–341

26. Shah JP (1990) Patterns of cervical lymph node metastasis from squamous carcinomas of the upper aerodigestive tract. Am J Surg 160:405–409

27. Woolgar JA (1999) Histological distribution of cervical lymph node metastases from intraoral/oropharyngeal squamous cell carcinomas. Br J Oral Maxillofac Surg 37:175–180

28. Razack MS, Silapasvang S, Sako K, Shedd DP (1978) Significance of site and nodal metastases in squamous cell carcinoma of the epiglottis. Am J Surg 136:520–524

29. Woolgar JA, Scott J (1995) Prediction of cervical lymph node metastasis in squamous cell carcinoma of the tongue/floor of mouth. Head Neck 17:463–472

30. Steinhart H, Kleinsasser O (1993) Growth and spread of squamous cell carcinoma of the floor of the mouth. Eur Arch Otorhinolaryngol 250:358–361

31. Moll R (1998) Cytokeratins as markers of differentiation in the diagnosis of epithelial tumors. In: Herrmann H, Harris JR (eds) Intermediate Filaments. Subcellular Biochemistry, Vol. 31. Plenum Press, New York, 205–262

32. Seifert G (2000) Orale Karzinome. In: Seifert G (ed) Oralpathologie III: Mundhöhle, angrenzendes Weichteil- und Knochengewebe. Springer, Berlin, 291–378

33. Broders AC (1941) The microscopic grading of cancer. Surg Clin North Am 21:947–962

34. Jakobsson PA, Eneroth CM, Killander D, Moberger G, Martensson B (1973) Histologic classification and grading of malignancy in carcinoma of the larynx. Acta Radiol Ther Phys Biol 12:1–8

35. Bryne M, Koppang HS, Lilleng R, Stene T, Bang G, Dabelsteen E (1989) New malignancy grading is a better prognostic indicator than Broders´ grading in oral squamous cell carcinomas. J Oral Pathol Med 18:432–437

36. Bässler R, Böcker W, Hermanek P, Pickartz H, Prechtel K, Schauer A, Schnurch HG, Stegner HE (1992) Die gegenwärtige Situation des Gradings beim Mammakarzinom. Pathologe 13:130–134

37. Bloom HJG, Richardson WW (1957) Histologic grading and prognosis in breast cancer. Br J Cancer 11:359–377

38. Moll R (1993) Cytokeratins as markers of differentiation: expression profiles in epithelia and epithelial tumors. Fischer, Stuttgart, 1–197

39. Mills SE, Gaffey MJ, Frierson HF (2000) Tumors of the upper aerodigestive tract and ear. Atlas of Tumor Pathology, 3rd Series, Fascicle 26. Armed Forces Institute of Pathology, Washington, 1–455

40. Burkhardt A (1980) Der Mundhöhlenkrebs und seine Vorstadien. Ultrastrukturelle und immunpathologische Aspekte. Veröff Pathol, Bd. 112. Gustav Fischer, Stuttgart, 1–271

41. Kannan S, Balaram P, Chandran GJ, Pillai MR, Mathew B, Nalinakumari KR, Nair MK (1994) Differential expression of cytokeratin proteins during tumour progression in oral mucosa. Epithelial Cell Biol 3:61–69

42. Su L, Morgan PR, Lane EB (1994) Protein and mRNA expression of simple epithelial keratins in normal, dysplastic, and malignant oral epithelia. Am J Pathol 145:1349–1357

43. Bosch FX, Schuhmann A, Kartenbeck J (2001) On the role of cell-cell adhesion in metastasis formation in head and neck cancer. In: Lippert BM, Werner JA (eds.) Metastases in head and neck cancer. Tectum, Marburg, 79–86

44. Schipper JH, Frixen UH, Behrens J, Unger A, Jahnke K, Birchmeier W (1991) E-cadherin expression in squamous cell carcinomas of head and neck: inverse correlation with tumor dedifferentiation and lymph node metastasis. Cancer Res 51:6328–6337

45. Shinohara M, Hiraki A, Ikebe T, Nakamura S, Kurahara S-I, Shirasuna K, Garrod DR (1998) Immunohistochemical study of desmosomes in oral squamous cell carcinoma: correlation with cytokeratin and E-cadherin staining, and with tumour behaviour. J Pathol 84:369–381

46. Williams HK, Sanders DS, Jankowski JA, Landini G, Brown AM (1998) Expression of cadherins and catenins in oral epithelial dysplasia and squamous cell carcinoma. J Oral Pathol Med 27:308–317

47. Warnke RA, Weiss LM, Chan JKC, Cleary ML, Dorfman RF (1995) Tumors of the lymph nodes and spleen. Atlas of Tumor Pathology, 3rd Series, Fascicle 14. Armed Forces Institute of Pathology, Washington, 1–544

48. Toker C (1963) Some observations on the deposition of metastatic carcinoma within cervical lymph nodes. Cancer 16:364–374

49. Nasser IA, Lee AK, Bosari S, Saganich R, Heatley G, Silverman ML (1993) Occult axillary lymph node metastases in "node-negative" breast carcinoma. Hum Pathol 24:950–957

50. Don DM, Anzai Y, Lufkin RB, Fu YS, Calcaterra TC (1995) Evaluation of cervical lymph node metastases in squamous cell carcinoma of the head and neck. Laryngoscope 105:669–674

51. van den Brekel MW, Stel HV, van der Valk P, van der Waal I, Meyer CJ, Snow GB (1992) Micrometastases from squamous cell carcinoma in Neck dissection specimens. Eur Arch Otorhinolaryngol 249:349–353

52. Woolgar JA (1999) Pathology of the N0 neck. Br J Oral Maxillofac Surg 37:205–209

53. Ferlito A, Devaney KO, Rinaldo A, Devaney SL, Carbone A (1999) Micrometastases: have they an impact on prognosis? Ann Otol Rhinol Laryngol 108:1185–1189

54. McDonald LA, Walker DM, Gibbins JR (1998) Cervical lymph node involvement in head and neck cancer detectable as expression of a spliced transcript of type II keratin K5. Oral Oncol 34:276–283

55. Hamakawa H, Fukizumi M, Bao Y, Sumida T, Onishi A, Tanioka H, Sato H, Yumoto E (1999) Genetic diagnosis of micrometastasis based on SCC antigen mRNA in cervical lymph nodes of head and neck cancer. Clin Exp Metastasis 17:593–599

56. Brennan JA, Mao L, Hruban RH, Boyle JO, Eby YJ, Koch WM, Goodman SN, Sidransky D (1995) Molecular assessment of histopathological staging in squamous-cell carcinoma of the head and neck. N Engl J Med 332:429–435

57. Carter RL, Bliss JM, Soo KC, O´Brien CJ (1987) Radical Neck dissections for squamous carcinomas: pathological findings and their clinical implications with particular reference to transcapsular spread. Int J Radiat Oncol Biol Phys 13:825–832

58. Snow GB, Annyas AA, van Slooten EA, Bartelink H, Hart AAM (1982) Prognostic factors of neck node metastasis. Clin Otolaryngol 7:185–192

59. Shingaki S, Saito R, Kawasaki T, Nakajima T (1985) Recurrence of carcinoma of the oral cavity, oropharynx and maxillary sinus after radical Neck dissection. J Maxillofac Surg 13:231–235

60. Kehrl W, Wenzel S, Niendorf A (1998) Einfluß verschiedener Formen des metastatischen Lymphknotenbefalls auf die Prognose von Plattenepithelkarzinomen im oberen Aerodigestivtrakt. Laryngorhinootologie 77:569–575

61. Wenzel S, Kehrl W, Bräsen J-H, Niendorf A (1998) Ein neues Schema zur Beurteilung des metastatischen Lymphknotenbefalls beim Plattenepithelkarzinom im HNO-Gebiet. Laryngorhinootologie 77:657–662

62. Micheau C, Cachin Y, Caillou B (1974) Cystic metastases in the neck revealing occult carcinoma of the tonsil: a report of six cases. Cancer 33:228–233

63. Thompson LD, Heffner DK (1998) The clinical importance of cystic squamous cell carcinomas in the neck: a study of 136 cases. Cancer 82:944–956

64. Micheau C, Klijanienko J, Luboinski B, Richard J (1990) So-called branchiogenic carcinoma is actually cystic metastases in the neck from a tonsillar primary. Laryngoscope 100:878–883

65. Regauer S, Mannweiler S, Anderhuber W, Gotschuli A, Berghold A, Schachenreiter J, Jakse R, Beham A (1999) Cystic lymph node metastases of squamous cell carcinoma of Waldeyer´s ring origin. Br J Cancer 79:1437–1442

66. Wenig BM (1993) Atlas of head and neck pathology. W.B. Saunders, Philadelphia, 1–412

67. Bhattathiri NV, Bindu L, Remani P, Chandralekha B, Nair KM (1998) Radiation-induced acute immediate nuclear abnormalities in oral cancer cells: serial cytologic evaluation. Acta Cytol 42:1084–1090

68. Tanner NS, Carter RL, Dalley VM, Clifford P, Shaw HJ (1980) The irradiated radical Neck dissection in squamous carci-noma: a clinico-pathological study. Clin Otolaryngol 5:259–271

69. Hamakawa H, Bao Y, Takarada M, Tanioka H (1998) Histological effects and predictive biomarkers of TPP induction chemotherapy for oral carcinoma. J Oral Pathol Med 27:87–94

70. Iro H, Waldfahrer F (1998) Evaluation of the newly updated TNM classification of head and neck carcinoma with data from 3247 patients. Cancer 83:2201–2207

71. Ellis GL, Auclair PL. Tumors of the salivary glands (1996) Atlas of Tumor Pathology, 3rd Series, Fascicle 17. Armed Forces of Institute of Pathology, Washington, 1–468

72. Hisa Y, Yasuda N, Tadaki N, Nishiyama Y, Fukushima T, Murakami Y (1992) Adenoid cystic carcinoma of the head and neck. A clinical review of 29 cases. Nippon Jibiinkoka Gakkai Kaiho 93:346–351

73. Minic AJ (1993) Unusual variant of a metastasizing malignant mixed tumor of the parotid gland. Oral Surg Oral Med Oral Pathol 76:330–332

74. Chen I, Tu H (2000). Pleomorphic adenoma of the parotid gland metastasizing to the cervical lymph node. Otolaryngol Head Neck Surg 122:455–457

75. Collina G, Eusebi V (1989) Pleomorphic adenoma with lymph-node metastases. Report of two cases. Path Res Pract 184:188–193

76. Freeman SB, Kennedy KS, Parker GS, Tatum SA (1990) Metastasizing pleomorphic adenoma of the nasal septum. Arch Otolaryngol Head Neck Surg 116:1331–1333

77. Schaafsma HE, van der Velden L-A, Manni JJ, Peters H, Link M, Ruiter DJ, Ramaekers FCS (1993) Increased expression of cytokeratins 8, 18 and vimentin in the invasion front of mucosal squamous cell carcinoma. J Pathol 170:77–86

78. van Dorst EB, van Muijen GN, Litvinov SV, Fleuren GJ (1998) The limited difference between keratin patterns of squamous cell carcinomas and adenocarcinomas is explicable by both cell lineage and state of differentiation of tumour cells. J Clin Pathol 51:679–684

79. Grau C, Johansen LV, Jakobsen J, Geertsen P, Andersen E, Jensen BB (2000) Cervical lymph node metastases from unknown primary tumours. Results from a national survey by the Danish Society for Head and Neck Oncology. Radiother Oncol 55:121–129

80. Batsakis JG (1981) The pathology of head and neck tumors: the occult primary and metastases to the head and neck, Part 10. Head Neck Surg 3:409–423

81. Moll R, Moll I, Gould VE (1996) Neuroendocrine-Merkel cells of the skin and their neoplasms. In: Lechago J, Gould VE (eds) Bloodworth´s Endocrine Pathology, 3rd ed. Williams & Wilkins, Baltimore, 641–661

82. Barnhill RL (2001) The biology of melanoma micrometastases. Recent Results Cancer Res 158:3–13

83. Woolgar JA, Scott J, Vaughan ED, Brown JS (1994) Pathological findings in clinically false-negative and false-positive Neck dissections for oral carcinoma. Ann R Coll Surg Engl 76:237–244

84. Pohris E, Eichhorn T, Glanz H, Kleinsasser O (1987) Immunohistological reaction patterns of cervical lymph nodes in patients with laryngeal carcinomas. Arch Otorhinolaryngol 244:278–283

85. Lennert K (1967) The significance of the unspecific inflammatory reaction in the cervical lymphatic system. In: Ruttiman A (ed) Progress in Lymphology. Proceedings of the International Symposium on Lymphology, Zurich, Switzerland, Thieme, Stuttgart, 293–294

86. Newland JR, Linke RP, Kleinsasser O, Lennert K (1983) Lymph node enlargement due to amyloid. Virchows Arch A Pathol Anat Histopathol 399:233–236

87. Newland JR, Linke RP, Lennert K (1986) Amyloid deposits in lymph nodes: a morphologic and immunohistochemical study. Hum Pathol 17:1245–1249

Diagnostic Techniques

B. M. Lippert

4.1 Introduction

The diagnosis of cervical lymph node enlargement has evolved over time and is generally well accepted, although often controversially discussed. In this chapter, we evaluate various examination procedures in regard to their necessity and timely sequence. We also examine various imaging techniques in view of their diagnostic importance and cost.

Cervical lymph node swelling is a condition that occurs very frequently. The origin is often viral or bacterial infections of the upper aerodigestive tract. However, the condition can also be caused by cervical masses due to metastases, solid tumors, cysts or vascular malformations. Using a combination of laboratory findings, including serology and bacteriology, and clinical diagnostic techniques leads to a reliable diagnosis in most cases.

For squamous cell carcinomas of the upper aerodigestive tract, the presence of lymph node metastases is an important prognostic factor [1]. Often only palpation is used to determine cervical lymph node swellings. Because of the low sensitivity of physical examination, a neck showing no metastases on palpation (clinical No neck) bears the risk of so-called occult metastases. Furthermore, many malignancies of the head and neck develop contralateral metastases, especially when the primary tumor is situated near the midline or has surpassed it [2].

Management of the clinical No neck is controversial. When the rate of occult metastases is higher than 20%, generally, an elective neck dissection is performed. The necessity of this is often determined independently from the results of imaging. In cases of smaller carcinomas, a so-called "wait and see" policy can be pursued instead of elective neck dissection. This approach seems to be appropriate if the probability of occult metastases is lower than 20%, and if there is a reasonable surgical option in the event of the later development of lymph node metastases. The risk of initially overlooking occult metastases can be reduced by the use of the appropriate imaging procedures [3]. If imaging confirms the palpatory No situation, the "wait and see" policy seems appropriate. This approach assumes, however, high reliability of imaging, as well as regular clinical follow-up at short intervals [1]. Nevertheless, one must bear in mind that about 25% of occult metastases in a No neck are micrometastases, and, therefore, no examination procedure can reach a sensitivity higher than 75% if the specificity is reduced simultaneously [4].

If clinical examination reveals obvious cervical lymph node enlargement, the number of unrecognized metastases is less important because generally all lymph node regions are resected by modified radical neck dissection. An exact description of the number and location of possible metastases is relevant only with a small primary tumor and only when selective neck dissection, with resection of certain lymph node regions, or radiotherapy, is performed. The identification of retropharyngeal or paratracheal lymph nodes by means of CT or MRI in cases where they are not accessible on palpation can also influence the therapeutic procedure [5]. Finally, patients with advanced cervical metastatic spread need to undergo imaging procedures in order to determine operability.

In light of the situations described above, the procedures used in the diagnosis of cervical lymph node enlargement will be described and their significance critically discussed, in particular as it applies to the determination of cervical lymph node metastases.

4.2 Inspection and Palpation

The first condition for the evaluation of lymph node swelling in the head and neck is a very carefully obtained patient history and physical exam, with information on duration of the swelling, change in size, presence or absence of pain, possibility of displacement, possible origins of the disease and any pretreatments.

Inspection and palpation form the basis of the medical examination and should be performed prior to any other type of examination. For examination of the neck, the patient should disrobe the upper part of the body and remove any jewelry. The patient should sit straight, due to the fact that the upright position promotes better cooperation and attention from the patient.

4.2.1 Inspection

The inspection of the external neck should be oriented at profiling structures, such as the sternocleidomastoid muscles and the laryngeal prominence. More extended swellings in the neck region may lead to asymmetries with resultant contour changes. Cervical lymph nodes are normally not visible in healthy adults, but they are occasionally seen in children, especially girls with thin skin.

During inspection of the neck, the physician must pay attention to swellings, changes of color and abnormal postures. Redness of the cervical skin indicates primarily an acute inflammatory process. It can also be an expression of malignant skin infiltration. The absolute and painless moving of the head in all directions must be examined, as well as the moving of shoulder, arm and hand. This serves to reveal lesions of the accessory nerve and/or the brachial plexus by infiltrative processes.

4.2.2 Palpation

For palpation of the head and neck, special care and clinical experience are required. The palpation of the neck is performed simultaneously on both sides, i.e., bimanually to compare the two sides. Usually the patient sits and the examiner stands in front of or behind the patient. For this examination, it is important to develop a strict systematic order in which to cover all cervical regions. The cervical lymph nodes are divided according to their anatomic localization and surgical control points. The classification describes especially 6 regions (1–6), which include the pre- and paratracheal region, as well as the mediastinal region (7a+b), the preauricular region (8) and the buccal region (9).

The palpation of single lymph node regions is performed with one hand, while the other hand guides the head of the patient or exposes the deeply situated tissue by counter pressure. For palpation of the supraclavicular lymph nodes, the patient should be asked to cough or strain, as these maneuvers will reveal palpable changes in the lymph nodes. The pre- and postauricular lymph nodes are mainly situated superficially and can be palpated with the fingertips.

The palpatory findings of the neck are often difficult to determine, due to the individual variation in the thickness of the covering layers. Usually, enlarged cervical lymph nodes are only palpable with certainty when they are larger than 10 mm. Frequently, the palpatory examination is complicated by surgical or radiotherapeutic pre-treatments (scarring, edema, fibrosis).

During palpation, the physician must pay attention to size, surface, form and consistency. He or she must also pay attention to the presence or absence of pain and to the mobility of the structures. Redness, warmth and pain indicate acute inflammations. The consistency of the palpated lymph nodes gives certain hints of possible diseases, but is not pathognomonic. A soft consistency might be a sign of a cystic transformation or a coagulation necrosis. Limited mobility indicates an accompanying inflammation or a malignant process with extracapsular spread and infiltration of adjacent structures. Scar tissue can mimic a tumor at inspection or palpation. Smaller nodes that are painful on palpation may indicate neuroma.

4.3 B-Mode Sonography

During the last two decades, ultrasonography has developed into an indispensable tool in the diagnosis of diseases of the head and neck region. Technical advances in sonographic equipment, as well as Doppler and color Doppler sonography, make the technique the imaging procedure of choice for the morphologic examination of cervical soft tissues. With a detection rate of 90–97%, B-mode sonography is a highly reliable tool in the detection of enlarged lymph nodes. Investigators have reported it to be superior to palpation (60%), computed tomography (83%) and MRI (83%) [6]. Its application is useful in differential diagnosis, surgical planning and the postoperative care of the neck.

For the patient, ultrasonography is free of side effects and can be rapidly performed. It is non-invasive, always available and very cost-effective. The examination can be repeatedly in a timely and organized manner. In contrast to computed tomography and magnetic resonance imaging, B-mode sonography is a dynamic examination method, i. e., the scanning levels can be chosen arbitrarily and adapted to the findings. By modifying the examination conditions, e. g., palpation, compression and Valsalva maneuver, a better differentiation of the structures is possible [6]. The so-called sonopalpation is a particularly useful evaluation tool if a defined cervical lymph node metastasis can be resected off a blood vessel wall, or if the wall is infiltrated.

Despite, or perhaps due to, the variability of sonography, certain preconditions must be fulfilled in order to achieve valid and reproducible results. Additionally, the accuracy of B-mode sonography is mainly influenced by the clinical and sonographic experience of the examiner [7]. For examination of the cervical region, high-resolution probes (5–7.5 MHz) with a width of about 1 cm and a length of 4–5 cm should be used. The use of a contact surface enables challenging areas like the paramandibular region to be depicted without significant artifacts.

The sonographic examination of pathologic transformations should always be performed at two levels, as only then is an exact determination of the extent of change possible. Findings must be described in clear relation to the surrounding structures. So-called landmarks, such as, for example, the sternocleidomastoid muscle or the common carotid artery, should always be included in the sonographic image. A pictograph for documentation of the position of the probe in relation to the neck is recommended. Documentation of the findings on a standardized examination sheet, and the use of video material, is essential for reproducibility and follow-up observations by different examiners.

Regarding their sono-acoustic properties, lymph nodes do not differ significantly from the surrounding fatty tissue. As a result, non-pathologically transformed lymph nodes cannot be described sonographically. The change of acoustic characteristics in the context of disease allows a sonographic depiction of lymph nodes only at a size of 4–5 mm.

The sonographic examination of lymph nodes is evaluated in terms of localization, size in transverse and longitudinal diameters, shape, echo characteristics, grouping/perfusion pattern and pulsatility as seen in the color Doppler [7].

In B-mode sonography, lymph nodes appear as echoless to mainly homogeneous structures. They are oval or round, mostly clearly limited and of different sizes. In the context of the whole clinical situation (symptoms, palpation and inspection), a certain percentage of sonographically and/or clinically detected lymph nodes can be accurately described. However, at this time, there are no certain sono-morphologic criteria, especially for lymph nodes smaller than 8 mm, that allow pathognomonic diagnosis or guarantee a precise differential diagnosis of malignancy. In order to ascertain the diagnosis, especially to exclude malignant diseases, almost always, a cytological examination is necessary.

4.3.1 Benign Lymphadenitis

Lymph nodes that are swollen because of bacterial or viral infections of the upper aerodigestive tract generally occur in the regional area of the infection. They appear sonographically as small (diameter < 20 mm) and solitary, or as a chain of nodes. Their shape is oval and sometimes bean-like. Occasionally, larger lymph nodes (diameter > 30 mm) can be observed, more so in children. Lymph nodes > 30 mm in diameter in adults are rarely benign. Regarding their sonographic characteristics, inflammatory lymph nodes are typically low-echogenic structures and can be easily separated from the surrounding tissue. In the center of the node, often a fine, linear higher-echogenic structure is revealed. It corresponds to the central fatty and connective tissues that delineate the low-echogenic sinus edge [7]. In the presence of an abscess in a lymph node, the sonographic image changes due to further inflammation. In this context, a confluence of single lymph nodes can often be observed. In total, the image can be described as inhomogeneous and spotty. Centrally low-echogenic or echoless areas are visible, with the dorsal amplification characteristic for liquids, as well as for more echogenic areas corresponding to cellular debris. An accompanying lymphadenitis is nearly always seen.

4.3.2 Malignant Lymphomas

Enlarged cervical lymph nodes occurring in the context of Hodgkin's or non-Hodgkin's lymphoma might be the first symptoms of the disease, or they can indicate an already advanced disease stage. Sonographic differentiation between Hodgkin's and non-Hodgkin's lymphoma is not possible. Cervical lymph nodes occurring in malignant lymphomas may develop in every lymph node region. In contrast to reactive lymphadenitis and also to lymphogenic metastatic spread, the location of pathologically transformed lymph nodes in the lymphomas does not depend on the lymphatic drainage region of the infection or primary tumor.

Sonographically, the lymph nodes appear as low-echogenic or echoless, self-limited masses, with a round or slightly oval form. Depending from the stage of the disease, the lymphomas occur solitarily or are arranged in groups. Frequently, both sides of the neck are affected. Generally, infiltration of the adjacent structures does not occur, although significant growth can lead to displacement and/or compression of larger cervical vessels [7]. In duplex sonography, abnormal drainage patterns with reduced perfusion can be observed; however, these findings are not specific [8]. If malignant lymphoma is suggested by sonomorphologic criteria and cytological result, excisional biopsy of at least one lymph node must be done for further histological examination and classification.

4.3.3 Lymph Node Metastases

4.3.3.1 Sonographic Criteria

It is characteristic of squamous cell carcinomas of the upper aerodigestive tract to develop early lymphogenic metastatic spread that primarily occurs in the regional drainage area of the primary tumor. As the tumor grows, the number of affected cervical lymph node stations increases. It is also possible for lymph node stations to be skipped. The metastatic spread generally occurs ipsilaterally. Bilateral lymphogenic metastatic spread can be observed when the tumor growth is near the midline or when the direction of the lymph vessels crosses the midline. The extent of the cervical lymphogenic metastatic spread is highly significant in determining patient prognosis and therapy. Therefore, early and reliable detection of cervical lymph node metastases is essential. An internationally accepted classification of the cervical lymph node metastases must be made according to UICC and AJCC criteria.

There is general agreement in the literature that B-mode sonography is the most sensitive method for detecting lymph node enlargement in primary staging [6, 7]. B-mode sonography is clearly superior to palpation, and, depending on the study and the comparative parameters, it is superior, or at least equal, to computed tomography and magnetic resonance imaging [1]. In conjunction with ultrasound-guided, fine needle aspiration cytology, the sensitivity of B-mode sonography is about 93–95 %, and the specificity is 87–93 % (▶ Table 4.1).

Table 4.1. Sensitivity and specificity of different lymph node sizes, in relation to the minimal axial diameter (modified according to van den Brekel et al. [2–4]

Size	Sensitivity (%)		Specificity (%)	
	N+	N0	N+	N0
5 mm	97	86	21	44
6 mm	96	78	21	58
7 mm	96	58	42	75
8 mm	92	42	58	81
9 mm	90	28	68	92
10 mm	86	17	74	96
11 mm	81	8	95	98

The sonographic assessment of lymph nodes considers localization, size, contour, delineation, density and the internal structure (▶ Fig. 4.1). Cervical lymph node metastases are generally low-echogenic, round or bean-shaped structures, with a diameter of more than 10 mm. Another criterion of malignancy is possibly the relationship between maximal and axial diameter, as well as the evidence of irregular central lymph node vessels [9].

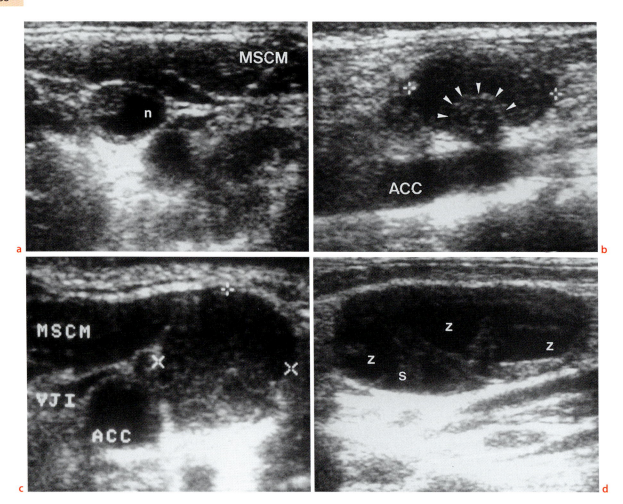

Figure 4.1 a–d

Sonographic findings of cervical lymph node metastases.
a Craniojugular transverse section with description of a lymph node metastasis with necrotic parts (*n*). **b** Lymph nodes with detection of tumor infiltration (*arrows*) in longitudinal section. **c** Lymph node metastasis situated at the anterior edge of the sternocleidomastoid muscle, well delineated. **d** Big, inhomogeneous lymph node metastasis with solid (*s*) and cystic (*z*) parts. *MSCM*, Sternocleidomastoid muscle; *VJI*, internal jugular vein; *ACC*, common carotid artery; *ACI*, internal carotid artery

Despite our knowledge of the guidelines discussed above, no clear sonomorphologic criteria typical for metastases have been established [6]. In the context of staging examinations, all enlarged lymph nodes must be suspect (▶ Table 4.1). This is very important because studies demonstrate that in 40 % of the cases, lymph nodes with a diameter of less than 10 mm are still found to be involved with cancer, with some showing extracapsular spread [10].

Obvious extracapsular growth with infiltration of adjacent structures, such as the internal jugular vein or the sternocleidomastoid muscle, easily prove the presence of malignancy. Although determination of malignancy based on sonomorphologic criteria alone is not justified, sonography delivers important information for patients suffering from malignancies of the upper aerodigestive tract. This includes information such as the number and size of lymph nodes and their relationship to adjacent structures, considerations that are very important in the determination of surgical treatment options [6].

Having the appropriate documentation in this context is essential. Potential metastases must be exactly defined as to their topography, and they must be documented according to their size. Furthermore, the surgeon must record whether lymph nodes should be examined by means of fine needle aspiration cytology and, if so, which ones. The status of the lymph node documented in this manner, together with the description of the localization and size of the primary tumor, helps to determine the extent of neck dissection. The exact documentation of all T1 carcinomas is of special importance, because, in these cases, the neck often remains untreated after functional resection of the primary tumor, and a "wait and see" policy in relationship to the neck is pursued with regular sonographic controls.

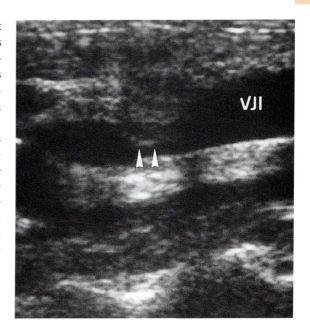

Figure 4.2

Sonographic image of infiltration of the internal jugular vein (*arrows*) by a lymph node metastasis. *VJI*, Internal jugular vein

4.3.3.2 Extracapsular Growth

Extracapsular growth of cervical lymph node metastases of squamous cell carcinomas of the head and neck results in a significantly poorer prognosis for the patient [10]. Clinical signs for extracapsular growth are skin infiltration, a reduced displacement up to fixation of the lymph node metastasis, visible infiltration of muscular structures and the infiltration of nerves with associated neurological deficits.

In spite of improved technical equipment (which includes color-coded duplex sonography), extracapsular extension in small lymph nodes (smaller than 10 mm diameter) cannot be depicted sonographically. Despite this, imaging procedures contribute enormously to the preoperative assessment of possible vascular invasion by cervical lymph node metastases (▶ Fig. 4.2), and sonography seems to be superior to MRI and CT [7].

Dynamic B-mode sonography with sonopalpation allows the examiner to assess the mobility of vessels in relation to adjacent structures. This is accomplished using manual displacement of the metastasis or by instructing the patient to swallow and using Valsalva maneuvers; either method enables the examiner to distinguish a metastatic-related compression of the internal jugular vein from an infiltration with thrombotic obliteration. Adherence to the internal jugular vein can be observed from a metastatic size of about 2.5 cm and up.

Sonopalpation can be very helpful in determining the surgical separation of tumor and artery, and the technique is possible in a patient exhibiting a fixed cervical lymph node metastasis. What makes it possible is that infiltration of the wall of the common carotid or the internal carotid artery becomes visible, due to the circumscribed interruption of the more echogenic vascular wall. If the arterial wall can be depicted uninterruptedly at two levels, the probability is very high that no vessel wall invasion is present. Infiltration is more probable if the lymph node metastasis contacts the artery for more than 3 cm, or if encircling of the vascular perimeter of more than 270° can be observed. Another indication is when the tumor cannot be displaced from the respective vessel using sonopalpation [7].

If there is a strong suspicion that the vessels have been invaded, arteriography, with examination of the cerebral circulation, must be done prior to planned surgery in order to avoid possible serious complications.

4.3.3.3 Lymph Node Metastases of Non-Squamous Origin

In addition to the lymph node metastases of squamous cell carcinomas of the upper aerodigestive tract, lymph node metastases from other tumor entities can be localized in the cervical soft tissue. Here, especially, carcinomas of salivary gland origin, malignant melanomas and carcinomas of the thyroid gland must be mentioned. Lymph node metastases from breast cancer or the urogenital tract are also occasionally observed. Regarding the sonomorphologic criteria, lymph node metastases of non-squamous carcinomas do not reveal specific differences. The use of color-coded duplex sonography to examine lymph node metastases of papillary carcinoma of the thyroid gland sometimes reveals very narrow, clew-shaped vessels in the lymph node stroma [8].

4.3.3.4 Follow-Up

B-mode sonography is very important in the follow-up of tumor patients. Palpation is often very difficult, due to surgical and/or radiotherapeutic prior treatment and the resulting scarring, fibrosis and edema. In these cases, sonography is essential for the early detection of locoregional recurrences. Recurrences are seen as low-echogenic masses and can be distinguished easily from the surrounding echogenic scar tissue [7]. However, scarring can also appear as low-echogenic, diffuse areas, which may hide recurrent metastasis. In particular, scar neuromas and suture granulomas must be considered in the differential diagnosis. In these cases, follow-up at short intervals with careful documentation and measurements, as well as aspiration cytology, can lead to diagnosis.

In small primary tumors with No necks, where the so-called "wait and see" policy is followed, or in cases where the patient has been pretreated with radiochemotherapy, the early detection of lymph node metastases is especially important, because, in these cases, a curative surgical therapy might still be possible [2].

The reader is reminded that sonographic assessment of cervical soft tissue can be very difficult, due to the extent of post-therapeutic fibrosis, the development of edcma, and the transformed anatomic situation after removal of the sternocleidomastoid muscle, submandibular gland or internal jugular vein. Limited mobility of the head and neck in some cases does not allow artifact-free examination with the ultrasound probes. In these cases, the reliability of sonography is even more dependant on the experience and expertise of the examiner.

4.3.4 Sonographic Differential Diagnosis of Enlarged Cervical Lymph Nodes

In order to assess correctly enlarged cervical lymph nodes by means of sonography, masses of other etiology must be included in the differential diagnostic evaluation.

In many cases the patient history, including age, general clinic considerations, laboratory parameters and characteristic sono-morphological aspects, allow the correct diagnostic evaluation of a cervical tumor. For further differential diagnostic clarification, sonographically controlled, fine needle aspiration cytology is very helpful.

4.3.5 Sonographically Controlled Fine Needle Aspiration Cytology

Increasingly during the past few years, sonography has been used in combination with aspiration cytology to improve the assessment of cervical tumors. In examinations by Mann et al. [7], fine needle aspiration cytology (FNAC) led to the correct diagnosis of malignancy in 90% of the cases, and in 66% of the cases, it led to a specific diagnosis. Core biopsy was reported to increase the sensitivity from 76% to 92%.

Fine needle aspiration biopsy is a diagnostic method that is very easy to use. It is also readily available, cost-effective and can be performed on an outpatient basis. It is minimally morbid for the patient and can easily be repeated if necessary. The advantage of ultrasound-directed FNA, in comparison to palpatory aspiration, is that the tumor is aspirated under vision. This is particularly important if the tumor is small and localized in the deeper cervical levels, where it cannot be assessed by palpation. Lymph nodes of size of 3–4 mm in diameter, or lymphomas situated very close to vessels, can be aspirated specifically. Furthermore, an assessment can be made as to whether the cellular aspiration was obtained from a solid or cystic part of the lymph node, which can be of significant diagnostic importance for necrotic lymph node metastases.

The basic difference between fine needle aspiration and core biopsy is that core biopsy is used to aspire a tissue cylinder sufficient for histological examination, whereas fine needle aspiration takes cells from the tissue aggregate so that they can then be diagnosed cytologically.

For FNA, a 20 ml syringe is used. This is fixed to a syringe holder that makes high suction possible using only one hand for aspiration (▶ Fig. 4.3). Needles of the size of 22 to 23 G with an external diameter of 0.7–0.8 mm are attached to the syringe. Cells or cell groups are aspirated from the tissue aggregate by

suction and an up and downward movement of the needle [6]. After discontinuation of the aspiration, the vacuum is broken while the cannula is still in the tumor (▶ Fig. 4.4). Thus, the theoretically possible seeding of tumor cells in the needle tract can be avoided.

For core biopsy, special aspiration cannulas (Tru-Cut system: 11.4 cm long, 14 G diameter) are used. Aspiration must generally be performed under sterile conditions. Local anesthesia is required, in contrast to FNA. Prior to the introduction of the aspiration cannula, an incision should be made with a scalpel to avoid adding small skin parts to the specimen. The biopsy specimen is fixed with formalin, and, after embedding in paraffin, it is examined histologically.

The results of FNA depend not only on the type and quantity of the aspirated material, but also on the experience of the pathologist assessing the specimens [11]. One primary source of error is choosing the wrong lymph node to be aspirated. Lymph node size and morphology help predict the metastatic behavior of the primary tumor. Similar to core needle biopsy, cytology represents only the part of the tumor where the cell aspiration has been performed. Aspiration of lymph node areas not harboring tumor cells, the aspiration of liquid parts or a very low number of tumor cells in the aspiration can lead to false negative results [3]. These difficulties occur most often in smaller (<5 mm) or necrotic lymph nodes.

The diagnostic significance of FNA is often limited to the differentiation of malignant and benign cases. This differentiation allows for diagnostic, as well as therapeutic, planning. Malignant lymphomas are difficult to diagnose cytologically because the assessment of the histo-architecture of a whole lymph node is of decisive differential diagnostic significance. Methodological limitations can also be observed for mesenchymal neoplasms, as well as for cystic or necrotic tumors [6]. Another problem is the evaluation of negative and, in particular, nonspecific results. In the event of a clinically persisting suspicion of malignancy, FNA should be repeated or a histological examination should be performed.

The complication rate from fine needle aspiration cytology and core biopsy is very low. The risk of seeding tumor cells of malignant tumors in the needle

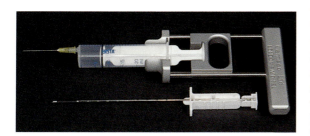

Figure 4.3

Tool holder with fixed syringe and needle for fine needle aspiration cytology as well as aspiration cannula (Sterican, B. Braun, Melsungen, Germany) for aspiration biopsy

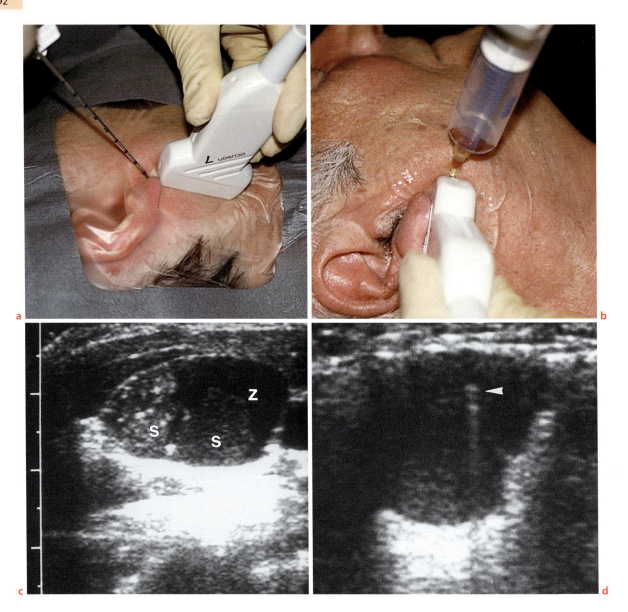

Figure 4.4 a–d

a Penetration of a needle under sonographic control. b Sonographically controlled fine needle aspiration of a parotid mass. c Lymph node metastasis with cystic (z) and solid (s) tumor parts. d Sonographic image of a lymph node with penetrated needle (arrow)

tract is considered to be very low [11]. Reports of this in the literature refer principally to the use of thicker needles [6].

Generally, the indication for FNA should be made generously to gain diagnostic advantage [7]. Due to the fact that smaller lymph nodes cannot be easily assessed sonographically in order to determine their malignant potential, and due to the fact that color-coded duplex sonography is not very helpful either in this situation [2], the assessment of smaller lymph nodes requires ultrasound-guided fine needle aspiration cytology in order to correctly choose the lymph nodes suspected of harboring metastases.

About 40% of cervical lymph node metastases have a diameter smaller than 10 mm [10]. Van den Brekel [2] recommends that lymph nodes from a size of 4 mm in the regions I, III, IV, V and VI, as well as lymph nodes from a size of 5–6 mm in the region II, be examined by FNA. In posttherapeutic follow-up, not only the absolute size of lymph nodes, but also their growth behavior, must be considered [2].

The sensitivity of sonographically controlled fine needle aspiration cytology for the clinical No neck is considered to be about 44–73% in the literature [12]. Due to the fact that false negative results are relatively rare, the specificity is near 100% [3]. Further optimization of the examination techniques, e.g., molecular-biological assessment of the cell aspirate by means of RT-PCR or improved detection of the sentinel lymph node by means of scintigraphic techniques, can possibly increase the sensitivity [1].

4.3.6 Future Technical Developments

4.3.6.1 Color-Coded Duplex Sonography

Doppler sonography is the basis for clinical examination and identification of blood vessels and their assessment regarding pathologic findings. Duplex sonography is a combination of traditional B-mode sonography with an additional pw Doppler. Whereas for the spectral pw Doppler, the time of the distribution velocity is measured at a specific point, the color-coded procedure analyzes the velocity at numerous points distributed over a chosen measurement window. The result is the spatial distribution of the average velocity and the flowing direction in the vessel. The simultaneous two-dimensional image with flashing of the Doppler window occurs over the B-mode image [8].

By means of color-coded duplex sonography, about 80% of enlarged lymph nodes reveal vessels. Depending on the examination conditions, vessels

with a diameter of up to 1 mm can be detected. Several studies indicate that the vascularization pattern of lymph nodes is an additional criterion for malignancy or benignancy [8].

The pathophysiologic basis for increased vascularization of malignant tumors and metastases is the induction of angiogenesis in the context of tumor neogenesis. By means of color-coded duplex sonography, the changed vascularization can be depicted and compared with that of benign lymph nodes. For evaluation, size, distance and drainage direction of the vessels that can be described in the lymph node stroma, the maximal systolic and minimal diastolic flowing velocities, as well as the pulsation index, are measured [13].

Westhofen et al. [8] described four types of lymph node vascularization characteristics:

1. lymph nodes without a depictable vascular pattern
2. lymph nodes with vascularization near the capsule, exterior to the lymph node stroma
3. lymph nodes with vessels that depart fan-shaped from the hilum
4. lymph nodes with solitary or conglomerate intranodal vessels of unordered direction

For chronic inflammatory lymphadenitis (▶ Fig. 4.5), the vascularization remains limited to the hilum area,

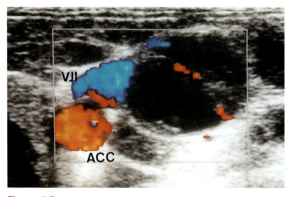

Figure 4.5

Benign lymph node in color-coded duplex sonography. The typical hilar perfusion pattern is depicted. *VJI*, Internal jugular vein; *ACC*, common carotid artery

as is seen in normal lymph node anatomy (hilar vascularization pattern). The arterial vessels run from the hilum of the lymph node fan-shaped into the stroma of the cortex [13]. A highly acute lymphadenitis shows a significant multiplication of the perinodal vascular pattern.

The finding of a heterogeneous vascularization pattern with borderline and irregularly running vessels (clear vascularization in the lymph node stroma and no vascularization in other regions) seems to be characteristic for the presence of a lymph node metastasis. This is caused by the tumor-induced vascular neoplasia, as well as by the displacement of regular vessels. The partly screw-like and narrowly lying vessels in the lymph node stroma are also reliable indicators of malignant growth. In relation to the size of the lymph node, they have a large diameter and are thus well depictable. Lymph node metastases generally show an increased resistance and pulsation index (Pourcelot index); however, in the literature the sizes vary significantly. Malignant lymphomas reveal irregular intranodal vascular convolutions [13]. Lymph nodes in Hodgkin's disease show an increased vascularization, both in the hilum and the stroma.

Regarding lymph node differentiation, the sensitivity is about 79% and the specificity up to 100% [8]. A significantly critical point, however, is the insufficient detection of smaller vessels, which impedes the assessment of smaller lymph nodes. Furthermore, in about 20% of the lymph nodes, no vessels can be revealed intranodally, rendering the method insufficiently sensitive.

The significance of the color-coded duplex sonography for the differential diagnosis of lymph node diseases, especially the differentiation of reactive lymphadenitis from cervical lymph node metastases, is not completely clear. The initial hope of significantly increasing the sensitivity by evaluating lymph node perfusion and establishing characteristic perfusion parameters has not yet been fully realized. Possibly the introduction of contrast enhancers can achieve a higher degree of accuracy.

4.3.6.2 Signal Amplification

Despite significant progress in technical equipment, vessels with small diameters and low flow, as well as vessels in deeply situated tumors, cannot always be detected by means of color-coded duplex sonography. In many cases, no vessels can be described, especially in smaller lymph nodes [13]. Because the smaller lymph nodes are difficult to assess for malignancy, an evaluation of their vascular pattern is of highest interest.

The use of the so-called signal amplification (ultrasound contrast enhancement) can reinforce the color-coded duplex signal. The physical basis for ultrasound contrast enhancers is that microscopically small vapor locks develop where the ultrasound waves disperse. The intravascular micro vapor locks lead to inhomogeneities where re-dispersion effects occur due to saltatory impedances. Furthermore, the encapsulated vapor locks start to vibrate which results in an increase of the contrast effect [14].

The contrast amplifiers usually used for color-coded duplex sonography are biologically inert substances. Levovist consists of palmitic acid-stabilized (0.1%) galactose microparticles (99.9%); Echovist consists of a monosaccharide galactose. After suspension in water, tiny adherent blebs develop (< 3-8 µm) as active parts that are able to amplify the color duplex signal up to 25 dB [14].

In the literature, there are only a few studies, and they contain small numbers of cases. Nevertheless, it may be concluded from these studies that the description of vessels becomes significantly clearer with signal amplifiers. The above-mentioned perfusion pattern for enlarged inflammatory lymph nodes and malignant processes becomes more evident for lymph nodes with a diameter greater than 10 mm. Possibly the signal amplifier is helpful for the often difficult distinction between postoperative scars (very low vascularization) and tumor or lymph node recurrences [14].

To what extent the application of signal amplifiers leads to an increased specificity of the color-coded duplex sonography in the diagnosis of enlarged cervical lymph nodes remains to be determined by larger prospective studies.

4.3.6.3 Digital Sonographic Procedures

Three-Dimensional Sonography

Conventional B-mode sonography is a two-dimensional examination tool. Three-dimensional ultrasound imaging is composed of information from many single levels and results in a three-dimensional image. The average level of thickness is 0.3 mm. The images can be turned in all directions, and single structures can be blown up. A real time description of a three-dimensional image is not possible due to computer limitations. A three-dimensional calculation of the volume is possible and can contribute to an improved depiction of the structure of tumor masses.

Clinical experience with three-dimensional sonography of the head and neck is very poor. Identical sensitivity and specificity concerning the preoperative diagnosis of cervical lymph node metastases can be shown with the use of B-mode sonography. However, when used to detect questionable vascular infiltration of the carotid artery, 3-D sonography has proven to be very useful [15]. Theoretically, it could also contribute to an improved sensitivity in ultrasound-guided fine needle aspiration cytology [6].

Panoramic Imaging Procedures

The conventional B-mode sonography allows only a description of a display detail that has already been determined. Panoramic imaging procedures allow the creation of ultrasound images with extended windows. The computer-assisted composition of many single images to provide a panoramic image can lead to a definition of larger organs or tumors similar to what is obtained through computed tomography or magnetic resonance imaging, except with more equivalent anatomic correlations. This procedure is also called "extended field of view" and was introduced in SieScape (manufactured by Siemens) into the clinical routine. The latest version of the panoramic imaging procedure also incorporates the color Doppler technique (Color SieScape).

Tissue Harmonic Imaging

"Tissue harmonic imaging" makes use of the non-linearity of sound created in tissue, and it allows the correction for defocusing, phase-shifting effects [6]. This new technology (Ultrasound System Elegra, produced by Siemens) improves spatial resolution by contrasting deeply situated tissue. Conventional B-mode sonography can thus be optimized, especially in obese patients and in cases of lymphedema or anatomic changes after surgical interventions. The technique involves the transmission of subsequent, inverted ultrasound impulses, which cause the regressive signals of the pulses and the linear echo to cancel each other out. The resulting images are better defined and sharper [16]. "Contrast harmonic imaging" allows the description of even the smallest vessels in color-coded duplex sonography, without motion artifacts or over-radiation of adjacent larger vessels. Initial experience with this technique is very encouraging [16].

Sono CT Real-Time Compound Imaging

In "sono CT real-time compound imaging," pulses, in addition to the vertical transmission of the probe, are sent and received. Via digital processing of the received signals with a very high computer capacity, an image is composed in real-time that is created from the single images of different sound angles and then summed up (compound technique). The resolution and quality of the image is improved with this technique, in comparison to the traditional B-mode imaging. Clinical experience in the head and neck region do not exist at this time.

4.4 Computed Tomography and Magnetic Resonance Imaging

Since their clinical introduction into the diagnostic routine, computed tomography (CT) and magnetic resonance imaging (MRI) have been used for the evaluation of enlarged cervical lymph nodes and tumorous masses. In addition to differential diagnostic applications, CT and MRI are performed to ascertain the exact localization and extent of cervical tumors, a determination that is not possible with palpation. These diagnostic entities help define the presence of infiltration in adjacent structures, and they also provide an assessment of surgical resectability.

Due to the fact that CT and MRI are significantly superior to palpation in terms of sensitivity, they are also used to stage examinations of head and neck malignancies. About 80 % of all patients suffering from head and neck malignancies receive CT or MRI. Besides an exact description of the primary tumor, CT/MRI allows evaluation of the stage of cervical lymph nodes. In particular, more deeply situated lymph node metastases can be assessed, including retropharyngeal lymph nodes, which are not accessible by palpation [17].

CT is generally preferred to MRI. It is more readily available, free from motion artifacts and easier to interpret by the head and neck surgeon. CT is indicated for all patients who suffer from claustrophobia or have other contraindications (e.g., cardiac pacemaker or metallic implantations) for magnetic resonance imaging [2].

4.4.1 Computed Tomography

CT scanning of the neck is performed routinely in axial fashion from the skull base to the clavicles with a maximal slice thickness of 5 mm. Depending on the specific region in question, the area should be examined in thinner slices of 1–3 mm. Native and contrast-enhanced scans can be performed. Due to the very short period of scanning, swallowing artifact can be avoided. The spiral CT, in particular, allows very short examinations. It also permits a determination of the slice thickness [2].

CT scanning is the procedure of choice for the assessment of possible bone infiltration. However, this assessment is limited by bone density artifacts or artifacts originating from metallic dental fillings, which, in spite of tilted tomography, cannot be avoided in the oral cavity. Newly developed software offers three-dimensional reassessment of the data, with the ability to depict the findings in virtual reality. It also

provides a description of the various reconstructed layers.

In the CT scan, normal lymph nodes are seen as well defined, generally long and oval masses. They reveal a homogeneous density comparable to vessels with hypodense values as seen in muscle. They can be distinguished from rotund vascular structures only after administration of intravenous contrast agents. A description of lymph nodes ≥ 5 mm is possible with the newer CT equipment; although this depends on the slice thickness specified. The diameter of benign lymph nodes is generally less than 10 mm, while lymph nodes in region II may be larger due to persistent tonsillar tissue.

After intravenous contrast enhancement, the density is higher in inflammatory diseases and malignant lymphomas than in metastases. Malignant lymphomas are most often well circumscribed, have a homogeneous density and do not reveal rim enhancement after contrast application. In lymph node metastases, central necrosis occurs early and presents as a hypodense area in the CT scan. Central necrosis and rim enhancement are nonspecific criteria that also occur in inflammatory lymph node diseases with necrosis or abscess formation.

4.4.2 Magnetic Resonance Imaging

In comparison to CT scanning, MRI better defines soft tissue due to its high tissue contrast capability. For the assessment of smaller cervical lymph nodes, a slice thickness of 3 mm is recommended, especially in the clinically most interesting regions, generally levels II and III [2]. The scans should always be performed in two levels from the skull base to the clavicle.

The contrast application of gadolinium-DTPA (Gd-DTPA) is helpful for the description of tumor necrosis within lymph nodes and also for better delineation of the primary tumor.

Lymph nodes can easily be discriminated from blood vessels, due to the absence of a signal generated by the intravascular blood flow. Typically, after contrast application, a signal augmentation in benign lymph nodes occurs. In contrast, the missing perfusion of necrotic tumor parts after Gd-DTPA application leads to an enhancement deficit. The infiltration of adjacent tissue, particularly muscles, becomes more obvious in the T1-weighted scan after contrast agent application. Another tissue differentiation can possibly be made by the so-called relaxometry, i.e., the determination of T1 and T2 time. Central necrosis, which is typically the case for lymph node metastases, leads to a prolonged T1 and T2 relaxation. This typically results in signal reduction in the T1-weighted scan and signal amplification in the T2-weighted scan. In short T1-weighted sequences, malignant lymphomas reveal a higher signal intensity, which corresponds to a short T1 relaxation.

An improved differentiation of benign and malignant cervical lymph nodes will be possible with MR lymphography. This technique requires the application of small iron oxide particles as contrast enhancers. These particles are absorbed in the macrophages of the reticulo-endothelial system of the lymph node's sinus and lead to a reduction of the signals in both T1 and T2-weighted sequences. Lymph node metastases lose the mechanism of phagocytosis, so that the accumulation of iron oxide does not occur and no reduction of the signal intensity is seen [18].

At present, very few patients have undergone this examination. When the examination is performed, the ferromagnetic contrast agent, Sinerem (or Combidex) is combined with low molecular weight dextrose in a dose of 2.6 mg FE/kg weight and intravenously applied. Fourteen to 36 hours after contrast agent application, the superparamagnetic iron oxide (SPIO)-MRI is formed, which makes it possible to better discriminate between malignant and benign tissue. (Lymph nodes that are too small for detection in the standard MRI, however, also cannot be seen in the SPIO-MRI.) The main disadvantage is that a second MRI scan after contrast agent application is necessary, which makes this technique expensive and time-consuming [18].

4.4.3 CT/MRI for Benign Cervical Masses

In cases of clinical suspicion of an inflammatory or benign disease, the indication for extensive examination procedures such as CT and MRI must generally reluctantly be made. In contrast, B-mode sonography is always an applicable technique, with low morbidity and expense to the patient.

Reactively enlarged cervical lymph nodes usually reveal better contrast- enhanced imaging than tumor tissue in CT scanning and MRI. Unfortunately, this different contrast description is not achievable with standard techniques, especially in the case of smaller lymph nodes. The reason for a reduced contrast enhancement can be fat tissue desaturation, which is frequently observed in inflammations or after radiotherapy. Other reasons include abscess formation or the spontaneous necrosis in lymph nodes, which simulates the image of metastases-associated necrosis [19].

Inflammatory lymph node diseases require CT when a phlegmonous extension or abscess is suspected. In contrast to sonography, CT allows the assessment of deeper cervical areas in the mediastinum.

4.4.4 CT/MRI for Lymph Node Metastases

In recent years, the accuracy of the various imaging procedures used in the detection of cervical lymph node metastases from carcinomas of the upper aerodigestive tract has been the subject of numerous clinical examinations [5]. Data concerning the sensitivity and specificity of CT, MRI, sonography and sonographically assisted fine needle aspiration have varied significantly (see ▶ Table 4.1). Although these imaging techniques all identify tumors in lymph nodes, sonography seems to be the most accurate. CT and MRI show comparable degrees of accuracy [5].

Because it influences the therapeutic approach, accuracy is important in the assessment of palpatory No neck [3, 12]. A comparison of imaging techniques for evaluation of the No neck is difficult not only because of the different criteria concerning size, but also because of the incidence of occult metastases and the clinician's influence on the results [3]. The rate of false negative results is highest in the clinical No neck, while the majority of false positive results occur in the N+ neck. The literature indicates that therapeutic decisions for the clinical No neck should not be based solely on findings assessed in CT or MRI. With CT, as well as MRI, approximately 40–60% of the occult metastases can be detected; however, the rate of false positive reports of lymph nodes is very high [2].

The accuracy of CT and MRI in the assessment of cervical lymph nodes depends to a large extent on the criteria defined for lymph node metastases [19, 20]. Characteristics for cervical lymph node metastases are a diameter of more than 10 mm, a rotund form, an alignment in groups and the detection of non-contrast enhanced areas within lymph nodes that originate from tumor necrosis, tumor keratogenesis or cystic areas within the tumor.

Radiologists define necrosis as the reduced and irregular contrast uptake. Only in rare cases do lymph node tissues infiltrated by the tumor accumulate more of the contrast agent than a lymph node that is reactively changed [2]. The detection of necrotic areas is a very reliable criterion for the presence of lymph node metastases. However, in smaller lymph nodes it is extremely rare or not seen at all [20, 21].

Computed tomography seems to be more appropriate than magnetic resonance imaging for the assessment of necrotic areas in lymph nodes. For an optimized description of necrosis, the administration of contrast agents is essential [19].

Due to the fact that the irregular contrast agent uptake in small lymph node metastases frequently cannot be depicted, the shape and size of the lymph nodes are of significant relevance for the assessment of the palpatory No neck. Generally, a round shape must be considered more suspicious than an oval or flat form. The size of the lymph node metastases varies according to the lymph node region. It is very difficult to define optimal criteria regarding size because small metastatic areas within a lymph node do not inevitably result in enlargement of the lymph node [9].

Size as a basis for the criterion "metastasis" is a compromise between sensitivity on one hand and specificity on the other hand. The definition of a small cutoff value means a high sensitivity with reduced specificity, and vice versa. Although the results of the imaging examination of the palpatory No neck are significant for determining whether to perform neck dissection or to wait, it is reasonable to use a very sensitive procedure in spite of the high number of false positive results [2].

In assessing the size criterion, it is important to notice from which patient population the data is obtained. The majority of data in the literature concerning lymph node sizes is based on studies that include patients with a positive cervical lymph node status. Van den Brekel et al. [3], however, were able to show that the sensitivity of a defined lymph node size in the clinical No neck is lower than in the N+ neck. Furthermore, the sizes of lymph node metastases vary significantly in the literature, the degree of variation equaling about 5 to 30 mm. Additionally, a gradation is visible depending on the lymph node region. Considering these results, it may be said that the majority of cervical lymph node metastases do not fall into the size category of 10 mm. Furthermore, in a study published in 1998, van den Brekel et al. [9] showed that it is essential to apply different size criteria in the different cervical regions. Using sonographic examinations, these authors were able to determine that a size of 7 mm is optimal for the palpatory No neck in the lymph node region II, whereas in all other neck regions lymph nodes with a minimal diameter of 6 mm must be considered suspicious for metastasis. The size of 10 mm is considered to be too high an indicator.

Some authors consult the quotient of the maximal and minimal axial diameter for further characterization. If the quotient is 1, as it is for round lymph nodes, it is considered to be suspect for metastases. The quotient of maximal axial and longitudinal diameter also can be included in the assessment. If the quotient is higher than 2, then in 80% of cases the nodes will be reactive [13].

Another criterion for the presence of lymph node metastasis is the detection of extracapsular growth with infiltration of adjacent structures. An extranodal growth is characterized by irregular lymph node edges and the absence of fine fatty layers in the CT/MRI [19].

Table 4.2. Lymph node classification based on radiologic-anatomic criteria according to Som et al. [20]

Level I	Lymph nodes above the hyoid, below the mylohyoid muscle and in front of the posterior edge of the submandibular gland
Level Ia	Lymph nodes between the medial limits of the muscle belly of the digastric muscle, above the hyoid and below the mylohyoid muscle
Level Ib	Lymph nodes lateral to the level IA and in front of the posterior edge of the submandibular gland
Level II	Lymph nodes situated from the skull base to the level of the hyoid. They are located dorsally to the submandibular gland and in front of the posterior edge of the sternocleidomastoid muscle
Level IIa	Lymph nodes arranged around the internal jugular vein (if the lymph nodes are located posterior they cannot be separated from the vein)
Level IIb	Lymph nodes situated behind the internal jugular vein (separated by fine fatty tissue)
Level III	Lymph nodes situated between the inferior edge of the hyoid and the inferior edge of the cricoid cartilage. They are located in front of the posterior edge of the sternocleidomastoid muscle
Level IV	Lymph nodes situated between the inferior edge of the cricoid cartilage and the clavicle. The lymph nodes are located in front of an imaginary line between the posterior edge of the sternocleidomastoid muscle and the posterior lateral margin of the anterior scalene muscle. They are situated lateral to the internal carotid artery
Level V	Lymph nodes situated from the skull base to the clavicle. The lymph nodes are located behind an imaginary line between the posterior edge of the sternocleidomastoid muscle and the posterior lateral margin of the anterior scalene muscle. They are situated in front of the anterior edge of the trapezius muscle
Level Va	Superior level 5: lymph nodes situated from the skull base to the inferior edge of the cricoid cartilage
Level Vb	Inferior level 5: lymph nodes situated from the inferior edge of the cricoid cartilage to the clavicle
Level VI	Lymph nodes situated between the internal carotid artery from the inferior edge of the hyoid to the beginning of the sternum
Level VII	Lymph nodes situated between the internal carotid artery below the superior edge of the sternum and the brachiocephalic vein
Supraclavicular lymph nodes	Lymph nodes situated above the clavicle and lateral to the internal carotid artery; above and medial to the ribs
Retropharyngeal lymph nodes	Lymph nodes situated 2 cm inferior to the skull base and medial to the internal carotid artery

The significance of CT and MRI for the assessment of capsular rupture is controversial in the literature. The accuracy for both procedures is about 70–90%. However, this data refers to larger lymph node metastases with infiltration of large vessels of the sternocleidomastoid muscle [19]. Van den Brekel et al. [9] do not consider extracapsular growth a reliable criterion because the detection of capsular rupture is primarily a histological diagnosis that cannot reliably be made in smaller lymph nodes by means of CT and MRI.

Som et al. [17] established anatomic scanning criteria for CT and MRI for the assessment and documentation of cervical lymph node metastases using the lymph node classification of the American Academy of Otolaryngology, Head and Neck Surgery and the American Joint Committee on Cancer (▶ Table 4.2). The precondition for such a classification is a standardized examination procedure. CT scanning should be performed either in axial direction with contrast enhancement, via continuous 3 mm slices from the skull base to the manubrium sterni, or using spiral CT techniques with reconstructed 2–3 mm slices. The slice thickness in the MRI should be less than 5 mm. The purpose of this radiologic lymph node classification is to provide more exact and reproducible documentation of lymph node metastasis. Such studies stand out in the history of randomized, multicenter analyses, due to the fact that the findings can be collected and evaluated independently of the examiner.

In 9–50 % of patients suffering from an oro- or hypopharyngeal carcinoma, retropharyngeal lymph node metastases occur. Retropharyngeal, and also paratracheal, lymph node metastases are usually very small (< 15 mm) and, consequently, difficult to assess clinically. Due to their location, these metastases either cannot be described at all, or they can be described only unreliably by means of B-mode sonography. As a result, CT or MRI is always indicated. The occurrence of retropharyngeal or paratracheal metastases leads to a significantly poorer prognosis. Early detection is essential in planning the therapeutic approach in order to extend the neck dissection or enlarge the radiation field [5].

The results of CT and MRI in the early diagnosis of lymph node recurrences are discouraging because the differentiation between tumor tissue and scar tissue or edema is too inexact. After radiochemotherapy, lymph node metastases reveal a central necrosis, or they are cicatricially changed. Both conditions are present, for example, in MRI in the T2-weighted scans with high signal. A contrast-enhanced scan 4–6 months after therapy can indicate recurrence [12]. Comparison with scans performed earlier is important. Therefore, several weeks after acute posttherapeutic tissue reactions subside, a baseline scan should be performed. This period is generally about 3–4 months after primary therapy.

Neither CT nor MRI can reliably differentiate reactively enlarged lymph nodes from metastases [5]. Morphologic criteria such as the irregularity of marginal structures or the description of smaller tumor areas within a lymph node will become more significant when better contrast-enhanced techniques and imaging procedures are developed [2]. With the exception of newer MRI techniques, which allow better contrasting with fat suppression, and accelerated scanning techniques for decreasing motion artifacts [3], there have been few improvements of diagnostic significance [2]. Three-dimensional CT reconstructions can be useful for an exact localization in the planning of radiotherapy of head and neck tumors, but they provide no advantage in the evaluation of malignant cervical lymph nodes [22].

4.5 Lymphoscintigraphy

The application of nuclear medicine techniques to imaging descriptions of malignant processes in the head and neck is an important addition to conventional methods. Previously treated patients with a clinical suspicion of local recurrence and/or cervical lymph node metastasis cannot be assessed reliably by means of morphologic changes alone.

The scintigraphic differentiation of malignant and benign growth generally is based on three mechanisms: specific metabolism of the tumor tissue to be detected (e. g., radioiodine uptake in cases of metastasis of a differentiated thyroid carcinoma), certain superficial characteristics of the tumor cell that can be detected by means of radioactively marked antibodies (e. g., anti-225.28-S-antibodies in malignant melanomas) and a malignancy-specific accumulation or uptake of certain radioactive tracer substances (e. g., persisting uptake of Thallium in malignant tissue).

4.5.1 Dynamic Scintigraphy of Lymphatic Drainage

For malignant melanoma and breast carcinoma, lymphoscintigraphy is a well established diagnostic procedure for the description of lymphatic drainage, including "sentinel lymph node" drainage [23]. In contrast to lymph angiography, no surgical preparation of lymphatic vessels is required. For lymphoscintigraphy, usually ^{99m}technetium (^{99m}Tc)-marked nanocolloid is applied. Due to its average particle size of 10–20 nm, ^{99m}Tc has an optimal tracking kinetic. The radiation exposure for the patient is low.

In the head and neck, lymphoscintigraphy has been used for the preoperative description of the lymphatic drainage of carcinomas. In this area, however, the detection of lymph node metastases by this method is less important because B-mode sonography represents a more reliable and less costly technique for routine staging. The purpose of lymphoscintigraphy when used with squamous cell carcinomas of the head and neck is primarily the determination of lymphatic drainage direction in order to obtain further information regarding the extent of neck dissection [23].

The direction of lymphatic drainage in the neck depends on the localization of the primary tumor. By means of lymphoscintigraphy, the physician can verify whether the metastatic spread is limited to the predominant lymphatic direction or whether other lymph node regions and/or the contralateral side must also be considered in the treatment strategy. This is especially important for the No neck because selective neck dissection should be performed in neck lymph node areas only when the chance of metastatic spread is high. Furthermore, in cases of advanced ipsilateral metastatic spread, and therefore potentially exhausted transport capacity of the lymphatic fluid, contralateral lymphatic spread can also be detected.

In up to 70% of the cases, the results of lymphoscintigraphy have shown a good description of ipsilateral and/or contralateral lymphatic drainage in relation to the location of defined cervical lymph node regions. In about 30% of the patients examined, no lymphatic drainage could be detected. The authors explain this discrepancy by reduced lymphatic drainage due to intraoperative tissue compression by the endoscopy instruments [23]. Other reasons might include suspended lymphatic drainage (due to tumor infiltration of the lymph nodes) as well as posttherapeutically transformed or completely missing lymph vessels. At this point, it must be stressed that the radionuclide is taken up in reduced quantity or not at all by the lymph nodes that are affected by a metastases and possibly have capsular rupture.

A distinct disadvantage of dynamic lympho-scintigraphy is that only tumor localizations in the region of the oral cavity and the oropharynx allow the application of the radionuclide without additional anesthesia [24].

Summing up the experiences collected to date, lymphoscintigraphy in the double tracer technique reveals the exact location of a described lymphatic drainage pathway in relation to the anatomic structures of the head and neck. Thus, it and can be useful in the preoperative diagnosis paradigm to augment other imaging procedures. For the primary detection of cervical lymph nodes, however, it is not appropriate.

4.5.2 Thallium-201 Scintigraphy

Another functional technique is thallium-201 scintigraphy (^{201}Tl SPECT). Originally, thallium chloride was used for scintigraphic measurements of myocardial perfusion. However, it also accumulates in malignant tissue. While the enhancement mechanism of increased uptake of the potassium analog thallium via furosemide-inhibiting potassium co-transport of the tumor cell has been proposed, the exact mechanism of accumulation in the tumor tissue is not clear. ^{201}Tl SPECT has been used in the detection of various malignancies, but in the head and neck region very few, and somewhat contradictory, results have been reported [25].

Regarding the description of the primary tumor, no advantages can be demonstrated compared with CT or MRI. ^{201}Tl SPECT is not appropriate for the staging of cervical lymph node metastases. A possible application of 201Tl SPECT may be in follow-up control after primary therapy for the early detection of possible residual cancer or tumor recurrences [25].

4.5.3 Sentinel Lymphadenectomy

The sentinel lymph node (SLN) concept is one of the most important advances in clinical oncology of the last decade. The principle of lymphatic mapping started with the assumption that a primarily lymphogenic spreading melanoma drains initially to the first (the so-called sentinel) lymph node in the regional lymphatic drainage region and from there further lymphogenic metastatic spread occurs.

The bases for the detection of the sentinel lymph nodes are the pre- and intraoperative scintigraphy of lymphatic drainage and the use of intraoperative gamma probe measurements in cases of clinically inaccessible lymph node metastases. After scintigraphic examination, the first draining lymph node is identified, removed and submitted to histopathologic evaluation. If the sentinel lymph node is not involved with cancer, an extended lymph node dissection can be avoided, which potentially may lead to a significant reduction in surgery-related morbidity. Sentinel lymphadenectomy is both diagnostic and therapeutic in that it reveals subclinical lymphogenic metastatic spread which might otherwise be missed, due to small tumor size and location, unless a neck dissection were done.

In summary, while sentinel lymphadenectomy seems to be a reliable staging procedure for malignant melanoma, breast carcinoma and also prostate carcinoma, for squamous cell carcinomas of the upper aerodigestive tract, little literature exists [24]. The technique and the actual significance of sentinel lymphonodectomy in the head and neck will be discussed further in Chap. 7.6.

4.5.4 Radioimmunoscintigraphy

A new and innovative technique for selective targeting of tumor cells, in particular for the identification of lymph node metastases, is radioimmunoscintigraphy (RIS) with monoclonal antibodies (MAbs). The technique involves the use of MAbs directed against tumor-specific or tumor-associated antigens labeled with radionuclide. Due to the radiation of the radionuclide, the tumor tissue can scintigraphically be visualized [26]. Usually 99mTc is used because of its short half-life.

The accuracy of RIS is influenced by the targeting antigen (specificity, inhomogeneous expression), as well as by the applied antibodies or antibody fragments themselves. Further factors influencing RIS are the histological tumor composition, the tumor vascularity and, finally, the antibody-adapted scintigraphic technique.

RIS is used for the detection of occult primary tumors, for further examination after unclear MRI or CT findings and in the assessment of residual or recurrent cancer after primary therapy [26]. For malignancies of the head and neck, little data exists. The reason for this is that the determination of the specific monoclonal antibodies to be used against squamous cell carcinomas of the upper aerodigestive tract is much more difficult than with other malignancies. To date, 30 MAbs have been described for squamous cell carcinomas of the head and neck [26].

The group at the Department of Otolaryngology, Head and Neck Surgery at the University of Amsterdam has the greatest experience in the field of radioimmunoscintigraphy. In a prospective clinical study, 49 patients with histologically proven squamous cell carcinoma of the upper aerodigestive tract were provided with MAb E48 IgG (24 patients), E48 F(ab')$_2$-fragments (15 patients) or U36 IgG (10 patients), and immunoscintigraphy was performed to detect possible cervical lymph node metastases. For comparison purposes, all patients underwent a physical examination, CT and MRI. After neck dissection, a comparative analysis of the procedures mentioned was performed based on the histological processing of the labeled lymph nodes.

In all patients, the primary tumor was detected immunoscintigraphically. In 66 surgically treated cases, yielding a total of 318 examined lymph node regions, RIS showed a sensitivity of 55% for all lymph node regions, and 69% for the ipsilateral sites. Thirty-five lymph node regions and 16 ipsilateral sites were considered false negative. The accuracy of RIS amounted to 87% for the lymph node regions and 72% for the ipsilateral sites. In comparison, the accuracy for palpation, CT and MRI was 87%, 86% and 88% for all lymph node regions and 82%, 82% and 77% for the examined ipsilateral neck sites. The lymph nodes considered as false negative were micrometastases with few tumor cells, lymph nodes with a diameter less than 20 mm and lymph nodes with significant necrotic cellular material (keratin or fibrin) [26]. Moreover, the usefulness of RIS was found to be limited due to insufficient spatial solution capacity.

The results of RIS for the detection of metastases was comparable to palpation, CT or MRI as far as sensitivity and specificity were concerned. Due to the high rate of false negative results, RIS is not currently recommended for the diagnosis of cervical lymph node metastases [26]. An interesting future consideration is whether early detection of smaller metastases and micrometastases will be possible with RIS in patients with No neck.

4.6 Positron Emission Tomography

Positron emission tomography (PET) is a non-invasive procedure for measuring biochemical processes in tissue. In contrast to morphologic imaging (such as CT/MRI), PET allows the description of function in organs and tissues. In PET scanning, the radiopharmaceuticals are labeled with a so-called positron- emitting radionuclide. These are extraordinarily transient elements occurring in organic material. The most common are ^{15}O ($t_{1/2}$: 2 min), ^{13}N ($t_{1/2}$: 10 min), ^{11}C ($t_{1/2}$: 20 min) and, as a substitute for hydrogen, ^{18}F ($t_{1/2}$: 110 min). The radiation resulting from decay of the PET nuclides can be measured using numerous detectors arranged in a circular array and calibrated according to complex reconstruction algorithms in section images [27].

Computed tomography and magnetic resonance scans can be fused with PET images for co-registration of morphologic and metabolic information; this allows an easier assignment of metabolic images to known tumorous masses and thus increases the benefits [28].

The application of PET in oncologic diagnosis is based on the biologic behavior of the tumors themselves. It is well known that tumors differ from normal tissue due to their extremely increased glucose metabolism. Tumors meet their increased energy demand in the face of insufficient vascularization (and thus low oxygen) by massively increasing anaerobe glycolysis.

The PET radiopharmaceutical that is most widely used today is the glucose analog 2-18F-deoxyglucose (FDG). As is the case with glucose, FDG is absorbed via the glucose transporter 1 in malignant cells, and

there it is metabolized by hexokinase to FDG-6-P. However, FDG-6-P is not a substrate for further metabolism by either glucose-6-P-isomerase or glucose-6-P-phosphotase and, therefore, accumulates in cells [29]. With FDG, the first step of glycolysis can be determined quantitatively. Due to the generally increased metabolism in malignant cells, other tracers, such as radioactively labeled amino acids, must be considered for potential use with PET [27].

Commonly, FDG-PET has been used for the description of the primary tumor [29] because tumors accumulate FDG more intensively than healthy tissue. Advanced carcinomas in the head and neck reveal sensitivities of up to 100 % [27]. The detection of smaller tumors (with a diameter of less than 1 cm) is much less reliable. Coupling PET with CT or MRI resulted in a diagnosis of 97 % of primary tumors that were later definitively identified by inspection or endoscopy, versus a diagnosis of only 77 % when MRI was used alone [29].

Due to these encouraging results, FDG-PET has been used for the detection of occult primary tumors in patients with manifest cervical lymph node metastases [28]. In cases of the so-called CUP syndrome (cancer of unknown primary origin), where cervical lymph node metastases occur as the first symptoms of the malignant disease, the majority of the metastases are the result of either squamous cell carcinomas or undifferentiated carcinomas. In spite of extended diagnostic techniques (including CT, MRI and, chiefly, panendoscopy with tonsillectomy, as well as laser surgical resection of the tongue base and excision of specimens from the nasopharynx), in 5–12 % of the patients the primary tumor cannot be found.

According to various other reports, the primary tumor could be detected in 30–50 % of patients suffering from the CUP syndrome. According to these studies, the values for sensitivity and specificity amounted to 50–74 % and 83–100 %, respectively [28, 29]. Because of this high detection rate, FDG-PET seems to be indicated for unknown primary cancers. Furthermore, FDG-PET allows the simultaneous scanning of all regions, which is very useful in cases of the CUP syndrome because in up to 40 % of the cases the primary tumor is situated outside the head and neck region.

Table 4.3. Sensitivity and specificity (%) of PET for detection of cervical lymph node metastases

	Number of patients (examined lymph nodes)	PET	CT/MRI
Bailet et al., 1992	8 (203)	Sens. 71 Spec. 98	Sens. 59 Spec. 98
Jabour et al., 1993	9 (256)	Sens. 74 Spec. 99	Sens. 71 Spec. 98
Braams et al., 1995	12 (199)	Sens. 91 Spec. 88	Sens. 36 Spec. 94
Laubenbacher et al., 1995	17 (521)	Sens. 90 Spec. 96	Sens. 78 Spec. 71
Benchaou et al., 1996	48 (468)	Sens. 72 Spec. 99	Sens. 67 Spec. 97
Myers et al., 1998	14	Sens. 78 Spec. 100	Sens. 57 Spec. 90
Kau et al., 1999	70	Sens. 87 Spec. 94	Sens. 88 Spec. 40
DiMartino et al., 2000	40	Sens. 82 Spec. 87	Sens. 82 Spec. 94

Histological processing of positive lymph nodes after neck dissection
Modified according to Lindholm et al. [15]

Studies concerning the significance of PET for lymph node diagnoses are very few [29]. The aim of PET is the improved differentiation between benign and malignant cervical lymph node enlargement, especially in the clinical N0 neck [30].

The results of previous studies are summed up in ▶ Table 4.3. In the detection of cervical lymph node metastases, PET proved to be as accurate as CT or MRI. The sensitivity amounted to 71–90%, while the specificity varied between 77–100%. Furthermore, some studies were able to show that PET could identify lymph node metastases that had been characterized as negative in CT or MRI scans [30]. Despite this, the diagnostic gain from PET in the description of metastatic lymph nodes is not considered that great, with a few exceptions [27].

In contrast to pretherapeutic diagnosis, PET seems to have some advantages in the posttherapeutic assessment of the status of cervical lymph nodes. Its sensitivity in revealing recurrent or residual lymph node metastases is estimated to be greater than 90% [29]. Because many of the patients with locoregional recurrences already suffer from distant metastases, whole-body PET can be used to reliably identify the locations involved. The procedure is therefore of significant importance in making further diagnoses and planning further therapy.

When interpreting FDG-PET, generally the limited specificity must be taken into account [27]. Besides the high accumulation of FDG in many malignant tumors, increased FDG uptake can occur in diverse benign processes if more glucose is needed due to pathophysiologic circumstances. This is the case in all inflammatory diseases. Additionally, pathophysiologic FDG accumulation is known to occur in major salivary glands and particularly in the lymphatic tissue of Waldeyer's ring. False positive results due to reactively enlarged lymph nodes, however, seem to occur more often in CT or MRI scans [28]. Additional morphologic scanning (CT or MRI), together, of course, with knowledge of the clinical signs, is essential for a correct interpretation of PET [27].

Based on these conditions, the indication for FDG-PET must be made very carefully and the results must be interpreted in view of all clinical information. In spite of prediagnostic patient selection, false positive findings of 10–15 % are reported in the literature [29]. The authors explain this by inflammatory states that are not clinically apparent. When interpreting the posttherapeutic PET, it must be remembered that inflammatory tissue changes in the area of the primary tumor, acute edema, mucositis or reactive lymph node swellings all can induce FDG uptake and thus lead to false positive results with PET. For this reason, it is best to perform FDG-PET no sooner than 4 months after the end of the primary therapy.

In summary, PET with the glucose analog FDG, is a functional procedure for description of increased glucose metabolism. Clinically, it can be used in the detection of the primary tumor and its cervical lymph node metastases. The significance of PET today is certainly the improved detection of an occult primary tumor in cases of the CUP syndrome, as well as in the posttherapeutic assessment of a primary site or lymph node recurrence. Due to its insufficient spatial resolution capacity, missing information concerning anatomic adjacent structures and, finally, also its high costs, PET is actually clearly inferior to conventional imaging procedures, including the sonographically guided aspiration cytology in preoperative primary tumor or lymph node staging [27]. New indications for PET may possibly result from its combination with radioimmunoscintigraphy.

4.7 Lymphography

Cervical lymphography is a radiological–angiographic procedure. In comparison to lymphoscintigraphy, lymphography is characterized by the ability to describe lymph nodes and vessels radiographically. There are two types of lymphography: one relies on a direct injection method; and the other relies on an indirect injection method.

In direct lymphography, a lymph vessel is identified after making a small incision, the lymph vessel is then cannulated and ink, or another contrast agent, is injected directly into the lymph vessel. The radiologic examination can be performed during each stage of injection. In direct lymphography, lymph collectors and trunks can be well described. The initial lymph vessel situated in the lymphatic drainage region, however, cannot be sufficiently assessed as a result of lymphatic valves that avoid retrograde accumulation in initial lymph vessels.

In indirect lymphography a tracer substance, e. g., ink, is injected intracutaneously, which leads to an increased interstitial pressure. If this pressure is superior to the endovascular pressure, the endothelial ending is pressed like the sides of a door into the vascular lumen. The ink, being present in the interstitium, flows into the lymph vessel via the separated interendothelial cellular contacts.

The significance of the indirect injection method is controversial. The injected particles may miss lymph vessels by penetrating into artificial tissue interstices. Even in the case of correctly performed injections, the dye can leave the lymph vessels via interendothelial openings and form vessel-imitating extravasations. The result is a limited description of the lymphatic network due to insufficient filling of the initial lymphatic system.

In spite of the sources of error, indirect lymphography performed with dye has its place in the examination of an organ-specific lymphatic system. The findings indicate the distribution and direction of lymph vessels. The importance of understanding the direction of lymphatic drainage cannot be overemphasized. This is because the initial lymph sinuses have no directional valves; as a result, reversal of the lymphatic flow is always possible. The direction of the lymphatic drainage can be determined more easily with fluorescence micro-lymphography and with indirect lymphography applying the directly magnifying micro-focus radiation method. In lymphangioadenography, a lymph node is identified and the contrast agent is directly applied to it.

Cervical lymphography is indicated for the clarification of lymph node metastases in order to determine the extent of surgery, especially in neck dissection. This is very helpful with midline tumors, as well as in follow-up after chemo- or radiochemotherapy. The lymph angiography (lymphatic blockade with contralateral vessels and displacement of adjacent vessels) and the lymphadenography (size of the lymph node, marginal, solitary or multiple filling defects) are assessed.

A benign lymphadenitis appears as an enlargement of lymph nodes. In comparison to the normal findings, the lymphographic image shows a coarseness of the storage structure, whereas lymph node metastases appear as normal-sized or enlarged lymph nodes with filling defects in the marginal sinus or central parts. Complete infiltrations occur only in advanced metastatic processes. The depiction of bypasses, lymph and venous anastomoses, as well as filling defects, with failure of one lymph node group, are frequently observed.

The complication rate of lymphography is very low. Due to difficult surgical preparation and the associated high technical skill and time, direct lymphography is not a routinely performed procedure for the identification of the cervical lymphatic system. Recently, results seen with the indirect subepidermal or subcutaneous application of water-soluble contrast agents seems promising. However, this procedure is not a substitute for non-invasive examination techniques like sonography, CT and MRI.

4.8 Lymph Node Biopsy

4.8.1 Lymph Node Extirpation

The lymph node extirpation (excisional biopsy) with subsequent histological examination is the most accurate diagnostic procedure for the assessment of cervical lymph node enlargement. The indications for excision of lymph nodes should be adhered to very strictly. Imaging procedures, including aspiration cytology, generally should precede surgical lymph node extirpation. However, excisional biopsy performed by a surgeon experienced in head and neck operations is minimally morbid. The risk of intraoperative trauma to nerves and vessels, although low, is significantly influenced by the location and nature of adjacent structures.

The indication for diagnostic cervical lymph node extirpation, including fine needle aspiration cytology, must be made after the imaging diagnosis in the following cases:

- clinical and/or cytologic suspicion of a malignant lymphoma for histological classification;
- cytologically doubtful findings in order to accurately exclude a malignant process;
- persisting enlarged lymph nodes in order to determine the presence or absence of malignancy;
- enlarged lymph nodes in children, as fine needle biopsy and/or needle biopsy can be problematic and cannot be repeated easily;
- melanomas not located in the head and neck region in order to exclude lymphogenic metastatic spread. (Additionally, in malignancies of the breast and the urogenital tract, the histological determination of possible hormone receptors is decisive for subsequent therapy planning);
- suspicion of a specific lymph node disease, for example, tuberculosis or sarcoidosis, in order to gain tissue for definitive diagnosis (histology, molecular biologic diagnosis);
- suspicion of the CUP syndrome with cervical metastatic spread. In this context, intraoperatively, a frozen section diagnosis should be performed in order to allow simultaneous modified radical neck dissection if the histological diagnosis so dictates;
- suspicion of a cervical lymph node recurrence after surgical and/or radiotherapy when diagnostic or possibly a therapeutic intervention can be simultaneously done;
- inoperability, to gain tissue for histological examination; and, on rare occasion:
- when an overly anxious patient (or parents of young children), desire to exclude a malignant disease and thereby relieve the accompanying psychological burden.

With excisional biopsy of cervical lymph nodes, the incision should be oriented according to Langer's lines. The incision can be extended for full neck dissection when cancer is confirmed in the frozen section examination. The extirpation of a lymph node should always be complete, i. e., with an intact capsule and, if necessary, also with adjacent fatty tissue. This way, the risk of possible metastatic spread is kept low, and the pathologist can assess sufficiently for extracapsular extension. A partial excision should be avoided for two reasons: first, because postoperative persisting fistulae may develop, and, second, because the prognosis worsens in cases of incisional biopsy, due to the subsequent infiltration of the skin and the change of the metastatic direction. A partial excision must be considered obsolete in view of suspected metastatic spread.

4.8.2 Scalene Node Biopsy

The biopsy of non-palpable lymph nodes from the omoclavicular triangle (supraclavicular fossa) takes into consideration the fact that diseases become manifest morphologically in the area of the big venous angle between the internal jugular vein and the subclavian vein. The scalene lymph nodes of the omoclavicular triangle filter orthograde the lymphatic flow of the thoracic duct. The lymph fluid drains from the left superior pulmonary lobe and the right lung to the lymph nodes of the right supraclavicular cavity, whereas the lymph nodes of the left triangle represent the afflux station for the whole body.

Excision of tissue in this area is performed via an incision placed parallel to the clavicle. Fatty tissue is excised in tutu and then examined histologically. The results of scalene node biopsy are influenced by the localization, the stage and the type of disease. Due to modern imaging techniques, the scalene node biopsy has lost its importance for the diagnosis of thoracic and mediastinal diseases.

4.8.3 Mediastinoscopy

In mediastinoscopy, the pre- and paratracheal lymph nodes, the superior and inferior tracheobronchial lymph nodes and the anterior mediastinal lymph nodes are identified via a skin incision in the lower midline neck. A special tubular endoscope can then be passed up to the bifurcation of the trachea. Mediastinoscopy can be used for differential-diagnostic clarification and assessment of operability of mediastinal tumors and metastases. However, it is very rarely used these days due to the high accuracy of CT and MRI. Mediastinoscopy should be performed by an experienced thorax surgeon.

4.9 Conclusion

Diagnostic procedures relating to enlarged cervical lymph nodes is a subject of some controversy, particularly in view of the development of more exact imaging techniques. In particular, basic history and physical examination techniques are still the first steps in diagnosis. In the majority of the cases (especially in cases of benign lymphadenopathies), a reliable diagnosis can be established based on laboratory findings.

Imaging techniques can also be indicated, primarily in inflamed lymph node enlargements for follow-up, or to exclude abscess formation requiring drainage. Undoubtedly, the procedure of choice is B-mode sonography. For the patient it is free of side effects, rapid, non-invasive, always available and also cost-effective. CT and/or MRI may also be indicated due to differential diagnostic considerations and also for the determination of the localization and extent of extended cervical tumorous masses.

The most important part of imaging procedures relates to the staging examinations for head and neck cancers. Proper diagnosis and therapy is of urgent significance in order to detect cervical lymph node metastases. If necessary, CT or MRI should be used to determine the extent of the primary tumor in order to define cervical lymph node status. Otherwise, at least in Europe, B-mode sonography is the initial method of choice for the detection of possible cervical lymph node metastases. With greater expertise and experience, this will likely also become true in America.

If the clinical suspicion for the presence of cervical lymph node metastases is justified, the total number of metastases is less important because generally all lymph node regions are excised with modified radical neck dissection. An exact description of the number and location of potential metastases by means of sonography or CT/MRI is only relevant in cases of small primary tumors, where a selective neck dissection could be performed with excision of certain lymph node regions, or when primary radiotherapy is used. Furthermore, imaging techniques can give information on the resectability of extended, fixed metastases with the possible involvement of the major cervical vessels. Dynamic lymphoscintigraphy can be performed in cases of massive unilateral metastatic spread in order to exclude contralateral lymphatic drainage.

If palpation gives no information about the presence of cervical lymph node metastases (clinical No neck), there is still the risk of occult metastases, depending on the size and location of the primary tumor. For assessment of the No neck, B-mode sonography, including sonographically assisted aspiration cytology, has a reliability of over 90%. In this context, it must be mentioned that sonography is a dynamic examination technique that depends largely on the exprerience of the examiner and the pathologist, as well as on the cooperation of the patient him- or herself.

If the classical imaging procedures do not reveal a clear finding in the context of tumor follow-up, PET can be helpful for differentiation between scar tissue and the recurrence of lymph node metastasis. If findings are unclear with imaging, including PET, then biopsy with possible further surgery may be indicated.

Improved sonography, CT and MRI techniques, as well as the new nuclear medicine procedures, have not yet been successful in differentiating between reactive and metastatically enlarged lymph nodes. All diagnostic procedures have their disadvantages in terms of their limited abilities to detect smaller tumor volumes. Due to these disadvantages, it is still difficult to decide if and to what extent the neck should be included in the primary treatment scheme in order to avoid possible undertreatment or overtreatment. Because of the fact that the incidence of micrometastases (smaller than 3 mm) in the clinical No neck amounts to up to 25%, no imaging procedure can achieve a higher sensitivity than 75% without simultaneously losing an appropriate specificity. Depending on the tumor location and size, the indication for selective neck dissection should be made generously in case of doubt.

References

1. Van den Brekel MWM, Reitsma LC; Leemans CR, Smeele LE, van der Waal I, Snow GB (1999) Patient outcome of a wait and see policy for the No neck using ultrasound guided cytology during follow-up. Arch Otolaryngol Head Neck Surg 125: 153–156
2. Van den Brekel MWM (2000) Lymph node metastases: CT and MRI. Eur J Radiol 33: 230–238
3. Van den Brekel MWM, Castelijns JA, Stel HV, Golding RP, Meyer CJ, Snow GB (1993) Modern imaging techniques and ultrasound-guided aspiration cytology for the assessment of neck node metastases: a prospective comparative study. Eur Arch Otorhinolaryngol 250: 11–17
4. Van den Brekel MWM, van der Waal I, Meyer CJLM, Freeman JL, Castelijns JA, Snow GB (1996) The incidence of micrometastases in neck dissection specimens obtained from elective neck dissections. Laryngoscope 106: 987–991
5. Van den Brekel MWM, Castelijns JA (2000) Imaging of lymph nodes in the neck. Seminars in Roentgenology 35: 42–53
6. Iro H, Uttenweiler V, Zenk J (2000) Kopf-Hals-Sonographie. Springer, Berlin
7. Mann W, Welkoborsky H-J, Maurer J (1997) Kompendium Ultraschall im Kopf-Hals-Bereich. Thieme, Stuttgart New York
8. Westhofen M, Reichel C, Nadjmi D (1994) Die farblose Duplexsonographie der Halslymphknoten. Otorhinolaryngologica Nova 4: 285–291
9. Van den Brekel MWM, Castelijns JA, Snow GB (1998) The size of lymph nodes in the neck on sonograms as a radiologic criterion for metastasis: how reliable is it? Am J Neuroradiol 19: 695–700
10. Alvi A, Johnson JT (1996) Extracapsular spread in the clinically negative neck (No): implications and outcome. Otolaryngol Head Neck Surg 114: 65–70
11. Knappe M, Louw M, Gregor TR (2000) Ultrasonography-guided fine-needle aspiration for the assessment of cervical metastases. Arch Otolaryngol Head Neck Surg 126: 1091–1096
12. Atula TS, Varpula MJ, Kurki TJ, Klemi PJ, Grenman R (1997) Assessment of cervical lymph node status in head and neck cancer patients: palpation, computed tomography and low field magnetic resonance imaging compared with ultrasound-guided fine-needle aspiration cytology. Eur J Radiol 25: 152–161
13. Steinkamp HJ, Mueffelmann M, Böck JC, Thiel T, Kenzel P, Felix R (1998) Differential diagnosis of lymph node lesions: a semiquantitative approach with color Doppler ultrasound. Br J Radiol 71: 828–833
14. Schade G (2001) Erfahrungen mit der Anwendung des Ultraschall-Kontrastverstärkers Levovist® bei der Differenzierung zervikaler Lymphome mittels farbcodierter Duplexsonographie. Laryngorhinootologie 80: 209–213

15. Klimek L, Schreiber J, Amadee RG, Mann W (1998) Three-dimensional ultrasound evaluation in the head and neck.. Otolaryngol Head Neck Surg 118: 267–271

16. Jecker P, Maurer J, Mann WJ (2001) Verbesserte Orts- und Kontrastauflösung in der Ultraschalldiagnostik durch Nutzung harmonischer Frequenzen. Laryngorhinootologie 80: 203–208

17. Som PM, Curtin HD, Mancuso AA (1999) An imaging-based classification for the cervical lymph nodes designed as an adjunct to recent clinically based nodal classifications. Arch Otolaryngol Head Neck Surg 125: 388–396

18. Hoffmann HT, Quets J, Toshiaki T, Funk GF, McCulloc TM, Graham SM, Robinson RA, Schuster ME, Yuh WT (2000) Functional magnetic resonance imaging using iron oxide particles in characterizing head and neck adenopathy. Laryngoscope 110: 1425–1430

19. Som PM (1992) Detection of metastasis in cervical lymph nodes: CT and MR criteria and differential diagnosis. Am J Roentgenol 158: 961–969

20. Don DM, Anzai Y, Lufkin RB, Fu YS, Calcaterra TC (1995) Evaluation of cervical lymph node metastases in squamous cell carcinoma of the head and neck. Laryngoscope 105: 669–674

21. Curtin HD, Ishwaran H, Manucuso AA, Dalley BW, Caudry DJ, McNeil BJ (1998) comparison of CT and MR imaging in staging of neck metastases. Radiology 207: 123–130

22. Franca C, Levin-Plotnik D, Sehgal V, Chen GT, Ramsey RG (2000) Use of three-dimensional spiral computed tomography imaging for staging and surgical planning of head and neck cancer. J Digit Imaging 13 (Suppl. 1): 24–32

23. Klutmann S, Bohuslavizki KH, Brenner W, Höft S, Kröger S, Werner JA, Henze E, Clausen M (1999) Lymphoscintigraphy in tumors of the head and neck using double tracer technique. J Nucl Med 40: 776–782

24. Werner JA, Dünne AA, Ramaswamy A, Folz BJ, Lippert BM, Moll R, Behr T (2002) Sentinel node biopsy in N0 cancer of the pharynx and larynx. Br J Cancer 87: 711–715

25. Gapany M, Grund FM (2000) Thallium-201 imaging for upper aerodigestive tract cancer. In: Mukherij SK, Castelijins (eds) Modern head and neck imaging. In: Baert AL, Heuck FHW, Youker JE (eds) Medical radiology – Diagnostic imaging and radiation oncology. Springer, Berlin-Heidelberg-New York, 107–110

26. Van Dongen GAMS, de Bree R, Roos JC, Quak JJ, Snow GB (2000) The value of radioimmunoscintigraphy for detection of lymph node metastases in head and neck cancer patients. In: Mukherij SK, Castelijins (eds) Modern head and neck imaging. In: Baert AL, Heuck FHW, Youker JE (eds) Medical radiology – Diagnostic imaging and radiation oncology. Springer, Berlin-Heidelberg-New York, 157–172

27. Lindholm P, Lapela M, Leskinen S, Minn H (2000) PET scanning of head and neck cancer. In: Mukherij SK, Castelijins (eds) Modern head and neck imaging. In: Baert AL, Heuck FHW, Youker JE (eds) Medical radiology – Diagnostic imaging and radiation oncology. Springer, Berlin-Heidelberg-New York, 87–105

28. Jungehülsing M, Scheidauer K, Damm M, Eckel HE (2000) 3[F]-fluoro-2-deoxy-D-glucose positron emission tomography is a sensitive tool for the detection of occult primary cancer (carcinoma of unknown primary syndrome) with head and neck lymph node manifestation. Otolaryngol Head Neck Surg 123: 294–301

29. DiMartino E, Nowak B, Hassan HA, Hausmann R, Adam G, Büll U, Westhofen M (2000) Diagnosis and staging of head and neck cancer. Arch Otolaryngol Head Neck Surg 126: 1457–1461

30. Myers LL, Wax MK, Nabi H, Simpson GT, Lamonica D (1998) Positron emission tomography in the evaluation of the N0 neck. Laryngoscope 108: 232–236

Principles of Surgery

5.1 History and Classification of the Surgical Treatment of Cervicofacial Lymph Node Metastases

5.1.1 History

In 1847, Warren reported on an experimental surgical resection of a carcinoma in the neck [1]. A more detailed surgical technique was described 33 years later by Kocher, who explained lymph node dissection from the submandibular triangle in the context of access to the operative treatment of carcinomas of the tongue [2]. In 1885, Butlin described dissection of the cervical lymph nodes in the context of resection of a carcinoma of the tongue. In a book entitled *Modern Surgery*, which appeared in 1887, the resection of cervical lymph nodes was described as part of the surgical therapy for epidermoid carcinoma of the head and neck. Descriptions of lymph node dissections, including resection of the internal jugular vein and the carotid artery, were published by Langenbeck. Unfortunately, both patients treated with this last method died postoperatively [3].

In 1888, the Polish surgeon, Franciszek Jawdynski (▶ Fig. 5.1), performed a surgical intervention [4, 5] that was similar to the technique described 18 years later by George Washington Crile (▶ Fig. 5.2), which was called neck dissection [6]. Jawdynski reported on 4 cases of extended radical en-bloc resection [7]. Perhaps because the article was published in a Polish journal, this contribution did not get much attention and remained obscure.

In 1901, Jacob Da Silva Solis-Cohen [8] explained the necessity of performing cervical lymph node dis-

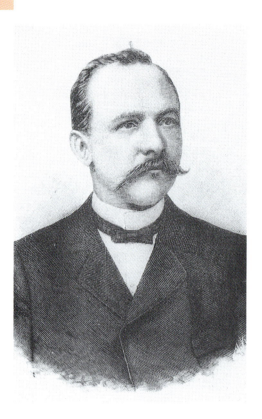

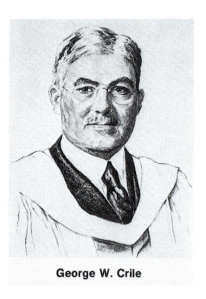

George W. Crile

Figure 5.2

George Washington Crile (1864–1934), who first described the so-called "radical neck dissection" in English literature thus promoting decisive progress in the treatment of metastatically affected cervical lymph nodes

Figure 5.1

Franciszek Jawdynski, surgeon from Poland, who first described the surgery technique later called, "radical neck dissection". (This photo was kindly provided by Prof. Dr. E. Towpik, Center of Oncology, Warsaw, Poland)

section with laryngectomy, independently of the danger of lymphogenic metastatic spread.

Radical Neck Dissection (RND). Decisive progress in the treatment of metastatically affected cervical lymph nodes was made by Crile who, in 1906, described RND [6] based on his experience in 132 surgeries. Crile called this surgical technique neck dissection (ND) and even this early used the term *comprehensive.*

In 1926, Bartlett and Callander [9] described less radical neck dissections with preservation of the accessory nerve, the internal jugular vein, the sternocleidomastoid muscle, the platysma, the stylohyoid

muscle and the digastric muscle. In 1933, however, the need to remove the accessory nerve was again indicated by Blair and Brown [10].

In 1945, Dargent [11] was the first surgeon to describe bilateral neck dissection as a curative treatment concept in carcinomas of the upper aerodigestive tract. He suggested preservation of at least the internal jugular vein.

In the 1940s and 1950s, the classical radical neck dissection again became more important. At that time, publications by Martin, who had great influence, underscored the importance of RND [13, 14].

In the 1960s, however, the principle of modified radical neck dissection came to the fore. This progress was due to Osvaldo Suárez (▶ Fig. 5.3), who, in 1963, described the so-called functional neck dissection that is based on the fascial compartments of the neck [15, 16]. Suárez's idea was predicated on the "small dissection," which had already been published by Silvestre-Begnis in 1944 [17]. This concept had its origin in publications by Truffert [18] and Pernkopf

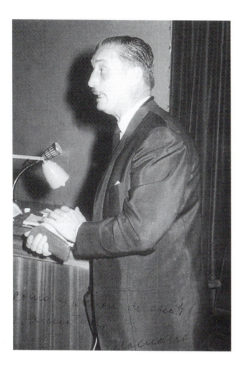

Figure 5.3

Osvaldo Suaréz, who first described a surgical technique which was later called, "functional neck dissection." This is a type of neck dissection based primarily on the fascial division of the neck. (This photo was kindly provided by Prof. Dr. J. Gavilán, Hospital "La Paz", Madrid, Spain)

[19], as well as those of the South-American surgeons, De Sel and Agra [20], and the Polish surgeon, Miodonski [21]. Supporters of the radical neck dissection often misunderstood the term, *functional*. They felt this neck dissection type was not sufficiently aggressive for lymphogenic metastatic spread, whereas Suárez indicated very early that the patient could maintain maximum function without diminishing the prognosis. It was Suarez, who, already in 1962, had stated that *the extent of cervical lymph node dissection had to be directed radically against the carcinoma, but not against the neck* [16].

The first description of functional neck dissection is often attributed to Ettore Bocca [22, 23] and not to Suárez. This is because Suárez published his results in the Spanish literature (5 years earlier than Bocca) [24]. The classic technique of functional neck dissection is still performed by supporters of this treatment approach [25]. Supporters of functional neck dissection describe the surgery as a more secure procedure, compared to selective neck dissection, with no increased morbidity. Opponents of functional neck dissection maintain that its performance in the case of an No neck – depending on the level – entails overtreatment of certain cervical lymph nodes [5, 26].

Limited dissection of specified cervical lymph node levels is based primarily on evaluations by

Table 5.1. Classification of neck dissection (according to Robbins [35]).

Neck dissection type	Dissected lymph node levels	Conserved structures
Complete neck dissection		
Radical	I–V	
Modified radical type I	I–V	NXI
Modified radical type II	I–V	NXI, VJI
Modified radical type III	I–V	NXI, VJI, MS
Selective neck dissection		
Supraomohyoidal	I–III	NXI, VJI, MS
Anterolateral	I–IV	NXI, VJI, MS
Lateral	II–IV	NXI, VJI, MS
Posterolateral	II–V	NXI, VJI, MS
Special types of limited selective neck dissection		
Anterior dissection	VI	NXI, VJI, MS
Submental	I	NXI, VJI, MS
Suprahyoidal	I–II	NXI, VJI, MS
Limited lateral	II–III	NXI, VJI, MS

NXI = accessory nerve; VJI = internal jugular vein; MS = sternocleidomastoid muscle

Lindberg [27] and Skolnik [28]. Identification of the most frequently affected lymph node groups in a given primary tumor is the basis for the decision to perform selective neck dissection, which must be attributed primarily to Ballantyne [29–31].

In addition to the terms, *radical neck dissection* and *functional neck dissection*, there are now numerous terms and surgical strategies that often lead to confusion (▶ Table 5.1). The high variability of neck dissection terminology is one of the main reasons for the inability to compare data on lymphogenic metastatic direction and frequency, as well as on treatment results. Given this state of affairs, it is of highest importance to standardize the nomenclature of neck dissection as reported in the medical literature in order to answer new scientific questions [32].

5.1.2 Neck Dissection Classification

To better understand the classification of neck dissection, it is essential to consider its development over the past two decades. Without doubt, the classification and nomenclature of selective neck dissection will become even more important in the future. In the past, selective neck dissection was performed mainly as a *staging* procedure. Obviously now selective neck dissection is also considered to have a possible *therapeutic function*, a concept that will undoubtedly become more and more important in the future.

One study of neck dissection (ND), which has often not been appreciated sufficiently, is the article published by Shah and co-workers in 1981 [33]. The authors favored the performance of radical ND as initially described by George Washington Crile in clinically positive necks. In cases of elective neck dissection, however, Shah and co-workers recommended the so-called *modified radical neck dissection* with preservation of the accessory nerve. Due to the metastatic behavior of carcinomas located in the oral cavity, the authors strongly objected to selective dissection in No necks of the main metastatic regions I to III as a staging procedure. Instead, they advocated a "wait-and-see" strategy that is directly related to the compliance of the patient, the experience of the re-

Table 5.2. ASA classification

ASA stage	Physical status
ASA 1	A normal healthy patient
ASA 2	A patient with mild systemic disease
ASA 3	A patient with severe systemic disease
ASA 4	A patient with severe systemic disease that is a constant threat to life
ASA 5	A moribund patient who is not expected to survive with or without the operation

sponsible surgeons and regular follow-up examinations at short intervals. According to these authors radical ND should be performed only in exceptional cases. Thus, the foundation for selective neck dissection was created.

The classification of radical neck dissection, modified radical neck dissection (syn.: functional neck dissection), as well as selective neck dissection, is now internationally accepted (▶ Table 5.2).

- The *classic radical neck dissection* (RND) is the standard procedure for dissection of the cervical lymph node levels I–V with simultaneous resection of the sternocleidomastoid muscle, the internal jugular vein and the accessory nerve.
- In *modified radical neck dissection* (MRND), levels I–V are also dissected, but with preservation of one or more non-lymphatic structures (accessory nerve, internal jugular vein or sternocleidomastoid muscle). Depending on the number of preserved structures, a distinction is made between MRND types I to III. MRND type I involves dissection of levels I–V with preservation of the accessory nerve. MRND type II includes dissection of levels I–V with preservation of the accessory nerve and the internal jugular vein, while MRND type III signifies the dissection of levels I–V with preservation of the accessory nerve, the internal jugular vein and the sternocleidomastoid muscle.
- In *selective neck dissection* (SND) one or more lymph node groups, which would be dissected in the case of modified radical neck dissection, remain untouched. The most frequently performed

types of selective neck dissection were classified as supraomohyoid ND (dissection of levels I–III), lateral ND (levels II–IV) and anterolateral ND (levels I–IV). Other types, such as anterior ND (level VI) and posterolateral ND (levels II–V), were also performed.

In the current classification of ND, published in 2000 [34], the basic structure of the ND types has not been changed. A differentiation is still made between radical neck dissection, extended RND, modified RND and selective neck dissection [5, 26].

According to the current classification, radical RND means the classic dissection of the cervical lymph nodes of levels I–V, including the accessory nerve, the internal jugular vein and the sternocleidomastoid muscle. The suboccipital lymph nodes, the periparotid lymph nodes (except for the infraparotid lymph nodes in the posterior part of the submandibular triangle), the malar lymph nodes, the retropharyngeal lymph nodes and the lymph nodes of the so-called anterior compartment are *not* involved in the surgical dissection.

The dissection of one or more additional lymph node groups and/or non-lymphatic structures, such as the carotid artery, the hypoglossal nerve, the vagus nerve or the paravertebral muscles, is called *extended radical neck dissection* (ERND).

As previously stated, with MRND, lymph node levels I–V are dissected and one or more non-lymphatic structures are preserved. The recommended description of modified radical neck dissection is no longer divided into MRND type I, type II and type III, but referred to as MRND with preservation by name of the non-lymphatic structure(s) that remain(s).

In the 1991 classification [35], the category of selective neck dissection was divided into supraomohyoid, anterolateral, lateral and posterolateral neck dissection. In the more recent, revised classification, this has been changed. Surgery is no longer referred to as supraomohyoidal neck dissection, but rather SND (I–III). The same applies for anterolateral neck dissection – now referred to as SND (I–IV), lateral neck dissection – now SND (II–IV), and posterolateral neck dissection – now SND (II–V). The types of neck dissection performed in cases of thyroid carci-

nomas adds another level (VI). If metastatic spread has already occurred in caudal direction, i. e., inferior to the upper margin of the sternum, the dissection of the upper mediastinum is called, SND VI with upper mediastinal lymph nodes. If the metastatic spread has advanced into level V, the neck dissection type is called SND (II–VI). For the sake of completeness it is important to mention that in cases of ND for thyroid carcinoma, general surgeons have traditionally divided the neck into compartments.

According to the current American classification [34], dissection of level I usually includes excision of the submandibular gland and, if the lymph nodes of the submandibular region are dissected, the neck dissection specimen. Special attention must be paid to the perivascular submandibular lymph nodes, where frequently metastases can be detected in cases of carcinomas of the anterior oral cavity and the floor of the mouth [15]. Dissection of the submandibular gland without including these nodes is not a complete oncologic resection.

In cases of RND, all ipsilateral lymph node groups in levels I–V are dissected, as well as the internal jugular vein, the sternocleidomastoid muscle and the accessory nerve. The following structures are not resected:

- suboccipital lymph nodes;
- parotid lymph nodes (except infraparotid lymph nodes);
- buccal lymph nodes;
- retropharyngeal lymph nodes; and
- paratracheal lymph nodes.

In RND, the surgeon must be aware that not all tissue containing lymph nodes should be dissected on the operated neck side. This became apparent in scintigraphic examinations of patients who still had residual lymph vessels and nodes after classic dissection of cervical soft tissues as described above.

Today, the greater reluctance to perform RND (including bilateral RND) can be explained by the high morbidity rate. A significant impairment after RND is the limited mobility of the shoulder and the pain that occurs because of transection of the accessory nerve. To avoid these problems, a technique described by Jones and Stell, which preserves the motor branches from the cervical plexus C3/C4 to the trapezius muscle, has been used to achieve better shoulder function. If bilateral RND cannot be avoided, it should be performed, if possible, in two sessions with an interval of about 4 weeks between the two surgical interventions [36]. However, even with staging operations, morbidity is only marginally reduced when this procedure is performed.

In modified RND, levels I–V are dissected, preserving the accessory nerve and/or the internal jugular vein and/or the sternocleidomastoid muscle. This technique, first described by Suárez [16] and referred to as functional ND, is no simple modification of RND. Functional ND identifies a surgical intervention based on specific anatomic relationships between lymphatic structures and the fascial system of the neck.

Concerning the possible oncologic significance of preservation of the accessory nerve, Mann et al. [37] performed a retrospective evaluation of 256 patients. They found that preservation of the accessory nerve had no influence on the recurrence rate or on the prognosis, provided that the preservation of the nerve was possible without limiting the thoroughness of lymphoid tissue resection, and provided the patient underwent postoperative radiotherapy.

The term *functional neck dissection,* originally coined by Suárez (as indicated above), still describes the dissection of levels I–V. In contrast, Bocca, in his first description of the dissection of levels II–V in laryngeal carcinoma, talked about *modified radical neck dissection.* The significant conceptual relevance of functional neck dissection is that, according to the definition, this surgery is oriented by the cervical fascial system. This surgical technique also, however, fits into the category of modified radical neck dissection, as the resection of lymphoid tissue is the same as in classic MRND. Of course, any discussion concerning the most appropriate terminology (modified radical neck dissection vs. functional neck dissection) has only historic significance, provided the meaning of the terminology is understood.

A related topic concerns the definition of functional vs. selective neck dissection. At this point, it is not our wish to initiate a debate regarding the princi-

ples or implications of these neck dissection types. This situation, however, makes clear the difficulty of standardizing neck dissection techniques when there is confusion regarding the correct nomenclature. Although supporters of functional neck dissection – due to the standardized surgical procedure based on the fascial system – are reluctant to face the necessity of differentiating between the single levels, the treatment concept of selective neck dissection is directly based on a division into the different cervical lymph node levels. However, this division must be non-ambiguous so that there are no significant differences in the extent of each level, as was the case in the classification of 1991 [35], where the extent of level II clearly varied between the skull base and the hyoid and the skull base and the carotid bifurcation. Meanwhile, new definitions of the single levels have been proposed for standardizing descriptions of limited operative cervical lymph node dissection.

The distinction between functional neck dissection and selective neck dissection would be less ambiguous if supporters of functional neck dissection in the N0 neck performed less extensive lymph node dissections. Such a change would address the criticism regarding possible over-treatment of neck levels that are probably not affected by metastatic spread. An example of this situation is the case of clinical T2N0 carcinoma of the anterior floor of the mouth or the mobile tongue where the question of the need to dissect levels IV and V is raised. Historical data, and more importantly, emerging lymphoscintigraphic studies, suggest that these levels need not be resected with this cancer when the neck is staged N0.

The studies performed by Lindberg [27] and Skolnik [28] form the basis for SND. Among the different possibilities described to date, the most commonly applied types include:

- SND (I–III);
- SND (I–IV);
- SND (II–IV);
- SND (II–V); and
- SND (VI) (Syn.: dissection of the anterior compartment).

Supporters of selective neck dissection refer to reduced morbidity vs. modified RND, and they subscribe to the idea that immunologically functioning lymph nodes not affected by carcinoma can function to avoid further metastatic dissemination of the disease [38].

SND (I–III). SND (I–III) is a common neck dissection method for the treatment of the lymphatic drainage of carcinomas of the anterior oral cavity. While Banerjee and Alun-Jones [39], at least in cases of supraomohyoid ND, require that frozen sections always be examined to determine whether RND is necessary, Medina [40, 41] rejected intraoperative frozen section with SND (I–III). He recommended instead an extension of the dissection to level IV in the event of enlarged lymph nodes and a continuation with SND (I–IV). This method is also supported by other authors.

Rassekh et al. [42] as well tried to answer the question of whether operative staging of the No neck by inspection and/or palpation can prognosticate the presence of metastases. They were able to show that intraoperative inspection and/or palpation alone has no more significance in making such a determination than the clinical staging procedure. On the contrary, they found that operative findings could be over-interpreted so that sometimes the surgical intervention was unnecessarily extended. In contrast, the intraoperative frozen section diagnosis as described by Manni and van den Hoogen [43] was found to achieve a higher significance. Manni (personal communication) sends the whole, carefully mounted ND specimen to frozen section examination and leaves the decision to the pathologist concerning which lymph nodes to examine. If metastases are detected, selective ND is extended to modified RND. In many cases, according to Manni, no further metastases are found. Obviously, a prerequisite for such an undoubtedly advantageous practice is an excellent working relationship between surgeons and pathologists, which, for various reasons, is not always the case.

SND (I–IV). This type of ND includes the dissection of levels I–IV. The point has already been raised concerning why level IV is not always included in SND (I–III), as the additional surgical effort seems small.

Those who object to including level IV point out that doing so strikes at the heart of the concept of limited dissection itself, and that the possible complication of a chyle fistula can occur, especially on the left side.

SND (II–IV). SND (II–IV) is also called *inter-jugular dissection* or *anterior jugular dissection*. This type of ND is often performed in cases of oropharyngeal or hypopharyngeal carcinoma, as well as in supraglottic laryngeal carcinoma, in which dissections are frequently performed bilaterally.

SND (II–V). SND (II–V) was first described by Rochlin [44]. It includes the systematic resection of the lymph nodes of the cranio-dorsal cervical region. This type of ND is mostly used in cases of malignant melanoma of the back of the head. Frequently, it becomes necessary to also dissect the lymph node groups listed below. The postauricular and suboccipital lymph nodes are of high oncologic importance for malignant tumors of the following regions:

- scalp;
- postauricular area;
- suboccipital region of the neck; and
- aerodigestive tract (this is rare).

Regarding the surgical technique, the thickness of the posterior flap is of decisive importance for this type of ND. A flap that is too thick and contains the superficial suboccipital lymph nodes can impair the success of the surgical intervention, whereas a flap that is too thin tends to necrose. These facts must be taken into account in the preparation for this type of surgery [45].

Suprahyoid Neck Dissection. The so-called suprahyoid neck dissection includes:

- lymph nodes of level I;
- subdigastric lymph nodes (also referred to as Kuttner's lymph node group); and
- lymph nodes of the cranial carotid triangle [46].

This type of ND has not been sufficiently validated for the treatment of lymphatic drainage in cases of squamous cell carcinomas of the upper aerodigestive tract [30, 41]. In patients suffering from carcinomas of the oral cavity, for example, locoregional recurrences were observed in 29.2% of the cases of N0 neck after suprahyoidal ND with en-bloc tumor resection, compared with only 0% and 3.5%, respectively, of the regional recurrences after modified RND or RND with en-bloc tumor resection [47].

Dissection of Levels II and III. This type of ND is often reported by Steiner's group [38] in their treatment concept of carcinomas of the upper aerodigestive tract. Their purpose, however, is not always diagnostic as they also apply SND (II and III) therapeutically. The validity of this limited dissection must be evaluated by further studies from other investigators, including sentinel node studies where the potential for spread to level IV can be appropriately assessed.

Dissection of the Anterior Compartment. The dissection of the anterior area (level VI), also called ND of the anterior area or anterior ND, is mostly applied in cases of thyroid carcinomas. This is usually defined as bilateral paratracheal dissection, and it is typically coupled with dissection of other neck levels, typically II–IV (unilateral or bilateral).

Transsternal Mediastinal Lymph Node Dissection. Finally, a particular type of limited selective ND will be mentioned. The lymph node-containing tissue of the upper mediastinum can be resected, e.g., in cases of recurrence at the tracheostoma, as a transsternal mediastinal lymph node dissection [1, 28].

This treatment is contraindicated when large vessels of the mediastinum are also affected, or when distant metastatic spread has occurred beyond this level.

The survival rate after transsternal mediastinal dissection is still very low. However, such a treatment measure can be accepted in selected cases when performed with palliative intention. Appropriate imaging of the mediastinum, usually by CT or even mediastinoscopy, is performed prior to transsternal mediastinal lymph node dissection in order to get the necessary information on surgical resectability [48]. The need to use mediastinoscopy for this purpose is less

now because of modern imaging techniques (see chapter on diagnostic techniques).

5.2 Decision Points in Neck Dissection

5.2.1 Pre- and Perioperative Care

The performance of ND implies the observation of definitive, partly individually defined, pre- and perioperative measures that will be explained below.

5.2.1.1 Facets of Preoperative Lymph Node Biopsy

The impact of cervical lymph node biopsy prior to definitive surgical treatment of the lymphatic drainage is controversial. McGuirt and McCabe [36] observed that the risk of wound recurrence in patients who underwent cervical lymph node biopsy prior to definite surgery was higher (20% vs. 13%). At the same time, there was an increased risk for developing regional recurrent metastases (33% vs. 20%) and distant metastases (40% vs. 25%). The increased rate of distant metastases was statistically significant in their studies. Other authors [49] did not observe such negative results in cases of preoperative lymph node biopsy. However, it is incontestable that fully excisional versus incisional biopsy must be done. In this context, the significance of the preoperative cytological diagnosis must also be mentioned. If FNA demonstrates cancer, then excisional biopsy with intraoperative frozen section and possible extension to ND is not needed.

5.2.1.2 Diagnostics of Therapeutic Carotid Occlusion

If there is a question of carotid artery infiltration by cancer, then a therapeutic carotid occlusion may be indicated. In order to assess preoperatively collateral cerebral blood circulation, multimodality testing is needed in order to estimate the hemodynamic risk of stroke prior to permanent occlusion of the internal carotid artery [50]. However, multimodality testing does not fully exclude the risk of stroke. Additionally, the risk of thromboembolism cannot reliably be assessed.

Preoperative studies should be done include:
- verification of cortical function (EEG);
- determination of cerebral perfusion (SPECT); and
- hemodynamic effects at rest and under endovascular balloon occlusion of the internal carotid artery, with evaluation of cerebrovascular reserve capacity.

In reference to cases involving the detection of limited cerebral perfusion, which carries a significantly higher risk of stroke, the procedure for the preoperative carotid occlusion described by von Schobel et al. [51] should be mentioned. With this technique, the common carotid artery is partially occluded supraclavicularly by means of a ligature placed initially under local anesthesia, and then, during a second session, followed by total occlusion with a completely tied second ligature.

5.2.2 Timing of Neck Dissection

The classic principle of en-bloc resection of carcinomas and regional lymph nodes is questionable in light of the evolving treatment of primary carcinomas of the upper aerodigestive tract by laser surgery. In this context, a question also must be raised concerning the most appropriate time for the surgical treatment of the lymphatic drainage after initial laser resection of the primary tumor.

Leemans compared the treatment results of patients suffering from carcinoma of the anterior oral cavity who underwent transoral tumor excision with subsequent discontinuous ND to patients treated with the so-called en-bloc therapy. It became obvious that the group undergoing discontinuous ND developed metastatic neck recurrences to a significantly higher extent (19%) than the group with en-bloc resection (5.3%). Because procedures performed in two areas that are not anatomically contiguous can contribute to tumor emboli being left behind, some au-

thors favor waiting two to three weeks if en-block resection is not initially done [52, 53].

Steiner hypothesized that delayed ND was justified by the fact that tumor cells which reside in the lymph vessels during surgery of the primary tumor may have the opportunity to reach the regional lymph nodes if they are later removed by ND. Steiner favors ND 4–8 days after surgery of the primary tumor, when the definite histological findings from the primary site are present. ND can, if necessary, occur simultaneously with a local revision or after 4–6 weeks (in cases of N0 neck), coupled with a microlaryngoscopic laser biopsy survey. Steiner prefers the latter procedure with patients who have to undergo very extended partial resection. We generally perform ND simultaneously with laser resection of the primary carcinoma. This is indispensable when the lymphatic drainage of the primary tumor is examined with sentinel node biopsy. If sentinel node studies are not done, then ND is sometimes postponed, usually due to logistical reasons rather than the hypotheses of single tumor cells draining from the primary cancer to the lymph nodes. However, we do not wait longer than ten days after tumor resection to perform ND in order avoid prolonging the initiation of postoperative radiotherapy when this is necessary.

5.2.3 Patient Age and Neck Dissection

In the not-so-distant future, the population of individuals beyond the age of 75 will be growing steadily in the western industrial nations. This population group will make heavy demands on the medical care system, including, of course, therapy of head and neck squamous cell carcinomas.

The age of the patient may play a decisive role in determining the risk of complications with ND if certain risk factors occur together [54]. To what extent age is an independent factor will be discussed in the following section.

The coexistence of an increased rate of malignancy and mortality with advanced age and the increasing number of older people in most countries worldwide represents a complex clinical problem [55]. This pertains especially to the therapies that have a decisive impact on patient prognosis. The prognosis of patients with carcinomas of the upper aerodigestive tract is definitively determined by the location of the carcinoma, the tumor extent and, in particular, the extent of lymphogenic metastatic spread. In geriatric patients, the prognosis is also influenced by factors related to age. This is because pulmonary, cardiovascular, renal, neural and endocrine functions are reduced by the aging process [56]. Additionally, older patients cannot cope easily with extreme stress, therapeutic complications are less tolerated and, not uncommonly, can be lethal.

Among the various treatment strategies, surgical treatment of the primary tumor and its lymphatic drainage in cases of carcinomas in the head and neck represents the most important therapeutic intervention. Surgical treatment is frequently combined with radio(chemo)therapy [57]. The planning of therapy for older patients is often limited by their advanced age [58]. Furthermore, advanced age itself is frequently associated with an incomplete diagnosis and reduced therapeutic options [59, 60]. Due to comorbidities, or the conviction that a standard therapy might not be well tolerated by these patients, they are often excluded from a potentially curative treatment regimen.

In the literature, the term, *advanced age*, is not clearly defined. Mainly patients beyond the age of 75 are labeled *old patients*. In geriatrics, the group of patients of advanced age consists of younger patients (between the age of 65 and 74), older patients (between the age of 75 and 84), and oldest patients (beyond the age of 85) [61].

In spite of the frequency and clinical relevance of the effect and tolerance of neck dissection in patients beyond the age of 65 suffering from carcinomas of the head and neck, predictive parameters are relatively unknown. This is especially true in locally advanced carcinomas of the upper aerodigestive tract with extended lymphogenic metastatic spread. Studies relating to surgical therapeutic outcome often neglect this group. Despite these historical precedents, it is our firm opinion that older patients must be offered the same treatment options as long as no contraindications are present.

Epidemiology. The percentage of people beyond the age of 65 within the population is increasing [62]. The risk of developing a malignant tumor is the highest for this age group [63, 64]. The frequency of malignant tumors increases nearly exponentially after the age of 40. About 50 % of all malignancies occur after the age of 65, with 33 % in the seventh decade or later. Given this age distribution, it is not astonishing that most of the tumor- related deaths occur in patients at an age of more than 65 years [62, 65, 66].

Squamous cell carcinomas of the upper aerodigestive tract occur mostly in the fifth and sixth decade. Fewer than 20 % of these carcinomas occur after the age of 65 [67]. Tobacco and alcohol abuse are the main risk factors for carcinogenesis in the head and neck [57]. Thus, numerous patients suffer from the consequences of long-lasting tobacco and alcohol abuse, including chronic emphysematous bronchitis, cor pulmonale, coronary heart disease, liver cirrhosis, alcoholic cardio-myopathy and encephalopathy. A considerable number of geriatric patients, however, do not report previous tobacco or alcohol abuse [68, 69]. All elderly patients, however, regardless of whether they suffer the consequences of substance abuse, suffer from age-related accumulations of spontaneous mutations, reduced effectiveness of DNA repair and reduced immune defense factors. This is reflected by a reduced p53 mutation rate in this age group, in contrast to younger patients in which tobacco use significantly increases the p53 mutation rate [67, 70].

Diagnostics. The effort to find a quick diagnosis of a malignant process at the initial stage of the symptoms is often missing in geriatric patients. The reason for this is often because the patient him- or herself waits to seek medical attention. However, the diagnostic intention of the caring physician must also be examined. The arguments stated in this context mostly refer to the advanced age, to age-related immune deficiency and to the comparably lower life expectancy of these patients [71]. Due to comorbidities like cardiovascular and pulmonary disease, and due to fear of mortality associated with the surgical intervention and postoperative complications, the treating physician frequently recommends incomplete diagnostic evaluations and limited palliative therapy for older patients suffering from malignant tumors [72].

In our opinion, all patients, regardless of age, should undergo a complete staging prior to the planning of the therapy [73]. Advanced age should not be a reason to refuse routinely performed panendoscopies for tumor staging and the exclusion of secondary carcinoma, which occurs in 7–10 % of the cases [61]. Although the discussion about basic aspects of the rationale for complete panendoscopies related to tumor location is not the topic of this chapter, some studies have shown that the frequency of multiple carcinomas increases with age [67, 74]. Certain methods of tumor diagnosis can, of course, be influenced by age-related physical limitations. As an example, MRI scanning may become impossible because of a hip joint prosthesis or a cardiac pacemaker, although positron emission tomography with 18-fluorodeoxyglucose may alleviate these drawbacks. Its value in the pre-therapeutic diagnosis of head and neck carcinomas is not fully known yet, but due to the examination's high sensitivity and diagnostic exactness, it can be a helpful measure for all patients, including those of advanced age [75, 76].

Therapy and Complications. The abandonment of curative treatment for cancer at advanced age often prolongs the suffering of these patients as well as their hospitalization, and it thus increases the related expenses of what becomes mostly long-term palliative therapy. In the same manner, therapy that is not timely may increase the rate of regional metastatic spread, which further deteriorates the prognosis of these patients [77]. Finally, progressive tumor growth in the upper aerodigestive tract is accompanied by increasing dysphagia and dyspnea, by pain, and by a higher risk of tumor-related bleeding. In cases of progressive deterioration of a patient's general condition, the risk of infections and cardio-pulmonary complications also increases. These factors also indicate the importance of adequate and possibly curative tumor therapy for this age group.

Even for older patients suffering from carcinomas with advanced lymphogenic metastatic spread, extended therapy with curative purpose should be considered, although some authors refuse such therapy

and consider age as an important prognostic factor [78–80]. Several studies have evaluated the prognosis of patients after an extended surgical intervention such as laryngectomy, laryngopharyngectomy, defect coverage by means of different flap reconstructions, or neck dissection followed by additional radiotherapy [81–84]. No significant increase in mortality in relation to an acceptable incidence of complications could be found. Regarding the frequency of postoperative complications in patients aged 70 and above who had undergone defect coverage by means of a myocutaneous flap, there were no statistically significant differences [17, 85]. Nor did the duration of surgery have an influence on the rate of complications in this age group. This factor is important because the therapeutic strategy of this patient group only rarely includes complex reconstructive surgery in order to minimize the intraoperative complication rate by reducing the duration of the intervention. The complication rate of patients after microvascular free tissue transplantation at advanced ages was similar to that of younger patients [86].

The incidence of postoperative complications in patients with a carcinoma of the upper aerodigestive tract is relatively similar in all age groups, whereas the type of complication is age-dependent. While older patients mainly contract pulmonary and cardiovascular diseases, younger patients often show complications in the area of the operative access [87, 88]. A correlation between the known existing diseases and postoperative complications could not reliably be proven for the group of older patients. Interestingly, it has been reported that cardiovascular and pulmonary complications do not occur more often in patients with historically known cardio-pulmonary diseases [82]. In the context of the above-mentioned studies, there was no data showing an increased postoperative complication rate after preoperative radiotherapy. Whereas some studies have reported on frequent wound complications in previously irradiated patients [89], others, like the study mentioned above, have not shown a relationship between wound complications and preoperative radiation in the evaluated age group [90, 91].

Especially in cases of malignant diseases of the head and neck, advanced age itself should not represent a contraindication for adequate surgical treatment [92, 93]. Often an effective and timely therapy can lead to a higher survival rate and a better quality of life. Progress in surgical and anesthesiology techniques, as well as improvements in intra- and postoperative monitoring, allow for optimized surgical treatment in older patients. In order to perform effective and well-tolerated therapy in geriatric patients, careful preparation, especially when cardiac and pulmonary diseases are present, should be effectuated after careful preoperative staging [53]. In the same way, individual medical and anesthesiology screening can lead to a possible improvement in the tolerance of narcosis [94, 95]. Preoperatively, cardio-pulmonary stabilization must be done, and the patient must be on a healthy diet to optimize the nutritional component. In addition, special attention must be paid to monitoring elderly patients before, during and after surgery.

Particularities of Anesthesia in Geriatric Patients. Progress in anesthesia and postoperative intensive care contributes significantly to the fact that now more important surgical interventions can be performed successfully on older patients. Although no systematically collected data exists on anesthesia-related morbidity or mortality in geriatric patients, especially in cases of tumor interventions with accompanying neck dissection, general experience in the perioperative care of geriatric patients is also valid for these indications. Even in cases involving cardiosurgical interventions with the use of cardiopulmonary bypass (coronary surgery, prosthetic valve replacement), the perioperative mortality is not associated with the age but, rather, mainly with the severity of the cardiac disease or with the severity of concomitant diseases (e.g., renal insufficiency with obligatory dialysis).

Naturally, concomitant diseases such as arteriosclerosis, emphysema, malnutrition and diabetes type 2 occur more often in geriatric patients. This is especially true for the head and neck oncologic patient population. Elderly smokers almost always have chronic obstructive lung disease. Their clinical status can easily be evaluated by simple endurance tests, such as climbing stairs followed by capillary blood gas analysis, or by simple examinations of lung function, which can be performed at the patient's bedside. Quite often, in addition to tobacco and alcohol abuse, severe problems with benzodiazepine abuse is present. Resulting postoperative withdrawal symptoms can also lead to increased perioperative mortality. In addition, variation in muscle and adipose tissue, as well as reduced metabolism, has an effect on thermoregulation. The body temperature of older patients, especially during extended interventions, can drop more quickly than that of younger patients, unless this is prevented. Additionally, attention must be given to appropriate bedding in order to avoid pressure sores due to the reduced soft tissue padding in geriatric patients.

The cardiovascular reserves of geriatric patients are limited. Besides reduced sympathetic activity, the compensatory reactions of the autonomous nervous system are impaired with stress and volume loss. The tolerance of a reduced number of oxygen carriers (color index) is impaired so that the indication for blood transfusion can occur sooner than in younger patients.

The reduced respiration of older patients on hypercapnia and/or hypoxia is even more reduced by anesthetics or sedatives, so that the risk of respiratory insufficiency is high, especially in the early postoperative stage. This problem has been minimized by the introduction of quick-acting and thus well controllable intravenous anesthetics (propofol, remifentanil) and volatile anesthetics (sevoflurane, desflurane).

Regarding the administration of modern as well as conventional anesthetics, however, physiological age-related changes must be considered because they require a reduction in the dose, compared with younger patients. These changes are mainly a reduced distribution volume, reduced hepatic and renal clearance, and higher sensitivity of the central and peripheral nervous system to anesthetics and muscle relaxants. Relatively uniform is the fact that an eighty-year-old patient needs about 30% less anesthetic than a twenty-year-old patient.

As is true in younger patients, the preoperative condition of geriatric patients correlates clearly with the perioperative morbidity. Generally, the American

Society of Anesthesiology (ASA) classification is used for assessment (▶ Table 5.2). While a seventy-year-old patient of ASA class 1 or 2 would probably have the same risk of severe postoperative complications as a younger patient, the risk for patients of ASA class 3 is increased by one third, and for patients of ASA class 4 the risk is twice as high.

Improved preoperative preparations (e.g., pulmonary physiotherapy), modern anesthetics that are discharged mainly organ dependently, and improved perioperative monitoring (relaxometry, pulsoximetry) have decreased significantly the perioperative risk in older patients. As a result, the risk is not significantly higher than in younger patients. If the particularities of advanced age are considered, the indication for surgery and anesthesia can be decided independently of the patient's age. For the assessment of the risk in terms of anesthesia, the severity of the concomitant diseases is the most important factor.

Prognosis. After comparing the overall results of surgical interventions with general anesthesia, the specialty of otorhinolaryngology has a lower perioperative mortality in this age group than elective operative interventions in other body regions [48, 96]. Patients can recover their preoperative mobility sooner after head and neck procedures than after surgeries in other parts of the body. Serious fluid displacement does not generally occur. Furthermore, head and neck operations are associated with relatively low infection rates, compared with surgical interventions in other body areas. Due to intact gastrointestinal absorption mechanisms, postoperative nutrition is possible, by oral means or by means of gavage or PEG feeding. In cases of tracheotomy, tracheopulmonary care is possible.

In one study, patients suffering from carcinoma in the upper aerodigestive tract who are older than 75 have a significantly lower mortality and complication rate after curative treatment than patients without curative therapy [97]. In another study, the 3-year-survival rate of both groups was 77% [98]. According to results obtained in a literature search, the 30-day mortality rate of older patients was, on average, 6% in cases of otolaryngological surgery with general anesthesia. Up to 50% of the causes of death in these

patients were related to pulmonary complications. Frequently, the main cause of death cannot be ascribed to the carcinomas or therapeutic complications [2].

Conclusion. The current state of knowledge for the determination of mortality and morbidity of geriatric patients suffering from carcinoma of the upper aerodigestive tract can be summarized as follows. First, it should be mentioned that the necessary preconditions to perform a thorough and meaningful analysis have not been sufficiently fulfilled in most cases. Very often data on the comorbidities of the patients are missing. In order to make the assessment that older patients are (or are not) at greater risk, studies would be required with a control group consisting of a younger patient population with carcinomas of the same location and with identical staging examinations, therapy types, concomitant diseases and risk factors [99]. In spite of these shortcomings, however, the present results allow the conclusion that individual and adequate therapy can lead to satisfactory treatment results in geriatric patients suffering from carcinomas of the upper aerodigestive tract when their operative treatment is well coordinated with anesthesiology.

5.2.4 Infectious Prophylaxis

Progress in the treatment of malignancies with extensive lymphogenic metastatic spread is possible due to improved anesthesia techniques, the possibility of blood transfusion and the development of broad-spectrum antibiotics.

The risk of postoperative wound infection is directly influenced by the kind of surgical intervention. Generally, a distinction is made between aseptic and septic wounds. "Aseptic" wounds are those created by the surgeon under permanently sterile conditions without prior infection. These wounds are closed at the end of the operation without subsequent bacterial contamination. An example of an aseptic intervention in otolaryngology is the resection of an uninfected branchial cleft cyst or lymph node biopsy. With aseptic conditions, the expected rate of postoperative wound infection is less than 5%. Perioperative antibiotic prophylaxis is generally not indicated in these cases [100].

In contrast, "septic" wounds are not only traumatic and/or preoperatively infected but also surgically caused wounds. Here, the pharyngeal mucosa is opened by the tumor surgical intervention. This procedure bears the risk of contamination of the cervical soft tissues with bacteria from the upper aerodigestive tract. The rate of postoperative wound infections is expected to be about 24–85% [100].

Several clinical investigations on the value of prophylactic antibiotic administration in oncologic head and neck surgery have revealed that prophylactic antibiotic administration can reduce the postoperative wound infection rate in comparison to placebo groups [101].

The pathogenesis of postoperative wound infection can generally be explained by contamination with saliva and other secretions from the upper aerodigestive tract during surgery or during the postoperative course [102]. There is a positive correlation between the occurrence of wound infections and bilateral or unilateral radical neck dissection, laryngectomy, primarily performed tracheotomy and radiochemotherapy. Furthermore, several comorbidity factors, such as diabetes mellitus or a previous infection, directly influence the rate of postoperatively expected wound infections.

The detected microbiological spectrum includes *Staphylococcus aureus* and *Staphylococcus epidermis*, alpha hemolytic streptococcus and, in particular, gram-negative organisms. Among these, *Klebsiella*, *Proteus mirabilis*, *Pseudomonas aeruginosa*, and *Enterococcus* and *Enterobacter* species should be mentioned. To avoid infection with these bacteria, the administration of second-generation cephalosporins (e.g., cefuroxime) has proven effective against a broad spectrum of gram-positive and gram-negative microorganisms [103]. Due to limited effectiveness with Enterobacteriaceae (*Klebsiella*, *Proteus*, *E. coli*) a combination of cephalosporin and metronidazole seems to be useful when the pharynx is opened [103].

In the 1990s, prospective randomized studies on antimicrobiologic prophylaxis in oncologic head and neck surgery demonstrated that a 7-day or even a 3-day antibiotic prophylaxis did not reduce the infection rate when compared to the perioperative antibiotic administration of clindamycin-cefonicid, or cefotaxime [104–106]. This fact was reconfirmed in a recently published, prospectively randomized evaluation [107]. It is important to keep in mind that the effectiveness of the perioperative, one-day antibiotic prophylaxis is directly related to the pharmacokinetics of the intravenously administered antibiotics. The intravenous administration of a cephalosporin and/or metronidazole should be performed 30 minutes prior to surgery in order to achieve sufficient blood and tissues levels at the point of opening the pharynx, i.e., when there is the highest degree of contamination [23, 103, 108]. With normal metabolism, the effectiveness of the antibiotics will last for about three hours. In cases of longer-lasting interventions, redosing with the antibiotic becomes necessary [109].

In our opinion, the absence of proven benefits for intravenous antibiotic therapy beyond 24 hours of administration in urologic, gynecologic, cardiologic and abdominal surgical interventions [104] does not apply to interventions involving opening of the pharynx. When the pharynx is opened, a 3–5 day combined antibiotic course of second-generation cephalosporin, or the second generation antibiotic together with metronidazole, is beneficial. This course is also supported by the literature [103]. Part of the reason that this is necessary is that continued contamination of the cervical soft tissues is possible after the immediate preoperative period if wound breakdown occurs. This potential complication is more likely in patients who have had previous irradiation, which is another reason that we support a longer period of postoperative antibiotic therapy when the pharynx is opened. As indicated previously, protecting against *Staphylococcus aureus* and anaerobic bacteria is especially important. Even in the presence of antibiotic coverage, and more so after such therapy ends, careful attention must be given to the evaluation of skin flaps, incision integrity and the occurrence of possible fluid collections. With respect to the latter, surgeons must be vigilant and, when necessary, open sites of possible fluid collection early and widely enough to lessen the chance of progressive tissue loss.

It must not be forgotten that the perioperative administration of antibiotics does not release the surgeon from the responsibility of traumatizing the surrounding tissue as little as possible in order to avoid devitalization. Furthermore, tissue ischemia arising from too tightly placed skin sutures should be avoided. The intraoperative placement of active drains should allow an optimized flow of serum and blood. In our opinion, the controversially discussed possibility of ascending infection via these drains should not lead to their removal too soon. In conformity with the literature, we recommend removal between the third and fifth postoperative day if the quantitated drainage is lower than 30ml over a period of 24 hours [100].

When active drains are used, it is wise to suture them in place in the operative bed with small, absorbable sutures, such as 5–0 or 6–0 rapidly absorbing gut sutures. This prevents the drains from being displaced and damaging either a major vessel or nerve, or an inner (pharyngeal) suture, and thereby increasing the chance of fistulization. Drains should be individually monitored for the amount of drainage and individually removed when this is appropriate. All drains which collect less than 10–15 ml of fluid over an 8-hour period can be removed after 24–48 hours. Drain outputs which are gradually decreasing only to later rise in output may indicate evolving fistulization or possibly a chyle fistula. If this occurs, an appropriate evaluation of the collected fluid must be done.

The first signs of a developing postoperative wound infection can be fever, leukocytosis and/or a cervical redness in the area of the wound. These are only possible indications of infection, however. Because the criteria are not specific, they must be judged critically according to their clinical development. Redness of the skin and induration can also occur as a consequence of traumatized tissue with interruption of the venous drainage and the cervical lymphatic flow. In the same way, a moderate leukocytosis with values up to 13.000/μl can be typical for the postoperative course following white blood cell demargination, which is a situation that does not require intervention [100].

In the event of manifest postoperative wound infection, a gram stain should be made from the infected wound and examined under a microscope in order to treat the patient appropriately. Coverage is dependent on culture and sensitivity testing. Purulent soft tissue infections must additionally be debrided and, if necessary, rinsed with an aseptic solution (e.g., Betadine solution) several times daily for a period of several days. The defect generally accompanying a postoperative wound infection in the area of the cervical soft tissue arises due to an infection-related thrombophlebitis that may lead to the development of extended pharyngocutaneous fistulae if the infection persists. Adequate therapy, however, leads to secondary wound healing due to granulation [100].

5.2.5 Operative Approaches

There are a number of different incisions used to perform neck dissection (▶ Fig. 5.4). The choice of incision type must be individualized for each patient.

Choice of incision type requires the consideration of the following factors:

- tendency of necrosis of the detached skin parts;
- planned extent of the tumor intervention;
- primary defect coverage in cases of more extended skin resections;
- blood supply of the flaps;
- overview of the entire operation field;
- additional performance of tracheotomy;
- possible excision of existing scars;
- potential for no skin incision when mucosal incisions suffice; and
- possibility of extension of the incision if additional cervical lymph node regions must be dissected.

An incision running on and along the carotid artery favors the occurrence of carotid artery exposure and possible rupture in the event of wound dehiscence. This is especially true in trifurcating incisions that bear a higher risk of wound healing disturbances. The most widespread incision types are explained below.

Y-incisions. For a number of years, the simple Y-incision [12] and the double Y-incision [1] have been the

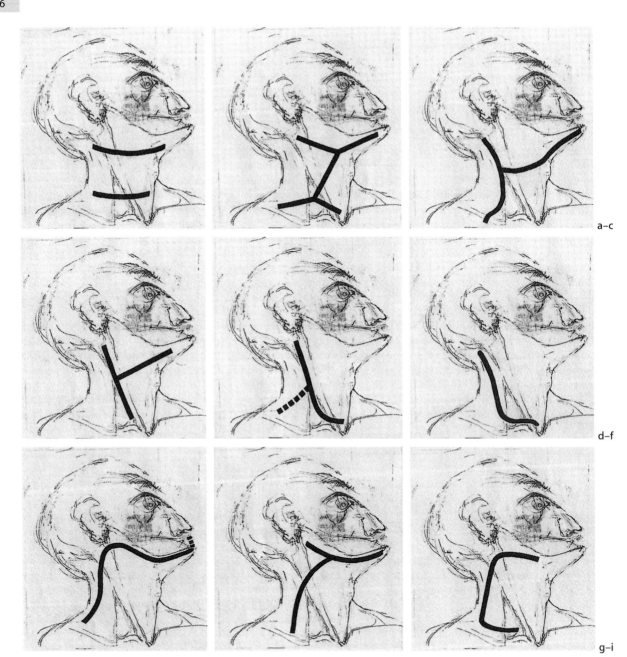

a–c

d–f

g–i

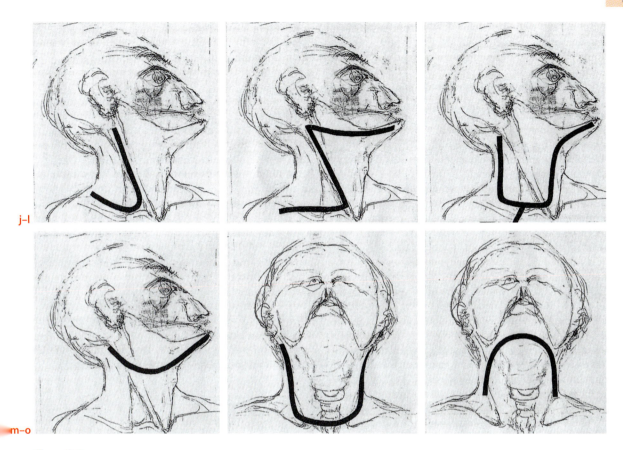

j–l

m–o

Figure 5.4 a–o

Incision types for neck dissection: **a** MacFee incision; **b** Martin incision; **c** the so-called 3/4-H-incision according to Hetter; **d** De Quervain incision, modified according to Roux-Berger; **e** Lahey incision; **f** modified hockey stick incision; **g** inverted hockey stick incision; **h** Schobinger incision; **i** Dietzel incision; **j** De Quervain incision; **k** Z incision; **l** Latshevsky incision; **m,n** U incision; **o** inverted U incision (from [77])

most frequently applied incisions for performance of RND [20]. The disadvantage of both incision types is the high risk of wound healing disturbances due to the trifurcations mentioned above. Significant necrosis can then lead to broad exposure of the carotid artery and an ensuing high risk of carotid rupture.

MacFee Incision. The so-called MacFee incision probably has the best chance of healing because this type of incision addresses the blood supply of the neck [1]. It leads to very good esthetic results as long as the in-

cisions are performed along skin lines, especially in pre-formed creases. Furthermore, this type of incision protects the carotid artery. The operative procedure is more difficult to perform in patients with short necks. Additionally, exposure of the operative field is often impaired so that intensive retraction by the assistant is required. The MacFee incision is preferred for patients suffering from a peripheral vascular disease or for patients who have undergone prior radiotherapy [110]. It is often used in younger patients undergoing neck dissection for thyroid cancer.

Hockey Stick Incision. Robbins [92] recommends the so-called inverted hockey stick incision in cases of modified RND or selective ND for the treatment of cervical lymph node metastases of carcinomas of the oral cavity and the oropharynx, surgical procedures that both require transection of the lower lip.

Pinafore Flaps. The pinafore flap is the most suitable type of incision if ND is combined with a total or partial laryngectomy [48].

To perform posterolateral ND, De Langen and Vermey [111] recommend a special incision technique.

Modified Pinafore Flap. A modified pinafore flap incision has been found to be suitable for resection of the cervical lymph nodes in cases of carcinoma of the oral cavity [92].

One of our favored incisions is an apron-type skin incision beginning below the mastoid tip. The incision initially runs along the anterior edge of the trapezius muscle to about 2 fingers above the clavicle in the middle of the neck. The incision is similar to the incision that is called the hockey stick incision in the American literature. It is suitable for MRND or SND, provided the horizontal section is performed further cranially in a cervical wrinkle.

An alternative approach we support is an incision starting 4 or 5cm below the mastoid tip and following a natural crease anteriorly across the neck. This allows excellent access to lymph node levels I – III. Access to level IV can easily be gained by dropping down an inferior limb "S-shaped" incision, which is placed posterior to the carotid artery system so that the trifurcation point does not overlay this vessel. If the lower lip must be transected to better access the oral cavity, then a vertical limb from the submental area can be made. This includes one or two "Z-shaped" portions to avoid scar contracture.

5.2.5.1 Radical Neck Dissection

The approach to radical neck dissection is described schematically in ▶ Fig. 5.5 a–d.

Skin Incision. Marking anatomic landmarks such as the maxillary angle, the upper edge of the sternum and the mastoid tip is helpful. After marking the planned incision, the arcuate skin incision is performed from below the mastoid tip along the anterior edge of the trapezius muscle until 2 finger breadths above the clavicle and then forward nearly to the midline of the neck. In comparison, a MacFee incision is performed when a pectoralis major myocutaneous flap is planned for defect coverage.

Preparation of the Skin Flap. The first step after skin incision is elevation of the skin flap, maintained under tension, generally including the platysma muscle, as it guarantees blood supply to the flap. The elevation of the skin flap is effectuated either by means of scissors, scalpel or the electric knife. Normally, the skin flap is first raised in ventral-caudal direction, then in dorso-caudal direction. In cases of radical ND, the external jugular vein is next transected. The ligature of this vessel can be performed with an absorbable suture (e.g., Vicryl 2/0) or with a non-absorbable material. The ligation of the internal jugular vein is performed according to the vascular diameter with a non-absorbable suture (e. g., Mersilene 2/0 or 0). The immense importance of correct ligation of the jugular vein cannot be underestimated. The general technique will be described at this point, and a more detailed description of the procedure provided later.

The internal jugular vein is ligated at its inferior or caudal end after clamping the vessel with two clamps parallel to the clavicle and one clamp in a cranial direction. Between this clamp and the middle clamp, the vessel is transected with scissors. Then the ligature is performed using a non-absorbable suture between the middle and inferiorly located clamp while slowly opening the middle clamp. Next, the suture is pulled through the vascular stub using an unattached needle and in this manner the knot is tied. After an additional ligature is placed caudally of the caudal

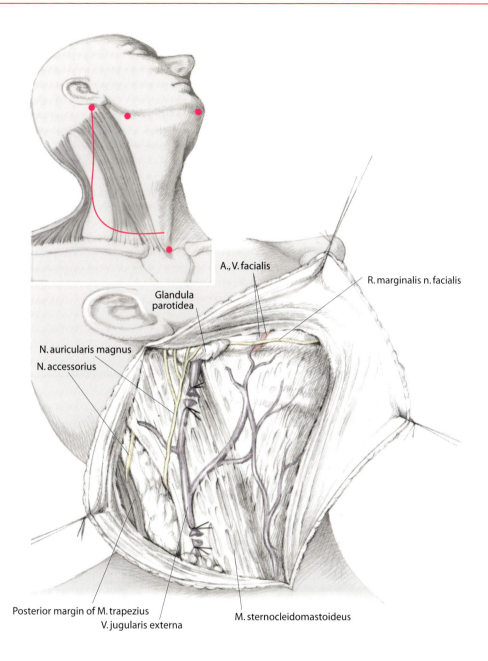

A., V. facialis

R. marginalis n. facialis

Glandula
parotidea

N. auricularis magnus

N. accessorius

Posterior margin of M. trapezius

V. jugularis externa

M. sternocleidomastoideus

Figure 5.5 a

a–d. Surgical procedure of radical neck dissection

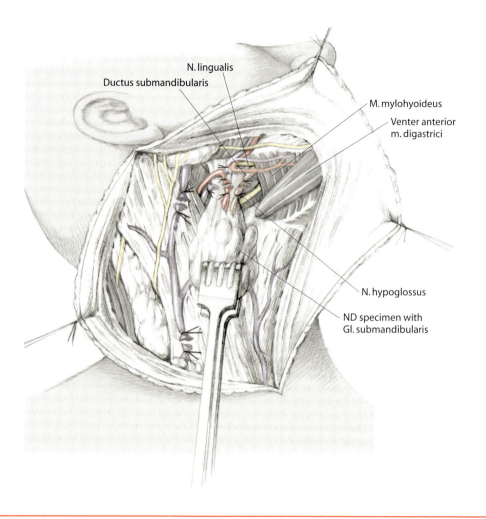

N. lingualis
Ductus submandibularis
M. mylohyoideus
Venter anterior
m. digastrici
N. hypoglossus
ND specimen with
Gl. submandibularis

Figure 5.5 b

clamp, both sutures are tied after removal of the caudal clamp and thus again fixed. The principle of cranial transection of the vessels is similar; the difference being that transection of the vessels is performed between the middle and caudal clamp. Regarding the supraclavicular removal of vessels, the stub of the internal jugular vein at the ND specimen with the still attached clamp is also ligated and fixed with the unattached needle. This is necessary to prevent the clamp from sliding, which could cause bleeding that might impair the surgery.

Another safe method for both cranial and caudal ligation of the jugular vein is based on the principle of "ligation to continuity." With this technique, the jugular vein is skeletonized, taking special care that the vagus nerve is not attached to the vein. A hemostat (typically, o thickness) is then passed under the vein, and sutures are positioned around the vein. One suture is then tied inferiorly, and the other suture superiorly, with a one–two-centimeter space between the sutures. Next, a suture ligature is placed immediately above the previously tied lower suture, using a non-cutting needle to penetrate the vein. After placing the first throw of the knot, the end of the suture without the needle is passed from under the vessel to the superior side. The suture is then further tied. A

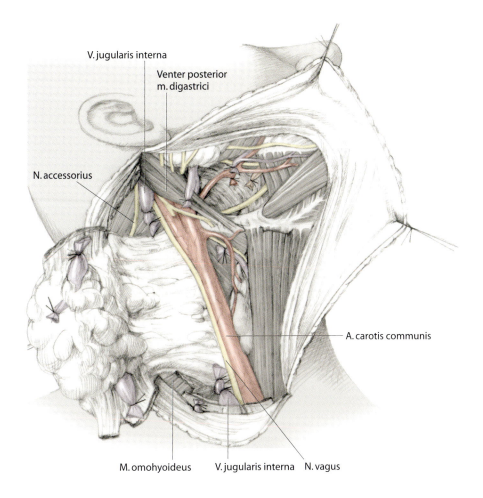

V. jugularis interna

Venter posterior
m. digastrici

N. accessorius

A. carotis communis

M. omohyoideus   V. jugularis interna   N. vagus

Figure 5.5 c

similar procedure is done on the upper area, except here the suture ligature is placed immediately below the free-tied upper o-ligature. After all four sutures are in place the vein is divided in the middle. The same procedure is applied when the jugular vein is transected cranially. With this technique, there is no risk of bleeding if a clamp on the vessel comes off prematurely.

The greater auricular nerve is transected after bipolar coagulation. Coagulation of the distal end of the greater auricular nerve is performed to avoid development of a neuroma. The skin flap is elevated up to the inferior parotid pole and the mandibular edge.

The marginal mandibular branch of the facial nerve and the facial artery are carefully protected. The skin flap can be fixed with two or three subcutaneously placed sutures using a clamp attached to the surgical drapes. Following this, the inferior flap elevation follows. The superficial fascia of the posterior triangle is opened so that the adipose tissue containing lymph nodes becomes visible. During this preparatory step, it is not uncommon to see the superficially running accessory nerve. The inferior skin flap should extend beyond the edge of the trapezius muscle by about 1cm.

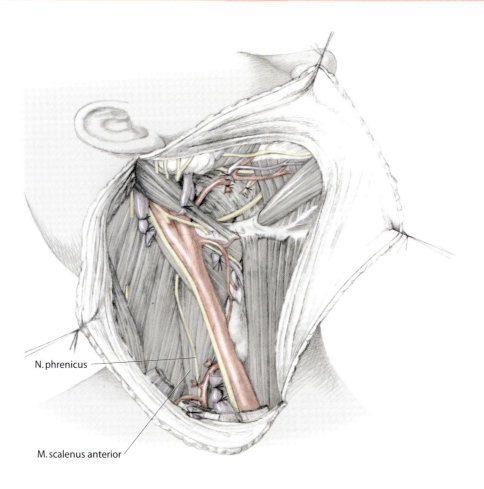

N. phrenicus

M. scalenus anterior

Figure 5.5 d

Dissection of Level I and the Submandibular Gland.
The dissection is performed in the area of the mandibular branch of the facial nerve. Careful attention must be paid to avoid accidental trauma to this nerve. The nerve generally crosses the facial artery and facial vein at the level of the lower edge of the mandible. This nerve branch should be identified and followed in dorsal direction for a short distance in order to mobilize it safely from the operative field in a superior direction. As a rule, the facial vein is ligated. By lifting the intermediate tendon of the digastric muscle, the hypoglossal nerve becomes visible and its course is followed in cranial direction. The descendant branch of the hypoglossal nerve traversing to the cervical ansa is later ligated at the level of the crossing of the internal and external branches of the carotid artery. The dissection is continued along the mandible to the submental edge of the anterior belly of the digastric muscle. The soft tissues between the anterior belly of the digastric muscle and the mandible are mobilized, and the dissection is performed submentally via the ventral belly of the digastric muscle to the raphe along the midline of the mylohyoid muscle. From the ventral direction, the dissection is generally performed toward the mylohyoid muscle to its free dorsal edge. For this purpose, the submandibular

gland is mobilized step-by-step in dorsal direction. During dissection, the lingual nerve and the secretory duct of the submandibular gland must be identified. This is easily accomplished by retracting the mylohyoid muscle superiorly once it is freed up at the anterior end of the submandibular gland. Wharton's duct is ligated with a non-absorbable suture (e.g., Mersilene 2/0) after its transection. Smaller branches from the facial artery that supply the gland are also ligated. During further dissection of the gland and associated adipose tissue, the hyoglossal nerve must be protected. This nerve runs parallel to and below the intermediate tendon of the digastric muscle and behind Wharton's duct on the hypoglossal muscle. To complete this step, the submandibular gland is resected along with the surrounding soft tissue containing lymph nodes from the facial artery distribution and delivered inferiorly at the main ND specimen.

Dissection of Levels II–IV. When necessary, the sternocleidomastoid muscle is removed from the mastoid process using the Bovie knife. This muscle is dissected free in the mentioned area to avoid accidental damage to structures covered by the muscle. If this procedure turns out to be difficult, the muscle is transected electro-surgically step-by-step from the exterior to the interior portion until all fiber bundles are loose. After complete transection of the sternocleidomastoid muscle, it is retracted laterally to reveal level II. The posterior belly of the digastric muscle is used for orientation as the cranial limitation. To expose the jugular vein, the posterior belly of the digastric muscle must be gently lifted. Prior to ligating the jugular vein, it must be delivered carefully from the surrounding soft tissue. Attention must be paid to the identification of the accessory nerve and the vagus nerve in the area of their exiting point from the jugular foramen in the region of the skull base. Internal jugular vein ligation is performed at the cranial removing stub, as already described, always fixed twice with a non-absorbable suture (e.g., Mersilene 2/0 or 0/0). Sutures are placed to avoid sliding of the knot. Finally, the cranial vascular stub is fixed with an unattached needle on the deep cervical fascia or the posterior belly of the digastric muscle. The caudal stub is ligated. The accessory nerve that often follows

a small branch from the occipital artery is also ligated and coagulated to avoid neurinoma at its proximal end. The adipose tissue of level II to level IV, containing lymph nodes that surrounds the vein, is removed from the carotid artery and its branches in caudal direction. The sternocleidomastoid muscle, as well as the omohyoid muscle, are transected at their sternal and clavicular end and added to the neck dissection preparation. As already mentioned, the jugular vein is removed about 1cm above the clavicle after double ligation and fixation. Care must be taken that the vagus nerve is not damaged accidentally. Especially on the left side, the opening of the thoracic duct into the internal jugular vein must be ligated completely and careful attention must be paid to aberrant lymphatic trunks, which must be ligated as well. It is not sufficient to simply divide these small lymphatic channels with either the bipolar or monopolar cautery. To do so without suture ligation increases the chance of developing a chyle fistula.

Dissection of Level V. Level V is normally dissected at the same time as levels II to IV, cranially in caudal direction as an en-bloc resection. The dissection is performed along the deep cervical fascia. Using this technique the skin branches of the cervical plexus are transected and coagulated. Because opening a deep layer of the deep cervical fascia leads to a situation where the phrenic nerve runs unprotected on the scalene muscle, the phrenic nerve must be protected meticulously. The en-bloc preparation is removed using clamps at the anterior edge of the trapezius muscle in order to avoid chyle fistulae, as well as bleeding from the branches of the transverse cervical artery. The accessory nerve is also coagulated and removed at the caudal-dorsal resection margin.

Closure of the Wound. After removing the en-block neck dissection specimen, the wound is rinsed with warm Ringer's solution. Suction drainage is implemented via a cutaneous puncture incision. The drainage tubing is fixed cutaneously by means of a 3.0 Vicryl suture at its exit. The subcutaneous closing of the wound is performed in the area of the platysma by means of 2/0 or 3/0 Vicryl. The skin margins are adapted with a 3/0 or 4/0 suture (e.g. Seralon).

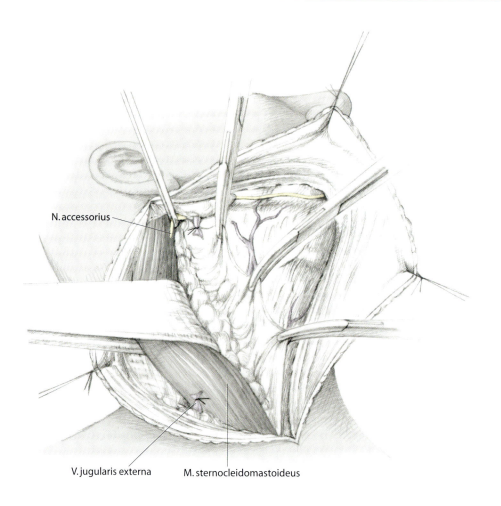

N. accessorius

V. jugularis externa   M. sternocleidomastoideus

Figure 5.6 a

a–d. Surgical procedure of modified radical neck dissection

5.2.5.2 Modified Radical Neck Dissection

The step-by-step procedure for modified radical neck dissection is described schematically in ▶ Fig. 5.6 a–d.

Elevation of the skin flap and other operative preliminaries are performed according to the above-mentioned procedure for radical neck dissection. The following section describes the essential elements involved in modified radical neck dissection.

Dissection of the Fascia of the Sternocleidomastoid Muscle. The fascia of the sternocleidomastoid muscle is included in the neck dissection specimen. Its dis-

section starts at the posterior edge of the muscle in anterior direction and involves the entire body of the muscle. Normally, it is performed sharply with the scalpel or with scissors.

Description of the Accessory Nerve. Generally, the accessory nerve runs in a dorso-caudo-lateral direction through the cranial part of the sternocleidomastoid muscle. Identification of the accessory nerve can usually be performed by bluntly splaying the adipose tissue covering the nerve with scissors at the medial side near the cranial third of the sternocleidomastoid muscle after its careful medialization and lifting by

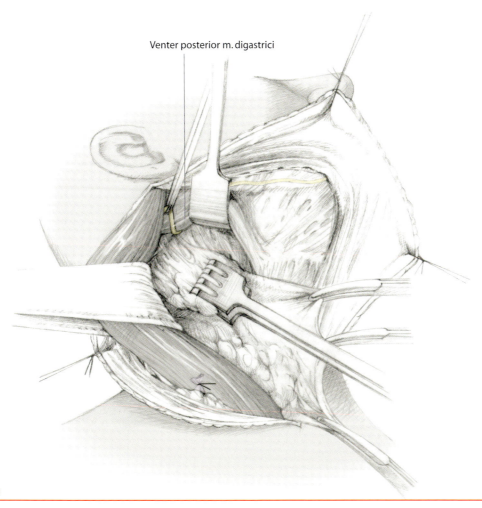

Venter posterior m. digastrici

Figure 5.6 b

means of a blunt hook. The nerve can also be identified at its exit, inferior to the jugular foramen and lateral to the internal jugular vein, especially if extended metastases are present. When the nerve is
identified, the surrounding adipose tissue is carefully
dissected until the nerve is isolated between the skull
base and the sternocleidomastoid muscle, and the
nerve is marked by means of a soft loop (e.g., ete-
loop) and carefully held. In using soft loops, great
care must be taken to avoid applying too much tension to structures that must primarily be protected.
After identification of the accessory nerve, the sternocleidomastoid muscle can be removed completely,

inferiorly to the neural exit from the adipose tissue
containing lymph nodes located underneath. The
nerve can then be lifted by means of a surgical
sponge that is held by a clamp.

Preparation of the Submuscular Recess. After identification of the accessory nerve, resection of the adipose tissue containing lymph nodes starts in the area
of the submuscular recess, the cranial part of level II
that is divided by the course of the nerve into levels
IIA and IIB. In order to completely resect the adipose
tissue of the submuscular recess containing lymph
nodes, the sternocleidomastoid muscle must be held

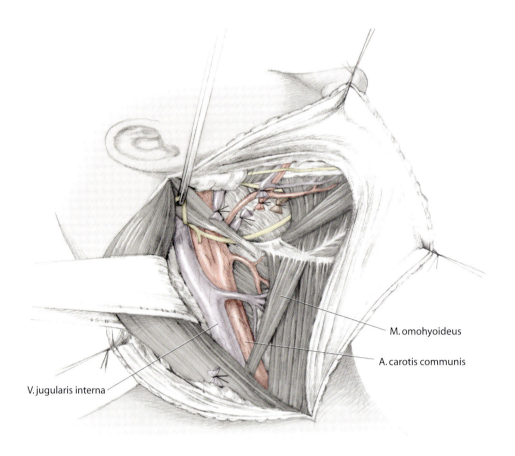

M. omohyoideus

A. carotis communis

V. jugularis interna

Figure 5.6 c

as far as possible in cranio-lateral direction. The site can then be opened by means of a hook that mobilizes the dorsal belly of the digastric muscle and the mandibular branch in cranial direction. The adipose tissue located on the underside of the sternocleidomastoid muscle is removed from the skull base and mobilized in caudal direction until it can be displaced completely below the accessory nerve in caudal direction. A precondition for this procedure is transection of the soft tissue at the border between levels IIA and IIB. To facilitate further inferior dissection, the cutaneous branches that can be identified at the posterior edge of the sternocleidomastoid muscle

from the cervical plexus must be transected in most cases and the nerve endings coagulated.

Dissection of level I and the submandibular gland is performed in the same manner as radical neck dissection.

Dissection of the Vascular Sheath and Levels II to IV. Lateralization of the sternocleidomastoid muscle allows dissection of the vascular sheath and ablation of the surrounding adipose tissue containing lymph nodes from cranial to caudal direction. Dissection behind the vascular sheath should be avoided in order to protect the sympathetic trunk and the superi-

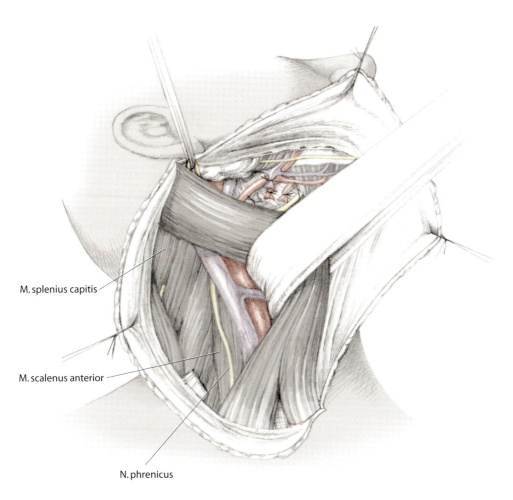

M. splenius capitis

M. scalenus anterior

N. phrenicus

Figure 5.6 d

or laryngeal nerve. The omohyoid muscle that divides levels III and IV can be removed at the lower edge at the clavicle and resected for inclusion in the neck dissection specimen. At the caudal resection edge, close attention must be paid to ensure that the adipose tissue of level V containing lymph nodes is removed en-bloc via clamps, followed by ligation to avoid the development of chylous fistulae.

Dissection of Level V. Because the already cranio-medially accessory nerve is isolated, its complete identification is performed in the area of the posterior triangle. The nerve can be observed in its course through the muscle or identified again in the posterior triangle. The tissue containing lymph nodes is mobilized from the splenius capitis muscle and the middle scalene muscle in the direction of the anterior edge of the trapezius muscle. At the dorsal resection edge of level V, the adipose tissue containing lymph nodes is removed in a manner similar to the caudal edge of level IV, applying clamps and ligatures. Due to the opening of the dorsal sheath of the fascia of the posterior triangle, which occurs in the dissection of level V, branches of the brachial plexus, of the phrenic nerve that runs on the scalene muscle, as well as the transverse cervical artery, are susceptible to damage.

Closing of the wound is performed in the manner already described.

5.2.5.3 Selective Neck Dissection

The surgical procedure for selective neck dissection is different from the neck dissection types already described in that only certain lymph node levels are dissected. The sternocleidomastoid muscle, the internal jugular vein and the accessory nerve remain in this type of neck dissection. When necessary, modifications can be made. For example, in the event of an oncological necessity to resect the accessory nerve, the appropriate intervention would be performed and described as "selective neck dissection (indication of the levels) with resection of N. XI."

Selective Neck Dissection (I–III)

In the case of SND (I–III), a Hockey stick or transverse cervical incision as already described is used. The dissection of the skin flap and the submuscular recess with description of the accessory nerve is performed in the manner also described above. After mobilization of the adipose tissue containing lymph nodes below the accessory nerve in caudal direction and lateralization of the sternocleidomastoid muscle, the dissection is continued until the border of level IV is identified. The critical points previously mentioned must be considered in order to avoid accidental damage to the neural structures. In principle, the surgical procedure of selective neck dissection types with regard to the dissection of level I does not differ from radical or modified radical neck dissection. Closing of the wound is performed as already described for RND.

Selective Neck Dissection (II–IV)

In the case of SND (II–IV), the incision is normally performed from below the mastoid tip along the posterior edge of the sternocleidomastoid muscle until 2cm above the thoracic outlet. Dissection of the skin flap and the submuscular recess with identification of the accessory nerve is performed in the same way as in MRND. Mobilization of the sternocleidomastoid muscle allows the further dissection of levels II–IV, with conservation of the internal jugular vein and protection of the neural structures. In some situations, the sternal head of the sternocleidomastoid muscle can be clamped and divided, and this part of the muscle can be retracted posterosuperiorly. Caution must be exercised not to damage the spinal accessory nerve where it exits the muscle posteriorly. Dividing and retracting the sternocleidomastoid muscle is especially helpful with neck dissection in thyroid cancers where level VI is also done. At the end of the dissection, the sternocleidomastoid muscle is reapproximated with 0-vicryl sutures in a horizontal mattress fashion. The omohyoid muscle dividing levels III and IV can be preserved. If it is removed, this intervention is generally performed without impairing function. The closing of the wound is performed according to the procedure described for RND.

Selective Neck Dissection (I–IV)

In case of SND (I–IV), the incision corresponds to the one described for MRND. The skin flap and the submuscular recess with identification of the accessory nerve are prepared in the same way as for MRND. The further dissection of levels I–IV is identical to the procedure described for SND (II–IV) and SND (I–III). The closing of the wound is performed as described for RND.

Selective Neck Dissection (II–V)

In the case of SND (II–V), the incision, the dissection of the skin flap and the submuscular recess with description of the accessory nerve, as well as level V, are all performed in the same manner as in MRND. Meticulous attention must be paid to the protection of the accessory nerve. The further dissection of levels II–IV is identical to the procedure described for SND (II–IV). The closing of the wound is the same as that described for RND.

References

1. Maves MD (1996) Transsternal mediastinal node dissection. In: Bailey BJ, Calhoun KH, Coffey AR, Neely JG (Hrsg) Atlas of head and neck surgery – otolaryngology. Lippincott, Philadelphia, 154–157

2. Kocher (1880) Ueber Radicalheilung des Krebses. Dtsch Z Chir 13:134–166

3. Regnault F (1887) Die malignen Tumoren der Gefäßscheide. Arch Klin Chir 35:50

4. Jawdynski F (1888) I. Przypadek raka pierwotnego szyi. T. z. raka skrzelowego volkmann'a. Wyciecie nowotworu wraz z rezekcyja tetnicy szyjowej wspolnej i zyly szyjowej wewnetrznej. Wyzdrowienie. Gaz Lek 28:530–535

5. Werner JA (2001) Historischer Abriss zur Nomenklatur der Halslymphknoten als Grundlage für die Klassifikation der Neck dissection. Laryngorhinootologie 80:400–409

6. Crile GW (1906) Excision of cancer of the head and neck with a special reference to the plan of dissection based upon one hundred thirty-two operations. JAMA 47:1780–1786

7. Towpik E (1990) Centennial of the first description of the en bloc Neck dissection. Plast Reconstr Surg 85:468–470

8. Solis-Cohen J (1901) The surgical treatment of laryngeal cancer. Trans Am Laryngol Assoc 22:75–87

9. Bartlett EI, Callander CL (1926) Neck dissections. Surg Clin North Am 6:481–505

10. Blair VP, Brown JB (1933) The treatment of the cancerous or potentially cancerous cervical lymph nodes. Ann Surg 98:650

11. Dargent M, Papillon J (1945) Les sequelles motrices de l'evidement ganglionnaire du cou. Lyon Chir 40:718–731

12. Werner JA, Dünne AA, Lippert BM (2001) Die Neck dissection im Wandel der Zeit. Onkologe 7:522–532

13. Martin H, Del Valle B, Ehrlich H, Cahan WG (1951) Neck dissection. Cancer 4:441–499

14. Myers EN, Gastman BR (2003) Neck dissection: an operation in evolution. Arch Otolaryngol Head Neck Surg 129:14–25

15. Gavilan J, Gavilan C, Herranz J (1992) Functional Neck dissection: three decades of controversy. Ann Otol Rhinol Laryngol 101:339–341

16. Suárez O (1962) Le probleme chirurgical du cancer du larynx. Ann Otolaryngol 79:22–34

17. Silvestre-Begnis C (1944) Consideraciones sobre el problema del tratamiento quirdrgico de los ganglios en los conceres de la laringe. Acta II Congreso Sudamericano ORL. Montevedio, Uruguay

18. Truffert P (1922) Le cou: anatomie topographique. Les aponevroses, les loges. Paris Arnette

19. Pernkopf FE (1952) Topographische Anatomie des Menschen. Vol. 3. Hals. Urban & Schwarzenburg, Wien, 1952:88–118

20. Del Dol JA, Agra A (1947) Cancer of the larynx: laryngectomy with systemic extirpation of connective tissue and cervical lymph nodes as a routine procedure. Trans Am Acad Ophthalmol Otolaryngol 51:653–655

21. Miodonski J (1954) Leczenie raka krtani. Czesc III. Otolaryngol Pol 8:93–102

22. Bocca E, Pignataro O, Sasaki, CT (1980). Functional Neck dissection. A description of operative technique. Arch Otolaryngol 106:524–527

23. Bocca E, Pignataro O, Oldini C, Cappa C (1984) Functional Neck dissection: An evaluation and review of 843 cases. Laryngoscope 94:942–945

24. Bocca E, Pignataro O (1976) A conservation technique in radical Neck dissection. Ann Otol Rhinol Laryngol 76:975–87

25. Prim MP, de Diego JI, Fernandez-Zubillaga A, Garcia-Raya P, Madero R, Gavilan J (2000) Patency and flow of the internal jugular vein after functional Neck dissection. Laryngoscope 110:47–50

26. Werner JA, Dünne AA, Lippert BM (2001) Die Neck dissection im Wandel der Zeit. Onkologe 7:522–532

27. Lindberg R (1972) Distribution of cervical lymph node metastasis from squamous cell carcinoma of the upper respiratory and digestive tracts. Cancer 29:1446–1449

28. Skolnik EM, Yee KF, Friedman M, Golden TA (1976) The posterior triangle in radical neck surgery. Arch Otolaryngol Head Neck Surg 102:1–4

29. Ballantyne AJ. Neck dissection for cancer. Curr Probl Cancer 1985 9:1–34

30. Byers RM, Wolf PF, Ballantyne AJ (1988) Rationale for elective modified Neck dissection. Head Neck Surg 10:160–7

31. Goepfert H, Jesse RH, Ballantyne AJ (1980) Posterolateral Neck dissection. Arch Otolaryngol 106:618–20

32. Weissler MC (1994) Technique of radical Neck dissection. In: Shockley WW, Pillsbury III HC (Hrsg) The neck. Diagnosis and Surgery. Mosby, St. Louis, 573–588

33. Shah JP, Strong E, Spiro RH, Vikram B (1981) Surgical grand rounds. Neck dissection: Current status and future possibilities. Clin Bull 11:25–33

34. Robbins KT, Denys D and the committee for Neck dissection classification, American Head and Neck Society (2000) The American head and neck society's revised classification for Neck dissection. In: Johnson JT, Shaha AR (Hrsg). Proceedings of the 5th International Conference in Head and Neck Cancer. Madison, Omnipress, 365–370

35. Robbins KT, Medina JE, Wolfe GT, Levine PA, Sessions RB, Pruet CW (1991) Standardizing Neck dissection terminology. Official report of the Academy's Committee for Head and Neck Surgery and Oncology. Arch Otolaryngol Head Neck Surg 117:601–605

36. McGuirt WF, McCabe BF (1980) Bilateral radical Neck dissections. Arch Otolaryngol Head Neck Surg 106:427–429

37. Mann W, Wolfensberger M, Fhller U, Beck C (1991) Radikale versus modifizierte Halsausräumung. Kanzerologische und funktionelle Gesichtspunkte. Laryngorhinootologie 70: 32–35

38. Ambrosch P, Kron M, Pradier O, Steiner W (2001) Efficacy of selective Neck dissection: A review of 503 cases of elective and therapeutic treatment of the neck in squamous cell carcinoma of the upper aerodigestive tract. Otolaryngol Head Neck Surg 124:180–187

39. Banerjee AR, Alun-Jones T (1995) Neck dissection. Clin Otolaryngol 20:286–290

40. Medina JE (1989) A rational classification of Neck dissections. Otolaryngol Head Neck Surg 100:169–176

41. Medina JE (1996) Radical Neck dissection. Supraomohyoid Neck dissection. Modified radical Neck dissection. Posterolateral Neck dissection. In: Bailey BJ, Calhoun KH, Coffey AR, Neely JG (Hrsg) Atlas of head and neck surgery – otolaryngology. Lippincott, Philadelphia, 140–153, 162–163

42. Rassekh CH, Johnson JT, Myers EN (1995) Accuracy of intraoperative staging of the No neck in squamous cell carcinoma. Laryngoscope 105:1334–1336

43. Manni JJ, van den Hoogen FJA (1991) Supraomohyoid Neck dissection with frozen section biopsy as a staging procedure in the clinically node-negative neck in carcinoma of the oral cavity. Am J Surg 162:373–376

44. Rochlin DB (1962) Posterolateral Neck dissection for malignant neoplasms. Surg Gynecol Obstet 115:369–373

45. Wustrow TP (1989) Zur Nomenklatur der verschiedenen Formen der Neck dissection. Laryngorhinootologie 68:529–530

46. Engleder R, Fries R (1992) Zur chirurgischenTherapie der Halslymphknoten-Metastasen bei Mundhöhlenkarzinomen. In: Vinzenz K, Waclawiczek HW (Hrsg) Chirurgische Therapie von Kopf-Hals-Karzinomen. Springer, Wien, 143–154

47. Johnson JT, Leipzig B, Cummings CW (1982) Management of T1 carcinoma of the anterior aspect of the tongue. Head Neck 4:209–212

48. Wax MK, Garnett JD, Graeber G (1995) Thorascopic staging of stomal recurrence. Head Neck 17:409–413

49. Jackson SR, Stell PM (1991) Second radical Neck dissection. Clin Otolaryngol 16:52–58

50. Keller E, Ries F, Grhnwald F, Honisch C, Roscanowski, Pavics L, Herberhold C, Solymosi L (1995) Multimodaler Karotisokklusionstest zur Bestimmung des Infarktrisikos vor therapeutischem Karotis-interna-Verschluss. Laryngorhinootologie 74:307–311

51. Schobel G, Hollmann K, Millesi W (1992) Über das Risiko der Mitresektion der Arteria carotis communis bzw. interna bei der Exstirpation von Tumoren im maxillo-facialen Bereich. In: Vinzenz K, Waclawiczek HW (Hrsg) Chirurgische Therapie von Kopf-Hals-Karzinomen. Springer, Wien, 269–282

52. Gluckman JL, Myer CM, Aseff JN, Donegan JO (1983) Rehabilitation following radical Neck dissection. Laryngoscope 93:1083–1085

53. Lampe HB, Lampe KM, Skillings J (1986) Head and neck cancer in the elderly. J Otolaryngol 15:235–238

54. Teymoortash A, Wulf H, Werner JA (2002) Chirurgie von Karzinomen der oberen Luft- und Speisewege bei Patienten im fortgeschrittenen Lebensalter. Laryngorhinootologie 81:293–298

55. Coebergh JW (1996) Significant trends in cancer in the elderly. Eur J Cancer 32:569–571

56. Stein M, Herberhold C, Walther EK, Langenberg S (2000) Einfluss von Begleiterkrankungen auf die Prognose von Plattenepithelkarzinomen im Kopf-Hals-Bereich. Laryngorhinootologie 79:345–349

57. Vokes EE, Weichselbaum RR, Lippman SM, Hong WK (1993) Head and neck cancer. N Engl J Med 328:184–194

58. Goodwin JS, Hunt WC, Samet JM (1993) Determinants of cancer therapy in elderly patients. Cancer 72:594–601

59. Fentiman IS, Tirelli U, Monfardini S, Schneider M, Festen J, Cognetti F, Aapro MS (1990) Cancer in the elderly: why so badly treated? Lancet 335:1020–1022

60. Wetle T (1987) Age as a risk factor for inadequate treatment. JAMA 258:516

61. Kennedy BJ (1988) Aging and cancer. J Clin Oncol 6:1903–1911

62. Yancik R, Ries LG (1991) Cancer in the aged. An epidemiologic perspective on treatment issues. Cancer 68:2502–2510

63. Cohen HJ (1994) Biology of aging as related to cancer. Cancer 74:2092–2100

64. Vercelli M, Parodi S, Serraino D (1998) Overall cancer incidence and mortality trends among elderly and adult Europeans. Crit Rev Oncol Hematol 27:87–96

65. Exton-Smith AN (1982) Epidemiological studies in the elderly: methodological considerations. Am J Clin Nutr 35:1273–1279

66. Levi F, La Vecchia C, Lucchini F, Negri E (1996) Worldwide trends in cancer mortality in the elderly, 1955–1992. Eur J Cancer 32:652–672

67. Koch WM, Patel H, Brennan J, Boyle JO, Sidransky D (1995) Squamous cell carcinoma of the head and neck in the elderly. Arch Otolaryngol Head Neck Surg 121:262–265

68. Leon X, Quer M, Agudelo D, Lopez-Pousa A, De Juan M, Diez S, Burgues J (1998) Influence of age on laryngeal carcinoma. Ann Otol Rhinol Laryngol 107:164–169

69. Nelson JF, Ship II (1971) Intraoral carcinoma: predisposing factors and their frequency of incidence as related to age at onset. J Am Dent Assoc 82:564–568

70. Brennan JA, Boyle JO, Koch WM, Goodman SN, Hruban RH, Eby YJ, Couch MJ, Forastiere AA, Sidransky D (1995) Association between cigarette smoking and mutation of the p53 gene in squamous-cell carcinoma of the head and neck. N Engl J Med 332:712–717

71. McKenna RJ (1994) Clinical aspects of cancer in the elderly. Treatment decisions, treatment choices, and follow-up. Cancer 74:2107–2117

72. Samet J, Hunt WC, Key C, Humble CG, Goodwin JS (1986) Choice of cancer therapy varies with age of patient. JAMA 255:3385–3390

73. Metges JP, Eschwege F, de Crevoisier R, Lusinchi A, Bourhis J, Wibault P (2000) Radiotherapy in head and neck cancer in the elderly: a challenge. Crit Rev Oncol Hematol 34:195–203

74. Carr RJ, Langdon JD (1989) Multiple primaries in mouth cancer – the price of success. Br J Oral Maxillofac Surg 27:394–399

75. Aassar OS, Fischbein NJ, Caputo GR, Kaplan MJ, Price DC, Singer MI, Dillon WP, Hawkins RA (1999) Metastatic head and neck cancer: role and usefulness of FDG PET in locating occult primary tumors. Radiology 10:177–181

76. Paulus P, Sambon A, Vivegnis D, Hustinx R, Moreau P, Collignon J, Deneufbourg JM, Rigo P (1998) 18FDG-PET for the assessment of primary head and neck tumors: clinical, computed tomography, and histopathological correlation in 38 patients. Laryngoscope 108:1578–1583

77. Werner JA (1997) Aktueller Stand der Versorgung des Lymphabflusses maligner Kopf-Hals-Tumoren. Eur Arch Otorhinolaryngol Suppl I, 47–85

78. Alajmo E, Fini-Storchi O, Agostini V, Polli G (1985) Conservation surgery for cancer of the larynx in the elderly. Laryngoscope 95:203–205

79. Huygen PL, van den Broek P, Kazem I (1980) Age and mortality in laryngeal cancer. Clin Otolaryngol 5:129–137

80. Kowalski LP, Franco EL, de Andrade Sobrinho J, Oliveira BV, Pontes PL (1991) Prognostic factors in laryngeal cancer patients submitted to surgical treatment. J Surg Oncol 48:87–95

81. Ampil FL, Mills GM, Stucker FJ, Burton GV, Nathan CO (2001) Radical combined treatment of locally extensive head and neck cancer in the elderly. Am J Otolaryngol 22:65–69

82. Harries M, Lund VJ (1989) Head and neck surgery in the elderly: a maturing problem. J Laryngol Otol 103:306–309

83. John AC, Vaughan ED (1980) Laryngeal resection in patients of seventy years and over. J Laryngol Otol 94:629–635

84. Singh B, Cordeiro PG, Santamaria E, Shaha AR, Pfister DG, Shah JP (1999) Factors associated with complications in microvascular reconstruction of head and neck defects. Plast Reconstr Surg 103:403–411

85. Bridger AG, O'Brien CJ, Lee KK (1994) Advanced patient age should not preclude the use of free-flap reconstruction for head and neck cancer. Am J Surg 168:425–428

86. Shaari CM, Buchbinder D, Costantino PD, Lawson W, Biller HF, Urken ML (1998) Complications of microvascular head and neck surgery in the elderly. Arch Otolaryngol Head Neck Surg 1998; 124: 407–411

87. Barzan L, Veronesi A, Caruso G, Serraino D, Magri D, Zagonel V, Tirelli U, Comoretto R, Monfardini S (1990) Head and neck cancer and ageing: a retrospective study in 438 patients. J Laryngol Otol 104:634–640

88. Clayman GL, Eicher SA, Sicard MW, Razmpa E, Goepfert H (1998) Surgical outcomes in head and neck cancer patients 80 years of age and older. Head Neck 20:216–223

89. Jun MY, Strong EW, Saltzman EI, Gerold FP (1983) Head and neck cancer in the elderly. Head Neck Surg 5:376–382

90. Bengtson BP, Schusterman MA, Baldwin BJ, Miller MJ, Reece GP, Kroll SS, Robb GL, Goepfert H (1993) Influence of prior radiotherapy on the development of postoperative complications and success of free tissue transfers in head and neck cancer reconstruction. Am J Surg 166:326–330

91. McGuirt WF, Davis SP III (1995) Demographic portrayal and outcome analysis of head and neck cancer surgery in the elderly. Arch Otolaryngol Head Neck Surg 121:150–154

92. Robbins KT (1994) Neck dissection: Classification and incisions. In: Schockley WW, Pillsbury III HC (Hrsg) The neck. Diagnosis and Surgery. Mosby, St. Louis, 381–391

93. Werner JA (2002) Lymphknotenerkrankungen im Kopf-Hals-Bereich. Springer, Berlin

94. Moorthy SS, Radpour S (1999) Management of anesthesia in geriatric patients undergoing head and neck surgery. Ear Nose Throat J 78:496–498

95. Trott JA, David DJ, Edwards RM (1982) Experience with surgery for head and neck cancer in a geriatric population. Aust N Z J Surg 52:149–153

96. Sisson GA, Straehley CJ, Johnson NE (1962) Mediastinal dissection for recurrent cancer after laryngectomy. Laryngoscope 73:1069–1074

97. Kowalski LP, Alcantara PS, Magrin J, Parise Junior O (1994) A case-control study on complications and survival in elderly patients undergoing major head and neck surgery. Am J Surg 168:485–490

98. Hirano M, Mori K (1998) Management of cancer in the elderly: therapeutic dilemmas. Otolaryngol Head Neck Surg 118:110–114

99. Linn BS, Linn MW, Wallen N (1982) Evaluation of results of surgical procedures in the elderly. Ann Surg 195:90–96

100. Grandis JR, Johnson JT (1996) The use of antibiotics in head and neck surgery. In: Myers EN, Suen JY (eds) Cancer of the head and neck. Third edition, Saunders, Philadelphia, 97–104

101. Schobel G, Hollmann K, Millesi W (1992) Prophylactic antibiotics in oral, pharyngeal, and laryngeal surgery for cancer: A double-blind study. Laryngoscope 83:1992–1998

102. Tabet JC, Johnson JT (1990) Wound infection in head and neck surgery: Prophylaxis, etiology and management. J Otolaryngol 19:197–200

103. Geyer G, Borneff M, Hartmetz G (1987) Perioperative Prophylaxe mit Cefuroxime und Metronidazole bei Patienten mit Kopf-Hals-Tumoren. HNO 35:355–359

104. Mustafa E, Tahsin A (1993) Cefotaxime prophylaxis in major non-contaminated head and neck surgery: one-day vs. seven-day therapy. J Laryngol Otol 107:30–32

105. Righi M, Manfredi R, Farneti G, Pasquini E, Cenacchi V (1996) Short-term versus long-term antimicrobial prophylaxis in oncologic head and neck surgery. Head Neck 18:399–404

106. Righi M, Manfredi R, Farneti G, Pasquini E, Cenacchi V (1996) Short-term versus long-term antimicrobial prophylaxis in oncologic head and neck surgery. Head Neck 18: 399–404

107. Coskun H, Erisen L, Basut O (2000) Factors affecting wound infection rates in head and neck surgery. Otolaryngol Head Neck Surg 123):328–333

108. Sous H, Hirsch I (1982) Experimental analyses assessing the bacterial activity of Cefmenoxime. 3rd Mediterran Congreß of Chemotherapy, Dubrovnik, Abstr Nr 190

109. Engemann R (1993) Possibilities for the use of 2nd generation cephalosporins in perioperative antibiotic prophylaxis. Infection 21: 17–20

110. Maran AGD, Amin M, Wilson JA (1989) Radical Neck dissection: A 19-year experience. J Laryngol Otol 103:760–764

111. de Langen ZJ, Vermey A (1988) Posterolateral Neck dissection. Head Neck 10:252–256

Radiation Therapy: Principles and Treatment

Radiation therapy plays an integral role in the management of primary squamous cell carcinoma of the head and neck. It may be used as the sole therapy in early stage disease or combined preoperatively with surgery. In more advanced stage disease, it may be combined postoperatively with surgery. There is also a role for elective neck irradiation in node negative patients, depending on the primary site. This chapter attempts to define the rationale behind radiation therapy and the techniques for administering irradiation in the relevant cases.

6.1 Elective Neck Irradiation

The indications for elective neck irradiation are very similar to those for elective neck dissection. They are based on the site and extent (T stage) of the primary tumor, as well as on the degree of histological differentiation. Mendenhall, et al. [1] defined low and high risk groups based on the following factors:

- low risk patients (those with less than 20 % risk of subclinical neck disease) included T1 lesions of the floor of mouth, retromolar trigone, gingiva, hard palate and buccal mucosa, as well as T1 and T2 lesions of the glottic larynx and suprahyoid epiglottis;
- high risk patients (defined as greater than 30 % risk of occult neck disease) included all patients with nasopharynx, pyriform sinus and base of tongue primaries, stage T2–4 soft palate, pharyngeal wall, supraglottic larynx and tonsil primaries and stage T3 and T4 lesions of all other sites.

Elective neck irradiation is recommended over elective neck dissection for patients whose primary site is being treated by primary radiation therapy. In 1991, Robbins, et al. [2] defined standardized terminology of the various anatomic levels of neck node metastases. The level II and III nodes, which are the most commonly involved subclinical nodes, are almost always included in the high dose radiation fields of the primary site using traditional radiation techniques. These regions typically receive the equivalent of 60 Gy over a period of six more weeks. The remaining N0 neck areas (typically the low neck, not included in the primary radiation field) are generally controlled by the administration of 40–50 Gy over a period of five weeks.

6.2 Postoperative Radiation of the Node Positive Neck

The need for postoperative radiotherapy will vary depending on a number of risk factors. Surgical treatment alone (neck dissection) of the node positive neck has been associated with an increased risk of recurrence and death from cancer in patients with N2 and N3 stage neck disease [3, 4]. The risk of failure clearly increases with the increasing number and size of the nodes [3, 4, 6]. Other risk factors that are associated with increased failure postoperatively include extracapsular extension of nodal disease [4, 5, 6], invasive cancer at the margin of resection [4, 7], perineural invasion [4, 8] and, lastly, extension of the tumor into soft tissues of the neck [4, 5, 6] and primary disease site [4, 9].

The risk of lymph node metastases increases depending on the site of the primary , poor histological differentiation, increasing size of the primary and the availability of capillary lymphatics [1]. Recurrent lesions carry a higher risk of nodal metastases as well.

Radiation for advanced neck disease (N2 or N3 stage) can be given either preoperatively or postoperatively. The sequence should depend on how the primary site will be treated and whether the nodal disease is to be completely resected. For example, a neck dissection with postoperative radiotherapy would be preferred if the primary site is to be treated with surgery. Preoperative radiotherapy would be preferred if the primary site is to be treated with radiation or if the neck nodes are fixed and cannot be completely resected. Postoperative radiotherapy ideally begins within 4–6 weeks after surgery, although at least one report shows no increased risk of neck failure if radiotherapy is initiated up to 10 weeks after surgery [4]. Typical postoperative doses consist of 60Gy in 30 fractions to 65Gy in 35 fractions over 6–7 weeks. Higher doses should be prescribed if residual disease is present in the neck or if margins of resection are positive [4, 10]. Split course radiation (i. e., a 1–2 week break in the radiotherapy mid-course) is clearly associated with an increase in failure [11].

Sequential chemotherapy, followed by radiotherapy in the postoperative setting, has not been shown to improve disease outcome in Intergroup Study 0034 [12]. This finding, together with reports of improved control in the simultaneous administration of chemotherapy and radiotherapy as the primary treatment for some head and neck sites, has lead to great interest in concomitant chemotherapy/ radiotherapy for high-risk patients in the postoperative setting. RTOG 9501 (also an Intergroup trial) was recently completed, which randomized high-risk patients to 60Gy of radiation with or without cisplatin chemotherapy (100 mg/m2 IV on days 1, 22, and 43). Local-regional recurrence as the first site of failure was higher in the radiation-alone arm, and distant metastases were less frequent in the concomitant chemotherapy-radiotherapy arm, but overall survival was not different in the two groups [13]. In contrast, a study by the EORTC presented one year earlier demonstrated both improved disease-free survival and overall survival in patients receiving concomitant cisplatin (100 mg/m2 on days 1, 22 and 43) and up to 66Gy in 2-Gy fractions, compared with patients receiving radiotherapy alone [14]. Both studies demonstrated a significant increase in acute toxicity in the postoperative chemotherapy-radiotherapy arms, compared with radiotherapy alone, but, thus far, neither the EORTC nor the RTOG studies have been published as full manuscripts.

6.3 Intensity-Modulated Radiation Therapy

Radiation therapy techniques have undergone a number of major changes in the past decade as a result of the availability of powerful computers for three dimensional (3D) treatment planning. These computer systems make possible the modern imaging technologies, computed tomography (CT) and magnetic resonance imaging (MRI), which are used to fully model the patient anatomy and tumor volumes in three dimensions (3D). Positron emission technology (PET) and PET-CT fusion techniques further enhance this ability. The more modern computer technology in latest generation medical linear accelerators allows computer control of multi-leaf collimators which can not only shape the fields to conform to the 3D anatomy but also modulate the beam intensity across the treatment field.

Conformal 3D treatment of tumors has recently evolved further into intensity-modulated radiation therapy (IMRT). With this treatment, the radiation beam can be optimized to maximize tumor dose and yet spare critical normal tissues. Head and neck tumors are particularly appropriate for treatment with IMRT because of the close proximity of the cancer or area at risk to numerous critical structures. These include salivary glands, spinal cord, brainstem and optic pathways. There is also a relative lack of internal organ motion, which makes this region of the body ideal for this treatment modality.

The ability to shape fields and treat the head and neck area using IMRT with very steep dose gradients makes knowledge of anatomy on CT and MRI critical. Much work has been done to define the normal nodal levels on imaging studies [15, 16, 17]. This is an evolving process, and the definitions continue to be updated by various groups. The routes by which cancer is spread in these varying imaging planes must also be precisely defined and this knowledge used in the development of radiation treatment plans for head and neck cancers.

Traditional treatment plans for head and neck irradiation have involved treatment to multiple target volumes, typically sequentially with differing doses. Field volume reductions follow treatment to larger volumes and result in higher total doses to smaller volumes of tissue. Critical structures (e.g., the spinal cord) are often shielded once a safe tolerance dose is reached, but in some cases permanent damage or dysfunction is not avoidable (e.g., salivary gland tissue). IMRT allows for the delivery of different doses to different areas of the treatment volume simultaneously. The numerous physical ways to obtain these differing doses of radiation using IMRT are beyond the scope of this chapter but are described elsewhere [18, 19].

Treatment with IMRT requires adequate immobilization of the patient during treatment sessions, which can run 20–30 minutes for a typical head and neck treatment utilizing 5–8 fields. For most patients, immobilization can be achieved using a thermoplastic mask system. Gilbeau and colleagues demonstrated a 0.22cm standard deviation of total displacement in patients using three different thermoplastic mask systems [20].

Target volume delineation for IMRT requires extensive knowledge of both the anatomy of the neck and the risk of spread (and spread patterns) within the anatomy in question. IMRT radiation treatment volumes have been defined by the International Commission on Radiation Units and Measurements (ICRU) in reports 50 and 62 [21, 22]. Gross tumor volume (GTV) and volumes of suspected microscopic spread make up the clinical target volume (CTV). Marginal volumes, which account for setup variations and organ and patient motion, are added to yield the planning target volume (or PTV). There are often multiple CTVs defined per patient. For example, in definitively irradiated cases, CTV1 would be defined as the gross tumor, clinically involved lymph nodes and adjacent high risk areas and would receive a higher radiation dose (e.g., 70 Gy in 35 fractions), and CTV2 would include prophylactically treated neck nodes and would receive a lower dose (e.g., 50–60Gy in 35 fractions). In the postoperative setting, CTV1 would include the primary surgical bed and the surgical beds of involved lymph nodes, while CTV2 would again define areas to be treated prophylactically. The margin added for set-up uncertainty and motion would then define PTV1 and PTV2, respectively.

Avoidance volumes and tolerance doses must also be delineated. The volumes are defined in a treatment

Table 6.1. Tolerance doses to whole organ radiation

Whole organ	Single dose (Gy)	Fractionated dose (Gy)*
Bone, cartilage	>30	>70
Brain	15–25	60–70
Lens of the eye	2–10	6–12
Mucosa	5–20	65–77
Muscle	>30	>70
Peripheral nerve	15–20	65–77
Parotid gland	–	24–32
Skin	15–20	30–40
Spinal cord	15–20	50–60
Thyroid	–	30–40
Vasculoconnective tissue	10–20	50–60

* Assumes 2 Gy per day fractions
Modified from: Rubin, P. The Law and Order of Radiation Sensitivity, Absolute vs. Relative. In: Vaeth, JM, Meyer, JL, eds. Radiation Tolerance of Normal Tissues: Frontiers of Radiation Therapy and Oncology, Vol. 23. Basel: S. Karger 1989: 7–40; and Eisbruch, A, Kim, HM, Terell, JE, et al. Xerostomia and its Predictors Following Parotid-Sparing Irradiation of Head and Neck Cancer. Int J Radiat Oncol Biol Phys 2001; 50: 695–704

planning CT of the patient using immobilization devices in the appropriate position and all available clinical and imaging information. Appropriate doses and fractionation are then prescribed to the volumes of interest. For example, the CTV of a primary nodal area may require 60Gy in 6 weeks, while the desired parotid gland dose may be less than a mean of 26Gy to the defined parotid volume during the same 6 weeks. Normal tissue tolerances have been explored in depth and are listed in ▶ Table 6.1. While the greatest potential advantage for treating patients with head and neck cancers with IMRT may be in preventing xerostomia associated with parotid dysfunction, the radiation oncologist must be skilled in not exceeding the tolerances of other critical tissues.

The volume irradiated using IMRT techniques should be defined just as one would define it with conventional techniques, i.e., according to the site of the primary, the extent of nodal disease and anticipated nodal spread patterns. The notable difference is that with IMRT more normal tissue may receive lower doses of radiation. The nodal volumes must therefore be identified carefully on CT slices. In addition to these volumes, the *retropharyngeal nodes must also be considered for treatment*. Borders include the base of the skull (cranial border), the cranial edge of the body of the hyoid (caudal border), the levator veli palatini (anterior border), prevertebral muscles (posterior border), the medial edge of the internal carotid and jugular vessels (lateral border) and the midline, medially [23].

A major concern in patients treated by IMRT is that by abandoning the conventional "wide field" radiation techniques, disease control will be lowered because of geographic misses. Data available to date fail to demonstrate this. At the Mallinckrodt Institute of Radiology, 126 patients received IMRT as primary treatment post-operatively between 1997 and 2000. A variety of sites were included and received approximately 70 Gy in 35 fractions. They resulted primarily in field failures in both definitively treated and post-operative patients [24]. A similar experience was reported at the University of Michigan among 58 patients treated with a parotid-sparing protocol for multiple head and neck tumor subsites [25]. Recently, data from the University of California, San Francisco,

Table 6.2. Classification of neck nodes

Robbins classification	Definition	CT boundaries
I A (submental) and I B (submandibular)	Bounded by post. belly of digastric muscle, Hyoid bone inferiorly, Body of mandible superiorly	**Cranial:** Mylohyoid muscle **Caudal:** Hyoid bone **Anterior:** Symphysis menti **Posterior:** Posterior edge of submandibular gland **Lateral:** Medial edge of mandible **Medial:** Lateral edge of anterior belly of digastric muscle
II (upper internal jugular)	Upper internal jugular nodes from level of hyoid inferiorly to skull base superiorly	**Cranial:** Cranial base **Caudal:** Bottom edge of lateral process of C1 **Anterior:** Post. Margin of submandibular gland or internal jugular vein **Posterior:** Posterior edge of sternocleidomastoid muscle (SCM) **Lateral:** Medial edge of SCM **Medial:** Medial edge of internal carotid and jugular vessels, paraspinal muscle, deep cervical muscles
III (middle internal jugular)	Extends from hyoid superiorly to cricothyroid membrane inferiorly	**Cranial:** Bottom edge of hyoid **Caudal:** Inferior margin of cricoid **Anterior:** Posterolateral edge of sternohyoid **Poster, lateral and medial:** see level II above
IV (lower internal jugular)	Cricothyroid superiorly to clavicle inferiorl	**Cranial:** Inferior edge of cricoid **Caudal:** Cranial border of clavicle or 2 cm superior to sternoclavicular joint **Anterior:** Posterolateral edge of SCM **Posterior:** Anterior edge of paraspinal muscle **Lateral and medial:** see level II
V (spinal accessory)	Posterior triangle nodes bounded by anterior border of trapezius (posterior). Posterior border of sternocleidomastoid (anterior) and clavicle (inferior)	**Cranial:** Skull base **Caudal:** Cranial border of clavicle **Anterior:** Posterior border of SCM **Posterior:** Anterior border of trapezius **Lateral:** Platysma muscle and skin **Medial:** Paraspinal muscle

Adapted from Robbins, KT, Medina, JE, et al: Standardizing Neck Dissection Terminology. Arch Otolaryngol. Head Neck Surg. 117: 601–605, 1991; Chao, KSC, Wippold, FJ, et al: Determination and Delineation of Nodal Target Volumes for Head and Neck Cancer Based on the Patterns of Failure in Patients Receiving Definitive and Postoperative IMRT. Int J Radiat Oncol Biol Phys. 57: 1174–1184, 2002; and Levendag, PC, Braalsma, M, et al: Selective Irradiation of the Neck: Validation of CT-Based Neck Nodal Delineation Rotterdam/Brussels Consensus Guidelines. Int J Radiat Oncol Biol Phys 54 (Suppl.):16, 2002

Table 6.3. Location of failure of patients treated with IMRT

	In field	Out of field	Marginal
Mallinckrodt (24)	74%	13%	13%
Univ. of Michigan (25)	59%	29%	12%
UCSF (26)	100%	0%	0%

has been reported with local control rates of 100% and 98% at 2 and 3 years [26]. These studies are summarized in ▶ Table 6.3.

Clinical experience and results from using IMRT to treat various head and neck sites is rapidly accumulating in the scientific literature. The following sections will address IMRT results in varying subsites of the head and neck.

6.3.1 IMRT in Nasopharynx Cancer

Surgical resection with acceptable margins is often not achievable in nasopharynx cancer because of its location immediately adjacent to the base of skull. Radiation therapy has been the mainstay of treatment for nasopharynx cancers, but local failures occur 25–69% of the time for T1-T4 lesions [27]. Recently, however, the Intergroup trial 0099 demonstrated a significant improvement in survival for patients treated with a combination of cisplatin (100 mg/m²) given on days 1, 22 and 43 of radiotherapy (70 Gy in 35 fractions), followed on day 1 by three courses of cisplatin (80 mg/m²) and fluorouracil (1000 mg/m²/day on days 1–4, given every 4 weeks), compared with the same dose of radiotherapy alone [28]. Three-year progression-free survival was 69% vs. 24%, favoring the chemotherapy arm, and overall survival was better as well. Other studies have failed to demonstrate this significant difference. Nonetheless, this procedure has become the standard of care in the United States for all but the very earliest stage nasopharynx cancers.

Because of the extensive volume requiring high doses of radiation and the conventional inclusion of the majority of salivary tissue, nasopharynx cancers provide an ideal situation for IMRT. The highest dose regions should include all gross disease defined by CT, MRI and physical examination, as well as the adjacent soft tissue and nodal regions. Elective nodal regions also require relatively high doses of radiation (50–60 Gy in 6 weeks). If possible, IMRT can allow the radiation therapist to avoid a significant portion of the parotid tissue, as well as limit the radiation dose to the brainstem, optic nerves and chiasm and temporal lobes of the brain.

The potential advantages of treating nasopharynx cancer with IMRT are being explored at a number of institutions. Cheng and coworkers have demonstrated the ability to spare the parotid gland while maintaining adequate coverage of the nodal and tumor areas at risk in 17 patients with nasopharynx cancer [29]. This has also been demonstrated by Hunt and coworkers in a cohort of 23 patients with nasopharyngeal carcinoma [30]. The University of California, San Francisco, has reported what is likely the largest series of patients with primary nasopharyngeal carcinoma treated with IMRT [31, 32]. A total of 67 patients were treated using three different IMRT techniques. Seventy-five percent of these patients also received concomitant cisplatin chemotherapy. Doses and fractionation are listed in ▶ Table 6.4. The local and locoregional progression-free survival at 4 years was 97 and 98%, respectively, and overall survival was 88%. The study also noted that the severity of xerostomia decreased over the first 2 years following IMRT, with over 60% of patients having no xerostomia and fewer than 10% having grade-2 xerostomia at the 24-month follow-up.

Researchers at the Washington University have also presented their experience using IMRT to treat nasopharyngeal cancer [33]. Nine patients in a larger series were treated with IMRT plus chemotherapy according to Intergroup 0099 [28]. The entire series

Table 6.4. UCSF doses for IMRT of nasopharynx cancer [26]

	Total dose	Daily fraction
Gross tumor and positive lymph nodes:	65–70 Gy	2.12–2.25 Gy
CTV (including adjacent spread areas):	60 Gy	1.8 Gy
Prophylactically treated lymph nodes:	50–60 Gy	1.8–2 Gy

also included 13 patients treated with conventional radiotherapy plus the same chemotherapy and 103 patients treated with conventional radiotherapy alone. Three-year progression-free survival was 90 % in the chemoradiotherapy group and 69 % in the radiation-alone therapy group. The patients receiving IMRT had significantly less moderate to severe xerostomia (defined as RTOG grade 2 or less).

6.3.2 IMRT of Oropharynx Cancer

The oropharynx contains a number of sites which commonly develop malignancy. These include the tonsillar fossa, faucial arch, soft palate and the base of the tongue. The lymphatic drainage of the oropharynx includes the subdigastric, upper cervical lymph nodes and parapharyngeal lymph nodes. Tonsillar fossa and base of tongue cancers have a high incidence of nodal metastases (60–70 %) at presentation. Early stage tumors in these locations may be treated with either surgery or radiation. More advanced lesions require post-operative radiation or treatment with concomitant chemoradiotherapy, which has been shown to achieve superior control compared with radiotherapy alone or induction chemotherapy followed by radiation [34, 35, 36]. One must remember, however, that morbidity is also increased using a chemoradiotherapy approach, and that this treatment must be used somewhat selectively.

A common long term effect of radiation in oropharyngeal cancer is the risk of xerostomia (as high as 75 %), as well as trismus (from radiation of the muscles of mastication). Theoretically, a significant portion of the contralateral parotid and even some of the ipsilateral parotid can be spared using IMRT. Chao and Ozygit reported the initial results of

IMRT in 42 cases of tonsillar fossa cancer treated at Washington University [37]. A variety of stages were represented and at brief follow-up (median 23 months), only five locoregional failures were observed (2 were salvaged with surgery). Chao and Ozygit reported no grade 3 or 4 late toxicity. Only five patients developed grade 2 xerostomia, and 16 patients had grade 1 long-term xerostomia. One patient developed trismus and another patient developed chronic serous otitis media.

Washington University has also reported its results in treating 15 patients with base of tongue carcinoma using IMRT [38]. Eight were treated definitively and seven postoperatively. With a median follow up of 22 months, there were two locoregional recurrences. Only 25 % developed moderate to severe xerostomia (RTOG grade 2 or higher), in contrast to their conventionally treated patients, of whom 75 % experience xerostomia. The authors observed no grade 3 or 4 late complications in their IMRT group.

Claus and coworkers in Ghent, Belgium, have reported on the feasibility of IMRT for oropharynx and oral cavity primaries [39]. They treated six patients with primary non-recurrent oral cavity and oropharynx carcinomas to test the practicability of IMRT in this group. They concluded that IMRT was feasible and well tolerated. Xerostomia was subjectively decreased and four of the six patients remained tumor-free after 5 months at follow-up. The same authors have reported on their experience retreating previously treated head and neck cancers. Although reirradiation was feasible, and normal critical tissue sparing could be accomplished, six of the eight patients treated relapsed within 4 months of the completion of IMRT.

6.3.3 IMRT of Paranasal Sinus Cancers

A number of authors have been intrigued by the potential of IMRT for treating a particularly challenging area of the head and neck, including the ethmoid and paranasal sinuses, the maxillary sinuses and, in general, the area surrounding the orbits and adjacent to the optic nerves, chiasm and optic pathways. Certainly, vision loss is one of the most devastating potential complications of radiation in this area, and most patients diagnosed with cancer here will need radiation as part of their treatment regimen.

Tsien, Eisbruch and coworkers, at the University of Michigan, replanned the treatment of 13 patients who had already been treated for locally advanced paranasal sinus tumors [40]. They examined multiple scenarios, including sparing only the contralateral optic pathway or attempting to spare both optic pathways. They concluded that IMRT offered significant advantages over conventional radiotherapy treatment from a dosimetry perspective, but that tradeoffs between dose (and therefore toxicity) to optic pathways and dose to the desired treatment volume may need to be made. They demonstrated better tumor coverage if only the contralateral optic pathway were spared, but emphasized that each clinical situation must be evaluated individually.

A report from the Royal Marsden Clinic also compared conventional three-dimensional radiotherapy plans with IMRT plans for six previously treated maxillary sinus patients [41]. They found significant advantages with IMRT using a 7-segment technique, which allowed them to spare the optic pathways and optimize dose to the tumor. They, too, found this to be a feasible treatment course in a busy radiotherapy clinic. Huang et al. have also implemented this technique with apparent sparing of critical normal structures in paranasal sinus tumors [42].

Preliminary reports of the treatment of ethmoid sinus cancers with IMRT show the capability of sparing the optic pathways. Specifically, Claus et al. described the treatment of 11 patients suffering from primary ethmoid sinus cancers with IMRT. Although their experience demonstrates the capability of sparing the optic pathways, the follow-up (as noted by the authors) was too short to allow a determination of clinical results [43]. Likewise, Lee, et al. planned the treatment of 10 patients suffering from ethmoid sinus cancers using IMRT and felt that the dose distribution and homogeneity was better with IMRT, compared with conventional 3D techniques [44]. Claus et al. also postulated that IMRT might help avoid dry eye syndrome after the treatment for sinonasal tumors. In all, they treated 32 patients using IMRT techniques [45]. Their median follow up was 15 months, and they noted minimal acute toxicity. They had no incidences of grade 3 or 4 dry eye syndrome or conjunctivitis. Zabel and coworkers in Heidelberg, Germany, planned the treatment for 13 patients with esthesioneuroblastoma using both 3D and IMRT techniques [46]. They noted that IMRT allows for more conformality in the treatment and postulated that the risk of complications could be minimized, and local control maximized, using IMRT.

6.3.4 IMRT in Other Situations

Intensity modulated radiotherapy has potential advantages at many other sites as well as those previously described. Munter and coworkers report a 92% 2-year survival, 93% local control and very little xerostomia in a population of 48 patients with a variety of head and neck primary tumor sites [47]. Nutting et al. performed a planning study of patients treated with external beam radiation for advanced thyroid cancers and noted the ability to decrease the spinal cord dose when using IMRT techniques, in contrast to three-dimensional treatment techniques [48]. There are also reports of the reirradiation of head and neck cancers using IMRT [39, 49]. Results of these studies are promising and show an ability to reirradiate without excessive normal tissue damage.
▶ Figure 6.1a–d shows an IMRT plan and dose distribution for a patient undergoing post-operative irradiation for a right-sided oral tongue cancer.

IMRT is likely the most profound advancement in radiation treatment over the past 20 years. Clinical data are accumulating rapidly, and there is great promise that the techniques involved will make radiation treatment of the head and neck region less morbid. In addition, clinicians may be able to escalate tu-

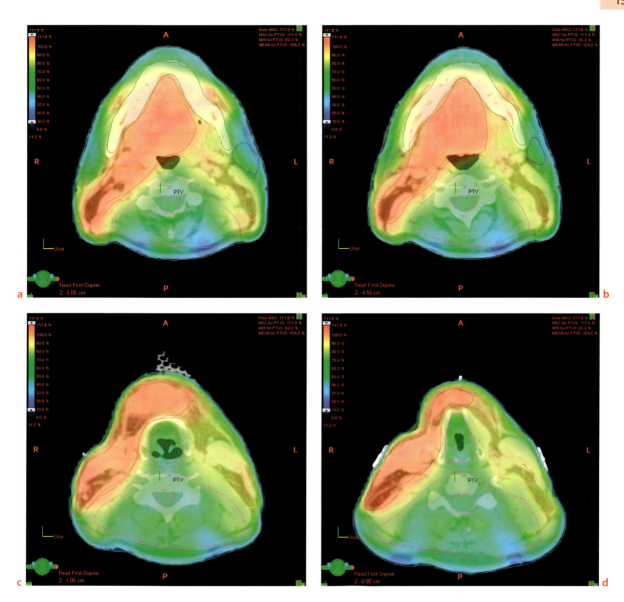

Figure 6.1 a–d

A 42-year-old man underwent resection and right neck dissection for a pathologically staged T1N0 oral tongue cancer. Five months later he developed a right submandibular mass which was resected and found to be metastatic disease in 2 submandibular lymph nodes. He was treated post-operatively to a dose of 60 Gy in 25 fractions to the right oral tongue and neck using a 6 field IMRT plan (outlined in *red*). The left neck received 50 Gy in the same time frame (outlined in *yellow*) with hopes of sparing dose to both parotids (*pink* outline on the *right* and *dark blue* on the *left*). A very steep dose gradient was achieved in (**a**) and (**b**) with sparing of the parotids and spinal cord. Lower in the neck one can see the continued highest dose to the right neck with slightly lower dose to the left neck and sparing of the spinal cord and larynx (**c**) and (**d**)

mor doses and, hopefully, increase control rates. One must be cautious, however, not to become cavalier in the use of IMRT. Extreme care must be taken in appropriately defining the anatomical regions requiring treatment and in not sparing normal tissue at the expense of undertreating cancer. The worst complication from cancer treatment is tumor recurrence.

The evolution of IMRT treatment in head and neck cancer will undoubtedly lead to a number of clinical research areas requiring exploration. One of these areas may include the question of whether one needs to treat all tissue "en bloc" in order to kill "in-transit metastases." Clearly, more conventional radiotherapy techniques treat wide fields and tend to include the tissues between the primary site and the nodal metastases. IMRT treatment may lead to shielding the primary site while treating the nodes, especially if the primary site is close to critical structures. Along with an anticipated decrease in radiation-induced toxicity, a comparison of elective neck IMRT, versus staging neck dissection, in N0 patients may be extremely valuable in the assessment of tumor control.

6.4 Future Potential Applications

IMRT has been well described for its application in primary sites of head and neck squamous cell cancers and the associated lymphatic drainage pathways. Radiation distribution delivered to primary sites and to surrounding tissues is beautifully illustrated in the figures that follow this chapter. "Radiation distribution delivered to primary sites and to surrounding tissues can be beautifully illustrated as was shown in the previous illustration."

From a surgical prospective, IMRT has the potential to make radiation "almost surgical," in that radiation can be delivered more precisely to targeted areas. The current thinking is focused on avoiding morbidity, especially from damage to vital organs such as the spinal cord, eyes and salivary tissues, where xerostomia continues to be the most significant patient morbidity. New ideas, such as the concept of ipsilateral neck irradiation for cancers typically treated bilaterally in lymph node drainage

areas, or the concept of delivering radiation only to regional lymph nodes when the primary cancer is well treated by surgery alone, have not yet really been addressed. The biggest concern for most radiation therapists in this regard will be the probability of field "misses," which will need to be addressed. A potential future benefit might be better field matching in cases of re-irradiation. Additionally, re-irradiation itself is currently gaining acceptance due to positive preliminary results, which will certainly be expanded upon in the by future uses of IMRT.

The concept of IMRT as "almost surgical" is perhaps best illustrated by revisiting statistics on the frequency of regional neck metastases, as previously described in this book, and then clarifying this concept through examples of potential uses.

Most current statistics on the probability of regional metastatic spread in head and neck cancer are based on studies done in large part prior to current imaging techniques; they include CT and MRI, but took place before the use of PET and before sentinel node studies. These statistics give good general baselines for the contemplation of therapy but their true reliability is still questionable.

Generally, when the historical data suggest that the probability of regional metastasis is greater than 20%, the potentially involved lymphatic drainage pathways are treated either by surgery or by irradiation. This certainly is a reasonable approach, but there are a number of examples where patients probably are overtreated.

As has already been mentioned in this book, most patients with infrahyoid supraglottic cancer, even when this condition is lateralized, are treated either surgically or radiotherapeutically on both sides of the neck. As also mentioned, De Santo and co-workers showed that if the ipsilateral neck when dissected was found to be pathologically free from metastatic cancer, the probability of contralateral neck spread was less than 2%. If these statistics are actually true, then many patients have unnecessary treatment to the contralateral N0 neck. It is at a minimum likely that this same principle could apply to the irradiation of both sides of the neck in a number of other lateralized head and neck primary cancers with bilateral clinical and radiological N0 necks.

One example relates to clinical T1N0 or T2N0 lateral mobile tongue cancer. Often when the primary site is treated by surgery, ipsilateral levels I, II and III (with or without level IV) neck dissection is done. If the primary site does not have threatening histological findings, and if the neck dissection specimen is pathologically N0, no further treatment is given. Conversely, if a patient has only the primary site treated by surgery, then almost always both sides of the neck are irradiated (including the primary site). The rationale for this approach is that, in the absence of confirming histological data, it is not really clear whether the contralateral neck has cancer or not. In this case, we do not have good data concerning the probability of contralateral neck cancer when the ipsilateral neck is also N0 by modern imaging techniques. Certainly, some necks may be pathologically positive even when clinically and radiologically N0. But the actual frequency of this is not very high. Again, it is clearly not known what the probability of contralateral spread is in this regard. If IMRT were used to treat the primary, and then used almost as a surgical modality to treat the ipsilateral neck, the contralateral neck could be spared irradiation. Opponents of such a philosophy point out that if cancer later develops in the untreated neck then survival may well be decreased, which is a reasonable objection. It is certainly not possible to make a dogmatic statement that anyone knows what the real probability of contralateral spread is in this setting. A prospective multi-institutional study might be able to address this.

Another example where IMRT may have a role relates to T1N0, or even T2N0 midline, floor-of-mouth cancer. If the primary site were treated by surgery, or even by irradiation, lymph node levels I, II and III on both sides could be treated using IMRT. These are the same areas bilateral selective neck dissection would also treat.

Another example relates to T2N0 oropharyngeal cancer. If the primary site were treated by surgery and a level I-IV neck dissection were done without finding any metastatic spread, then, potentially, the retropharyngeal area, probably including the primary site, could be treated by irradiation alone. The con-

tralateral neck in this situation very likely could be spared.

Consider the example of a T2N2b supraglottic carcinoma originating in the area of the aryepiglottic folds. From the De Santo data, it is clear that both sides of the neck need to be treated. Because the ipsilateral neck cancer is advanced (N2b), most patients with this diagnosis would receive supraglottic laryngectomy with ipsilateral or bilateral neck dissection and postoperative irradiation to both sides of the neck and probably to the primary site as well. It certainly seems well justified to treat both sides of the neck (ipsilateral by surgery in addition to irradiation, and the contralateral neck by at least one modality), but there is really no data showing that the primary site must also be treated. It is certainly well known that when open supraglottic laryngectomy is performed, coupled with postoperative irradiation, patients struggle enormously with postoperative swallowing problems. When the primary site, together with both sides of the neck, is treated primarily by irradiation, patients additionally struggle with issues of glottic competence or even potential glottic obstruction. IMRT could be used in a circumstance like this to treat the neck unilaterally or bilaterally as needed, while avoiding irradiation to the primary site with its attendant morbidity.

A final example relates to unknown primary site cancers metastatic to the neck. Irradiation to all potential head and neck primary sites, including the nasopharynx through the piriform sinuses, and bilateral neck irradiation is remarkably morbid. Already a number of institutions do not treat to this full extent, but instead tailor irradiation to the neck affected by cancer and some of the potential primary sites, often excluding the piriform sinus. The use of IMRT would be more precise in tailoring such a therapy.

There are many similar examples. The question is whether head and neck surgeons and radiation therapists will address this area. The addition of IMRT to the treatment options for head and neck cancer patients brings a new perspective to these considerations. Hopefully, future prospective, randomized, multi-institutional studies can be done to thoughtfully address this issue. It seems only reasonable that therapy should not be purely "traditional," but rather appropriately selective as determined by emerging concepts backed by studies addressing the relevant issues.

References

1. Mendenhall WM, Million RR (1986) Elective Neck Irradiation for Squamous Cell Carcinoma of the Head and Neck: Analysis of Time Dose Factors and Causes of Failure. Int J Radiat Oncol Biol Phys 12:741–746

2. Robbins KT, Medina JE, Wolfe GT, Levine PA, Sessions RB, Pruet CW (1991) Standardizing Neck Dissection Terminology. Arch. Otolaryngol Head Neck Surg 117:601–605

3. Shah JT, Cendon RA, Farr HW, Strong EW (1976) Carcinoma of the Oral Cavity: Factors Affecting Treatment at the Primary Site and Neck. Am J Surg 132:504–507

4. Amdur RJ, Parsons JT, Mendenhall WM, Million RR, Stringer SP, Cassissi NJ (1989) Postoperative Irradiation for Squamous Cell Carcinoma of the Head and Neck: An Analysis of Treatment Results and Complications. Int J Radiat Oncol Biol Phys 16:25–36

5. Johnson JT, Barnes EC, Myers EW, Schramm VL, Borochovitz D, Sigler BA (1981) The Extracapsular Spread of Tumors in Cervical Node Metastases. Arch Otolaryngol 107:725–729

6. Peters LJ, Goepfert H, Ang KK, Byers RM, Maor MH, Guillamondegui O, Morrison WH, Weber RS, Garden HS, Frankenthaler RA, Oswald MJ, Brown BW (1993) Evaluation of the Dose for Postoperative Radiation Therapy of Head and Neck Cancer: First Report of a Prospective Randomized Trial. Int J Radiat Oncol Biol Phys 26:3–11

7. Looser KG, Shah JP, Strong EN (1979) The Significance of Positive Margins in Marginally Resected Epidermoid Carcinoma. Head Neck Surg 1:107–111

8. Carter RL, Tanner HS, Clifford P, Shaw HJ (1979) Perineural Spread in Squamous Cell Carcinoma of the Head and Neck: A Clinico-pathologic Study. Clin Otolaryngol 4:271–281

9. Farr HW, Arthur K (1972) Epidermoid Carcinoma of the Mouth and Pharynx. J. Laryngol. Otol 86:243–253

10. Marcus RB Jr, Million RR, Cassissi NJ (1979) Postoperative Irradiation for Squamous Cell Carcinoma of the Head and Neck: Analysis of Time-dose Factors Related to Control Above the Clavicles. Int J Radiat Oncol Biol Phys 5:1943–1949

11. Mendenhall WM, Million RR, Bova FJ (1984) Analysis of Time-dose Factors in Clinically Positive Neck Nodes Treated with Irradiation Alone in Squamous Cell Carcinoma of the Head and Neck. Int J Radiat Oncol Biol Phys 10:639–643

12. Cooper JS, Scott CB, Laramore GE, et al (1993) Sequential Adjuvant Chemotherapy for Advanced Head and Neck Cancer. Johnson JT and Didolker, MS eds. Head and Neck Cancer, Volume III. Elsevier Science Publishers

13. Cooper JS, Pajak TF, Forastiere AA, Jacobs J, Saxman SB, Kish JA, Kim HE, Cmelak AJ, Rotman M, Machtay M, Ensley JF, Chao KC, Schultz CJ, Lee N, Fu KK (2002) Patterns of Failure for Resected Advanced Head and Neck Cancer Treated by Concurrent Chemotherapy and Radiation Therapy: An Analysis of RTOG 95–01/Intergroup Phase III Trial. Int J Radiat Oncol Biol Phys 54:2

14. Bernier J, Domenge C, Eschwege F, Ozsahin M, Matuszewska K, Moncho V, Greiner RH, Giralt J, Kirkpatrick A, van Glabbeke M (2001) Chemo-Radiotherapy, as Compared to Radiotherapy Alone, Significantly Increases Disease-Free and Overall Survival in Head and Neck Cancer Patients After Surgery: Results of EORTC Phase III Trial 22931. Int J Radiat Oncol Biol Phys 51 (Suppl.):1

15. Gregoire V, Coche V, Cosnard G, Hamoir M, Reychler H (2000) Selection and Deliniation of Lymph Node Target Volumes in Head and Neck Conformal Radiotherapy. Proposal for Standardizing Terminology and Procedure Based on the Surgical Experience. Radiother Oncol 56:135–150

16. Nowak PJCM, Wijers OB, Langerweard FJ, Levendag PC (1999) A Three-Dimesional CT-Based Definition fro Elective Irradiation of the Neck. Int J Radiat Oncol Biol Phys 45:33–39

17. Eisbruch A, Foote RL, O'Sullivan B, Beitler JJ, Vikram B (2002) Intensity-Modulated Radiation Therapy for Head and Neck Cancer: Emphasis on the Selection and Delineation of the Targets. Seminars in Radiat Oncol 12:238–249

18. Verhey LJ (2002) Issues in Optimization for Planning of Intensity-Modulated Radiation Therapy. Seminars in Radiat Oncol 12:210–218

19. Low DA (2003) Physics of Intensity-Modulated Radiation Therapy for Head and Neck Cancer. In: Chao KS, Ozyigit G, eds. Intensity Modulated Radiation for Head & Neck Cancer. Philadelphia: Lippincott Williams & Wilkins. 1–17

20. Gilbeau L, Octave-Prignot M, Loncol T, Renard L, Scalliet P, Gregoire V (2001) Comparison of Setup Accuracy of Three Different Thermoplastic Masks for the Treatment of Brain and Head and Neck Tumors. Radiother Oncol 58:155–162

21. ICRU Report 50: Prescribing, Recording and Reporting Photon Beam Therapy. Bethesda, MD: International Commission on Radiation Units and Measurements, 1–72, 1993.

22. ICRU Report 62: Prescribing, Recording and Reporting Photon Beam Therapy (Supplement to ICRU Report 50). Bethesda, MD: International Commission on Radiation Units and Measurements, 1–52, 1999.

23. Chao KSC, Wippold FJ, Ozyigit G, Tran BN, Dempsey JF (2002) Determination and Delineation of Nodal Target Volumes for Head and Neck Cancer Based on the Patterns of Failure in Patients Receiving Definitive and Postoperative IMRT. Int J Radiat Oncol Biol Phys 57:1174–1184

24. Chao KS, Low DA, Perez CA, Purdy JA (2000) Intensity-Modulated Radiation Therapy in Head and Neck Cancers: The Mallinkrodt Experience. Int J Cancer 90:92–103

25. Dawson LA, Anzai Y, Marsh L, Martel MK, Paulino A, Ship JA, Eisbruch A (2000) Patterns of Local-regional Recurrence Following Parotid Sparing Conformal and Segmental Intensity-Modulated Radiotherapy for Head and Neck Cancer. Int J Radiat Oncol Biol Phys 46:117–126

26. Lee N, Xia P, Fischbein P, Akazuma P, Akazuma C, Quivey JM (2002) Target Volume Delineation in Intensity-Modulated Radiation Therapy (IMRT) for Head and Neck Cancer and Correlation with Patterns of Failure. Int J Radiat Oncol Biol Phys. 54 (Suppl.):17

27. Chao KS, Ozyigit G (2003) Nasopharynx In: Chao, KS, Ozyigit, G, eds. Intensity Modulated Radiation Therapy for Head & Neck Cancer. Philadelphia: Lippincott Williams & Wilkins. 68–84

28. Al-Sarraf M, LeBlanc M, Giri PG, Fu KK, Cooper J, Vuong T, Forestiere AA, Adams G, Sakr WA, Schuller DE, Ensley JF (1998) Chemoradiotherapy Versus Radiotherapy in Patients With Advanced Nasopharyngeal Cancer: Phase III Randomized Intergroup Study 0099. J Clin Oncol 16:1310–1317

29. Cheng JCH, Chao KSC, Low D (2001) Comparison of IMRT Techniques for Nasopharyngeal Carcinoma. Int J Cancer 96:126–132

30. Hunt MA, Zelefsky MJ, Wolden S, Wolden S, Chui CS, LoSasso T, Rosenzweig K, Chong L, Spirou SV, Fromme L, Lumley M, Amols HA, Ling CC, Leibel SA (2001) Treatment Planning and Delivery for Primary Nasopharynx Cancer. Int J Radiat Oncol Biol Phys 49:623–632

31. Sultanen K, Shu HK, Xia P Akazawa C, Quivey JM, Vohey LJ, Fu KK (2000) Three-dimensional Intensity-modulated Radiotherapy in the Treatment of Nasopharyngeal Carcinoma: The University of California-San Francisco Experience. Int J Radiat Oncol Biol Phys 48:711–722

32. Lee N, Xia P, Fishbein NJ, Akazawa P, Akazawa C, Quivey JMl (2001) Intensity-modulated Radiotherapy in the Treatment of Nasopharyngeal Carcinoma: An Update of the UCSF Experience. Int J Radiat Oncol Biol Phys 53:12–22

33. Chao KSC, Cejnic M, Perez CA, et al. Superior Functional Outcome with IMRT in Locally Advanced Nasopharyngeal Carcinoma. Proc Am Soc Clin Oncol 924

34. Calais G, Alfonsi M, Bardet E, Sire C, Germain T, Bergerot P, Rhein B, Tortochaux J, Oudinot P, Bertrand P (1999) Randomized Trial of Radiation Therapy Versus Concomitant Chemotherapy and Radiation Therapy for Advanced-Stage Oropharynx Carcinoma. J Natl Cancer Inst 91:2081–2086

35. Brizel DM, Albers ME, Fisher SR, Scher RL, Richtsmeier WJ, Hars V, George SL, Huang AT, Prosnitz LR (1998) Hyperfractionated Irradiation With or Without Concurrent Chemotherapy for Locally Advanced Head and Neck Cancer. N Eng J Med 338:1788–1804

36. Wendt TG, Grabenbauer GG, Rodel CM, Thiel HJ, Aydin H, Rohloff R, Wustrow TP, Iro H, Popella C, Schalhorn A (1998) Simultaneous Radiochemotherapy Versus Radiotherapy Alone in Advanced Head and Neck Cancer: A Randomized Multicenter Study. J Clin Oncol 16:1318–1324

37. Chao KSC, Ozyigit G (2003) Tonsillar Fossa and Faucial Arch In: Chao KS and Ozyigit G eds. Intensity Modulated Radiation Therapy for Head & Neck Cancer. Philadelphia: Lippincott Williams & Wilkins. 100–113

38. Chao KSC (2003) Int J Radiat Oncol Biol Phys, in press

39. Claus F, Duthoy W, Boterberg T, De Gersem W, Huys J, Vermeersch H, De Neve W (2002) Intensity Modulated Radiation Therapy for Oropharyngeal and Oral Cavity Tumors: Clinical Use and Experience. Oral Oncol 38:597–604

40. Tsien C, Eisbruch A, McShan D, Kessler M, Marsch R, Frass B (2003) Intensity-modulated Radiation Therapy (IMRT) for Locally Advanced Paranasal Sinus Tumors: Incorporating Clinical Decisions in the Optimization Process. Int J Radiat Oncol Biol Phys 55:776–784

41. Adams EJ, Nutting CM, Convery DJ, Henk JM, Dearnaley DP, Webb S (2001) Potential Role of Intensity-modulated Radiotherapy in the Treatment of Tumors of the Maxillary Sinus. Int J Radiat Oncol Biol Phys 51:579–588

42. Huang D, Xia P, Akazawa P, Akazawa C, Quivey JM, Verhey LJ, Kaplan M, Lee N (2003) Comparison of Treatment Plans Using Intensity-mosulated Radiotherapy and Three-dimensional Conformal Radiotherapy for Paranasal Sinus Carcinoma. Int J Radiat Oncol Biol Phys 56:158–168

43. Claus F, De Gersem W, De Wagter C, Van Severen R, Vanhoutte I, Duthoy W, Remouchamps V, Van Duyse B, Vakaet L, Lemmerling M, Vermeersch H, De Neve W (2001) An Implementation Strategy for IMRT of Ethmoid Sinus Cancer With Bilateral Sparing of the Optic Pathways. Int J Radiat Oncol Biol Phys 51:318–331

44. Lee SW, Kim GE, Suh CO, Chu SS, Lee KK, Moon SR (2002) Intensity Modulation Technique Using the Complementary Boost-fields for Ethmoid Sinus Cancer. Clin Oncol 14:241–249

45. Claus F, Boterberg T, Ost P, De Neve W (2002) Short Term Toxicity profile for 32 Sinonasal Cancer Patients Treated with IMRT. Can we avoid dry eye syndrome? Radiother Oncol. 64:205–208

46. Zabel A, Thilmann C, Thilmann C, Zuna I, Schlegel W, Wannenmacher M, Debus J (2002) Comparison of Forward Planned Conformal Radiation Therapy and Inverse Planned Intensity Modulated Radiation Therapy for Esthesioneuroblastoma. Br J Radiol 75:356–361

47. Munter MW, Thilmann C, Hof H, Didinger B, Rhein B, Nill S, Schlegel W, Wannenmacher M, Debus J (2003) Stereotactic Intensity Modulated Radiation Therapy and Inverse Treatment Planning for Tumors of the Head and Neck Region: Clinical Implementation of the Step and Shoot Approach and First Clinical Results. Radiother Oncol 66: 313–321

48. Nutting CM, Convery DJ, Cosgrove VP, Rowbottom C, Vini L, Harmer C, Dearnaley DP, Webb S (2001) Improvements in Target Coverage and Reduced Spinal Cord Irradiation Using Intensity-modulated Radiotherapy (IMRT) in Patients with Carcinoma of the Thyroid Gland. Radiother Oncol 60: 173–80

49. Chen YJ, Kuo JV, Ramsinghani NS, Al-Ghazi MS (2002) Intensity-Modulated Radiotherapy for Previously Irradiated, Recurrent Head-and-neck Cancer. Med Dosim 27:171–176

50. Richard JM, Sancho-Garnier H, Micheau C, Saravane D, Cachin Y (1987) Prognostic Factors in Cervical Lymph Node Metastases in Upper Respiratory and Digestive Tract Carcinomas: Study of 1713 Cases in a 15-year Period. Laryngoscope 97:97–101

Surgical Treatment Concepts

7.1 The Role of Neck Dissection in the Treatment of Squamous Cell Carcinomas of the Upper Aerodigestive Tract

In this chapter, currently applied surgical treatment concepts for the lymphatic drainage of malignant head and neck tumors will be discussed. The numerous reports in the literature on this topic indicate a great deal of controversy regarding appropriate strategies. This problem can also be explained by the numerous more or less accepted varieties of neck dissection that have been augmented by additional limited selective neck dissection types (e.g., isolated dissection of levels II and III in cases of pharyngeal carcinoma with No or even with N+ neck). This broad treatment spectrum makes it very difficult at present to elaborate a generally accepted therapeutic concept for the management of the lymphatic drainage in cases of head and neck malignancies. Our purpose is to report on generally accepted treatment concepts or surgical therapies for the No neck, the N+ neck and lymph node metastases in cases of unknown primary cancer. We will use this information as a basis for discussion of the newer types of limited neck dissection.

Objective of Neck Dissection. Before holding a discussion about possible treatment concepts in cases of the No neck, two distinct objectives of ND must be mentioned.

- First, ND can be performed as an *operative staging procedure*. This concept, which often includes selective ND types, is applied if postoperative radiotherapy is planned in the event that lymphogenic metastatic spread is detected. On occasion, the subsequent dissection of cervical lymph node regions that had not been resected during the primary intervention is performed.

- Second, ND can be performed with *curative intention*. In this case, generally MRND is performed as a definitive treatment of the cervical lymphatic drainage. Currently, more and more communications are being published which suggest that selective ND types are appropriate for this purpose.

The following reflections on the indication, spectrum and the type of ND must consider which of these two intentions are to be pursued. Prior to discussing the importance of the individual ND types, however, considerations on the treatment of the No neck and on the indication for elective ND must be made.

7.1.1 Clinical N0 Neck

From the current point of view, the term *clinical No neck* means the palpatory and sonographic absence (or, the absence as determined by other forms of imaging such as CT or MRI) of cervical lymph nodes in the cervico-facial region. Such a situation, however, must not belie the fact that in about 30 % of the cases, cervical lymph node metastases nonetheless exist, a situation that is also called subclinical or occult metastases. The probability of occult metastases is related to a number of factors and increases in cases of deep tumor infiltration or lymphangitic carcinomatosis.

Elective treatment of subclinical lymph node spread can be performed surgically or radiotherapeutically. Due to the fact that the treatment results of elective radiotherapy seem to be comparable to elective ND [1, 2], the decision for the treatment of the cervical lymphatic drainage should be related to the therapy of the primary tumor. The recurrence rate, i. e., late metastases after prior elective radiotherapy, amounts to less than 5 % in the literature. However, such a rate must be considered cautiously, given that no data concerning the location or the extent of the primary cancer is mentioned. Opponents of primary radiotherapy indicate, among other things, a possible systemic effect on the immune system from irradia-

tion. Furthermore, fibrosis to some degree can be observed after radiotherapy, and this can also reduce the ability to assess recurrent metastases. Another argument against elective radiotherapy that must be mentioned is the significantly limited possibility of treating potential secondary carcinomas that develop metachronously in 10–40 % of the patients [3]. All the questions surrounding radiotherapy will not be discussed in view of the fact that controversies concerning the benefit of surgery for the No neck are already enormous, and additional discussion would only serve to dilute the significance of radiotherapy. Additionally, there is the problem that therapeutic success or failure is much more clear after surgery, as the actual lymph node status is known with the pathological evaluation of the resected specimen, whereas the assessment of success with radiotherapy depends on the reliability of the clinical and imaging diagnosis to detect metastasis, or on the assumption of statistical probabilities for cancer spread in the No neck.

At the heart of the discussion concerning the significance of elective ND in cases of the clinical No neck is the question of the presence or absence of occult lymph node metastases. The suspected incidence is from 12 % to over 50 %, with a mean of 33 % [4, 5], and it depends largely on the location of the primary tumor. For this reason, elective ND is considered superior by numerous authors in the event that the probability of occult lymph node metastases is 20 % or more. In our opinion, this often cited percentage must be questioned because it originates from findings that were based at the time on palpation alone without current imaging advances.

Our understanding of the process of invasion and metastases has improved, but our ability to detect occult metastatic disease or metastatic potential prior to the development of occult disease still lags behind. This underscores the importance of understanding the molecular metastatic process and using that understanding to develop marker panels with which to predict the presence and location of active metastatic disease and occult metastases. Even though a great deal of work has been done to discover prognostic markers of nodal metastases in head and neck cancer, much progress still needs to be made [6]. The determination of the metastatic probability, i. e., of individual risk, is related to several factors. In addition, there are numerous histological and molecular-biological factors that can be examined in view of their influence on the lymphogenic metastatic process. It has been shown that the infiltration depth of the tumor seems to correlate with metastatic frequency. There are numerous other risk factors that have been examined, however, in mostly small, inhomogeneous, patient populations. Thus, it is currently difficult to recommend well-defined histological or molecular guidelines for routine clinical use. Nevertheless, there seems to be a clear relationship between the density of the lymph vessels [7] and, in particular, the lymph collectors in the area of the primary tumor, as this relates to the extent of the resulting lymphogenic metastatic spread [8].

As already mentioned, the treatment of clinically or radiologically present cervical lymph node metastases is much less controversial than the treatment of the No neck or the clinically negative contralateral neck. In the following paragraphs, we will present our concept for operative intervention in a clinical and radiological No neck.

If the primary tumor is approached transcervically and resected, there are no convincing arguments against resecting regional lymph node stations that are included in the surgical approach (e.g., SND for oral cavity cancer), as the morbidity is low. Conversely, adjacent lymphatic stations are not resected with T1 or T2 true vocal cord cancers approached by open techniques. In rare instances of advanced T2 carcinomas of the vocal cords that are poorly differentiated, selective neck resection could be considered as part of an open approach. The experience of the surgeon with significant input from the patient is needed in this unusual situation.

Another primary location that is controversial in the literature concerns the necessity of lymph node dissection in cases of carcinoma of the lower lip with limited extent. The lymphogenic metastatic frequency of T1 carcinoma of the lower lip amounts to about 4–15 %. Given this low risk of occult metastatic spread in a clinical No neck, a wait-and-see strategy is favored after resection of the primary cancer. In cases of T2 carcinoma of the lower lip, the metastatic probability increases to 16–35 %, which would deem an

elective cervical lymph node dissection appropriate (SND with levels I–III). The inclusion of level III is controversial. The dissection of levels I and IIa, however, with extirpation of the submandibular gland(s), is less so.

With the exclusion of early glottic or lip cancer, all locations of primary cancer in the area of the upper aerodigestive tract can justify SND if the primary cancer is treated surgically. The extent of SND is based on tumor location, taking into account whether the carcinoma is situated unilaterally or reaches (or even crosses) the midline. The extent of SND depends largely on the location of the primary tumor.

In order to evaluate the most reasonable strategy in the suspected No neck, the question of rising costs must be considered. In this regard, it should be remembered that histological examination of the resected ND specimen leads to a higher degree of certainty for the assessment of the probable metastatic status than clinical examination or imaging alone; hence, a combined approach serves as a better guideline for the indication of postoperative radiotherapy. Also in this context, the high rate of occult metastases in the case of an No neck in carcinomas of the upper aerodigestive tract (up to 30 % in some locations) must be included in the discussion.

Given that there are only a few critical studies that are prospective and randomized for the surgery of the No neck, we can only present a more or less subjective strategy that is based on the literature and on our own experience. When considering possible elective ND, several considerations must be taken into account, including the operative therapy of the primary cancer, the estimated probability of already beginning but occult lymphogenic metastatic spread and, finally, the role of the surgeon if a wait-and-see strategy is an option [9].

The results presented recently at the *International Symposium on Metastases in Head and Neck Cancer* by Snow and associates [10] revealed clearly that a reasonable wait-and-see strategy could be performed in the follow-up of previous transoral tumor resection, at least in cases of carcinoma of the oral cavity. Their results, which are supported by an publication from Kaneko et al. [11], also pointed out that late metastases cannot be excluded, that the physician performing the pre- and postoperative sonography must be extraordinarily well trained and, furthermore, that the level of compliance on the part of the patient must be very high. If the treating physician has any doubts regarding these last mentioned points – compliance of the patient or experience of the sonographer – the question must be asked whether a staging surgical treatment should be performed in the first place. This is especially true for American physicians or any physician without a high degree of experience with ultrasonography. Identification of occult cervical lymph node metastases is critical in the decision regarding further treatment measures (esp. radiotherapy), and, for most physicians, selective neck dissection (versus ultrasound evaluation) is certainly more clear-cut. The diagnostic use of selective neck dissection undoubtedly engenders less controversy than the concept of therapeutic selective neck dissection.

An argument against elective ND is that, even with a 30 % risk of occult metastases, a large percentage of the patients (70–80 %) undergo surgery without benefit. [12] As a result, an intact lymph node system is removed that could work as a barrier against the cancerous disease. Furthermore, the high morbidity and mortality accompanying elective RND, in contrast to the notably lower morbidity with selective ND types, must be considered.

As previously mentioned, an advantage of elective ND, versus radiotherapy, is that the histological examination of the ND specimen gives important information directing subsequent therapy and prognosis. At the same time, the indication for SND includes not only the possibility of an optimized staging procedure, but also a therapeutic purpose. The indication for an optimized survival rate after SND with the No neck becomes more and more important in comparison to the wait-and-see attitude. This is not surprising, considering the fact that the rate of occult metastases detected with SND amounts to about 25 % [13]. The significance of the therapeutic function of SND was demonstrated in a study performed by Hosal and coworkers [14]. The authors were able to show that SND is appropriate for the elective treatment of the clinical No neck, independent of the location and the extent of the primary tumor situated in the upper aerodigestive tract. SND led to local control in 97 % of the No patients and in 96 % of the pN+ patients without extracapsular tumor growth. The rate of late metastases to lymph nodes outside the levels dissected by means of SND amounted to only 0.7 % (2/270), making clear how effective this treatment concept is. The results also explain the repeated, but statistically irrelevant, differences in the survival rates of patients with No necks and those with N1 neck without extracapsular spread. In interpreting these results, it must be acknowledged that the low recurrence rate is certainly in part related to the actual SND performed by the authors. Patients treated with SND generally underwent dissection of levels IIa and IIb, as did patients treated for carcinoma of the oral cavity level IV. The treatment results make it clear that such an SND (levels I-IV), when viewed from a staging as well as a therapeutic perspective, is as effective as MRND. The decrease in the extent of ND from MRND to SND, with conservation of at least one level, may seem too progressive for supporters of a therapeutic purpose for elective ND. However, it demonstrates that, at least in certain cases, it is possible to avoid the currently performed complete dissection (RND) or MRND in a limited N+ neck.

Clearly more non-traditional is the use of classic SND in cases of the N+ neck (including cases with more than one cervical lymph node metastasis), as has been shown by Steiner's group for several years now. Although Steiner's results seem promising [4, 15], a general acceptance of transformed treatment strategies can only be achieved by prospective, randomized studies. Appropriate application of the sentinel node concept in such a prospective multi-institution setting would be especially helpful.

Concerning the question of the treatment results after elective full therapeutic ND in cases of the No neck, no conclusive determination can currently be made based on prospective studies. The same is true for the clinical significance of micrometastasis, whose long-term value will have to be verified by prospective follow-up trials [16–18]. However, as indicated above, some studies have found no statistical differences in survival rates between therapeutic and elective ND [5]. In contrast, there are other studies that show a significant deterioration in the survival rate if clinically manifest metastases develop and are treated after the initial therapy [19–21].

At least two randomized clinical studies have examined the value of ND in cases of No neck in carcinomas of the floor of the mouth and the mobile tongue. In one of the studies [5], the patients were divided into two groups after interstitial radiotherapy for carcinoma of the floor of mouth or the tongue. One group underwent initial elective RND, and the second group underwent therapeutic ND – but only in cases of the later development of lymph node metastases. In the group of elective RND, 49 % of the patients had cervical lymph node metastases, whereas 53 % of the patients in the second group developed an N+ neck. A significant prognostic difference could not be shown. In a second study [22], patients suffering from a T1No or T2No carcinoma of the mobile tongue were divided into two groups. One group underwent only hemiglossectomy, and the other group underwent hemiglossectomy and elective RND. With a median follow-up of 20 months, no prognostically significant differences were apparent. More prospective randomized studies, especially with regard to other primary site locations, are needed. Unfortunately, in light of current studies, few solid conclusions can be drawn.

We feel strongly that radical neck dissection should not be done in the No neck. Our recommendations regarding the extent of SND for the different sites is shown in ▶ Table 10.1. Pathological lymph nodes in oropharyngeal squamous cell carcinomas are more frequent at level I than at level IV [23], but are rarely found in level I A [24]. The absence of metastases in level I A, and usually in level I B, does not justify a modified radical neck dissection [15]. Dissection of level I B in laryngeal carcinomas is indicated only in the presence of clinical, radiographic or cytologic evidence of metastatic disease [25]. Dissection of level I A is indicated for carcinomas of the upper lip, chin, cheek and skin of the nose [26]. Dissection of level II B, IV and V requires further discussion. This is because results of histopathological investigations suggest that nodal metastases in the submuscular recess (level II B) are rare in head and neck cancer patients [27], but not uncommon in non-squamous cell carcinomas. For the latter, the addi-

tional time requirement and the morbidity associated with dissection of the supraspinal accessory nerve component of level II B are justified in the case of thyroid or parotid gland cancer [28]. The rate of the late occurrence of metastasis in level IV after previous level I, II and III dissection for early floor-of-mouth, mobile tongue, and cheek primary cancers is low, and this perhaps justifies not initially dissecting level IV. Conversely, the extra time and morbidity seen with initially adding level IV is not excessive. For this reason, many surgeons, perhaps especially in America, prefer to always include level IV. Until prospective studies are done, there can be no justifiable conclusions in either regard. Dissection of the superior part of level V is not necessary in most head and neck cancers, but should be considered in selected cases of skin cancer of the posterior cephalic area (retroauricular region, occipital scalp) [29].

In the following section, some special situations concerning carcinomas localized in the head and neck region will be discussed, situations that physicians deal with time and again.

7.1.2   Contralateral N0 Neck in the Case of an Ipsilateral N+ Neck

7.1.2.1   Anterior Oral Cavity

Due to the high density of lymph vessels in the anterior oral cavity, about 30 % of patients develop clinically detectable lymphogenic metastatic spread. Because of the high number of lymph collectors of the tongue, patients suffering from squamous cell carcinomas in this area have the possibility of occult metastatic spread in up to 60 % of the cases [30]. Primary tumors located near the midline must always lead to the assumption of occult contralateral lymph node metastases. Among all malignant tumors of the anterior oral cavity, cervical lymph node metastases occur most often in cases of carcinomas of the tongue. Twenty to fifty percent of patients develop cervical lymph node metastases in the further course of their disease, even in cases of small primaries [31]. The significance of the cervical lymph nodes in the overall treatment concept must not be underestimated. Due to the fact that the therapeutic success after elective ND seems to be higher than after so-called salvage treatment [32], in cases of already proven ipsilateral lymphogenic metastatic spread, the contralateral neck side should be treated with at least SND (I, II A ± III) even in clinically and radiological N0 contralateral necks.

7.1.2.2 Oropharynx

Depending on the location of the primary tumor, 44–78% of the patients suffering from oropharyngeal carcinomas already have lymphogenic metastatic spread on the occasion of their first presentation [5]. This occurs most often in the area of level II and with decreasing frequency in levels III and IV. About 12% of the patients develop lymphogenic metastases in level I. The incidence of retropharyngeal lymphogenic spread must also be considered.

Due to the high density of lymph vessels in the oropharynx, an already developed ipsilateral metastatic spread should indicate a high probability of occult contralateral metastatic spread. This is especially true in cases of carcinomas of the palatine tonsil, where already-detected clinical metastatic spread in the draining contralateral lymph nodes occurs in up to 22% of the patients [33]. This is why, in cases of ipsilateral metastatic spread, the elective treatment of the contralateral neck side with SND (I-III) is reasonable.

7.1.2.3 Supraglottis

Within the area of the upper aerodigestive tract, the region of the supraglottis has a particularly high density of lymph collectors, with significant crossing of the midline. Thus, carcinomas localized in this area must be expected to develop early occult lymphogenic metastatic spread to contralateral lymph nodes. The strategy of including the contralateral neck side in the surgical treatment concept for supraglottic carcinomas of the larynx is based on the possibility of contralateral lymphatic spread. Patients who develop neck recurrence after successful primary cancer sur-

gery generally undergo bilateral neck dissection with performance of elective ND of the contralateral neck side, including Levels II–IV.

In 1990, Lawrence DeSanto and associates published a very thoughtful paper concerning the "second" side of the neck in supraglottic cancer [34]. They started with a group of 247 patients, 222 of whom had neck dissection, either unilateral (188 patients – 77%), or simultaneous bilateral dissection (34 patients – 14%). Patients were analyzed during a twelve-year period with the minimum follow up being either the time of death or three years after the last patient was enrolled. Of particular interest in this review was the fact that, of the patients who were shown at the time of unilateral neck dissection to be ultimately pathologically free of cancer, only one patient later developed contralateral neck disease. Conversely, of 90 patients who underwent unilateral neck dissection and were found to have pathologic cancer in the neck, 31 of these 90 patients developed contralateral neck spread.

Patients who underwent delayed dissection on the second side of the neck due to recurrent cancer had both a higher rate of death from disease in the neck and from distant metastases. From these observations it seems very clear that patients who are pathologically positive on the ipsilateral side of the neck should be treated on the contralateral side. DeSanto and coworkers argue that such treatment should be surgical, although irradiation to a clinically and radiologically N0 neck would also confer effective treatment in over 90% of patients. An especially interesting observation in this paper is the fact that only one out of 98 patients who were pathologically negative in the ipsilateral neck later developed contralateral disease.

Many surgeons worldwide advocate bilateral simultaneous neck dissection, even in initially N0 necks [35], but also a unilateral approach is recommended for clinical N0 necks [36]. If DeSanto's reported observations are true and the ipsilateral N0 neck is ultimately proven to be pathologically N0, then almost 98% of patients are over-treated by the second neck dissection. Conversely, if subclinical disease is found pathologically in the ipsilateral neck, then these patients should very reasonably be treated on the contralateral side with a second neck dissection or IMRT (radiation therapy). It will often not be practical to do frozen section analysis of the full ipsilateral neck dissection specimen to determine whether a simultaneous contralateral neck dissection could be done. If, in fact, disease is found in the N0 neck at permanent pathological review, then a delayed dissection or IMRT radiation could be given to the other side. Appropriate contralateral dissection could then be done, and unnecessary irradiation or neck dissection could be avoided.

Another very interesting question concerns whether this same principal can be applied to other aerodigestive tract sites when patients present with N0 necks. Beyond the supraglottic larynx, patients with oral cavity, oropharyngeal and hypopharyngeal cancers all have a high propensity for bilateral neck spread. If these patients present with cancers in the direct midline of the floor of the mouth, for example, or in the middle of the base of the tongue, then it is very difficult to know which side of the neck to first dissect. As a result, these patients need bilateral neck dissections until such time as sentinel node studies or other, newer technologies can address this issue. Conversely, if patients have disease that is more lateralized, then the ipsilateral neck could be treated by modified radical neck dissection or appropriate selective neck dissection. If there were no cancerous lymph nodes in the full neck dissection specimen, then, presumably, the contralateral neck would not need to be treated. While DeSanto's data suggests that this may, indeed, be a valid approach, his methodology has not been studied for the other aerodigestive tract sites. A carefully designed prospective multi-institutional study could profitably address this question.

7.1.2.4 Glottis

Carcinomas of the glottis only metastasize when the tumor has found an access to the lymph collectors in the area of the vocalis muscle or via Broyle's tendon in a prelaryngeal direction. Although the optimal treatment concept for advanced glottic carcinomas is debatable, the authors agree that treatment of the

lymphatic drainage should be based on the therapeutic concept for the primary tumor. With surgical treatment of the primary cancer, surgical intervention of the ipsilateral neck side is recommended for T3 and T4 carcinomas of the larynx according to the clinical N status [9].

Embryologically, lymph vessels are directed mainly alongside the pharyngeal arches. In the event of tumor invasion into adjacent parapharyngeal spaces, e. g., penetration of a laryngeal carcinoma in anterior direction, lymph node metastases must be suspected in absolutely atypical and also contralateral areas. Because of this, it seems reasonable to perform a contralateral ND (SND II–IV) in cases of advanced laryngeal carcinoma involving the anterior commissure or when tumor infiltration into the thyroid gland or into the preepiglottic space is found.

7.1.2.5 Hypopharynx

Due to the density of lymph collectors in the area of the hypopharynx and the increased risk of contralateral occult metastatic spread, treatment of the contralateral clinical N0 neck in cases of hypopharyngeal carcinoma should include SND as part of the initial treatment of the cervical lymphatic drainage [3, 37]. In view of the main drainage regions, a SND II-IV should be performed. In this context, the observations of Johnson et al. [14] need to be mentioned. According to this group, a high rate of contralateral metastases occurs in patients suffering from carcinoma infiltrating the medial wall of the piriform sinus. When carcinomas extend to the piriform sinus apex, Weisler [38] recommends that a hemithyroidectomy be performed on the side of the tumor. Theoretically, the ipsilateral paratracheal lymph nodes are also at risk of at least the occult spread of carcinoma.

7.1.3 Verified Lymph Node Metastases (N+ Neck)

7.1.3.1 N1 and N2 Neck

In the event of verified lymphogenic metastatic spread, the basic question that must be addressed is whether the neck side containing metastases should be treated surgically by selective ND or by comprehensive ND. The potential of curative selective ND in cases of the N1 neck without extracapsular spread has already been described. Selective neck dissection, when used for N+ disease in combination with postoperative radiochemotherapy, yields survival and recurrence results comparable to those of radical neck dissection and modified radical neck dissection in combination with irradiation [39]. However, it must be remembered that currently selective neck dissection is not widely accepted as a verified curative procedure for N+ necks. Although it will probably be established as such in the future, this may be many years from now. Currently, the most accepted surgical therapy in cases of verified lymphogenic metastatic spread of squamous cell carcinomas of the upper aerodigestive tract is modified radical ND, with possible conservation of all three non-lymphatic structures.

The well-described and currently widespread therapeutic concept of MRD must not belie the fact that even today there are countries in which radical ND is routinely performed in cases of one cervical lymph node metastasis. If contralateral metastatic spread is present, then, four weeks later, staged contralateral radical ND is advocated. This approach is often based on regional peculiarities – for example, among other things, the presumed lower morbidity of staged dissection or the likelihood of poor patient compliance with follow-up examinations.

RND, MRND and SND do not include treatment of the Delphian node, but the clinician must remove this node when there is clinical or radiological evidence of its involvement. The presence of metastasis in the Delphian node is an independent adverse prognostic factor in laryngeal and hypopharyngeal cancer [40].

7.1.3.2 Fixed Lymph Node Metastases

Various approaches are commonly used in the management of the neck in patients presenting with advanced nodal disease: surgical resection of the primary tumor and neck dissection followed by radiotherapy; radical radiotherapy with planned neck dissection regardless of nodal response; radical radiotherapy with surgery only for those with clinically persistent or recurrent disease or radical radiotherapy combined with chemoradiation therapy.

The treatment of fixed cervical lymph node metastases only rarely leads to a cure. The final rate of cure is reduced to less than 5% in cases of advanced lymphogenic metastatic spread in neck levels IV or V. Based on this knowledge, the indication for surgical treatment of an N3 neck, for example, is realistically made with palliative intention. Finally, the surgical treatment of fixed lymph node metastases causes special problems. With fixation to skin, wide local resection is surgically easy, but intra- and subcutaneous tumor spread is rarely cured.

Normally, in the case of infiltration of the prevertebral fascia and deep cervical muscles by lymph node metastases, no curative surgical resection is possible. In such cases, the application of radioactive iodine elements or the performance of brachytherapy (▶ Fig. 7.1 b) following extended RND may be indicated.

Vascular Infiltration. The treatment of lymph node metastases that have infiltrated the common or internal carotid artery leads to special diagnostic questions which must be clarified preoperatively (see Chap. 5.2.1.2). If carotid artery resection is indicated, then a decision concerning reconstruction or ligation of the artery should be made.

In cases where resection of the carotid artery seems to be a high risk due to the results of the balloon occlusion test, an alternative may be ultimate ligation of the artery after previous step-by-step occlusion of the vessel with successive resection of the infiltrated part of the carotid artery. In order to reconstruct the carotid artery, a saphenous vein or vascular prostheses, simultaneously covered by a pectoralis major flap [2], can be used (▶ Fig. 7.1 a, b).

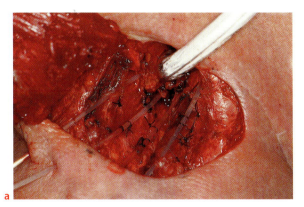

a

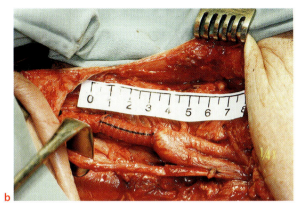

b

Figure 7.1 a, b

Treatment options for fixed cervical lymph node metastases. **a** In case of verified infiltration of the carotid artery, the infiltrating lymph node metastasis can be resected with the carotid artery, and the vessel can be reconstructed with a prosthesis. The patient, a 75-year-old at the time of surgery, survived the intervention more than 10 years tumor-free. **b** In the case of infiltration of the deep cervical muscles additional brachytherapy with intraoperatively applied applicators is possible

According to a retrospective analysis of 156 cases [41], the mortality rate after ligation of the carotid artery can be reduced significantly from 15–21% [41] to 3–6% if a step-by-step occlusion of the carotid artery is performed over a period of more than 13 days prior to tumor resection so that sufficient collaterals can develop.

Well-known neurologic complications [42] after carotid ligation are

- encephalomalacia leading to death;
- organic psychic syndromes;
- persisting hemiparesis; or
- passing focal neurological deficit(s).

7.1.3.3 Neck Dissection Following Primary Radio(Chemo)Therapy

In the treatment of advanced carcinomas of the upper aerodigestive tract, primary radio(chemo)therapy is more frequently being chosen. Often, pre-therapeutic verified cervical lymph node metastases persist for more than 8 weeks after termination of radiotherapy. In a five-year study of 88 patients, Boysen and co-workers [43] prospectively evaluated the results of combined radiochemotherapy and surgical treatment of the lymphatic drainage 4–6 weeks after primary radiochemotherapy. After termination of primary radiochemotherapy, the neck became N0 in 26% of the patients. Histologically, however, 22% of these patients still had viable tumor tissue in the neck dissection specimen. The remaining 74% of the patients had palpable tumor tissue remaining after termination of primary radiochemotherapy. Histologically, viable tumor tissue was found in 60% of these patients. The detection of viable tumor tissue after termination of the primary radiochemotherapy was found to be independent of the N status. While 39% of the patients with N1 or N2a neck disease had viable tumor in the neck dissection specimen, 53% of initial N2b, N2c or N3 neck still had cancer. The rate of persisting viable tumor tissue with increasingly higher lymphogenic metastatic status can explain the poor prognosis of these patients. On the basis of the results of this evaluation, primary radiochemotherapy should always be planned in combination with subsequent surgical treatment of the lymphatic drainage [44–47]. This fact emphasizes the importance of close cooperation between head and neck surgeons and their colleagues in radiotherapy in order to achieve an individually optimized treatment plan, i.e., consisting of primary radiochemotherapy followed by surgery, versus initial surgery followed by postoperative radiochemotherapy.

Our concept includes unilateral or bilateral ND about 6–8 weeks after the finish of radiation in all patients who were initially N2b, N2c or N3, in order to eliminate any doubt concerning the complete treatment of lymph node metastases. N1 patients who become clinically and radiologically N0, based on ultrasound or CT scanning, should be carefully observed. If these imaging studies are equivocal, then PET scanning may be very helpful. Patients with positive PET scans need neck dissection, whereas PET-negative patients can be further observed. The benefit of this concept has not yet been demonstrated by prospective studies. From our point of view, intense evaluations of the frequency of clinically relevant, persisting lymph node metastases are necessary to further clarify this difficult problem.

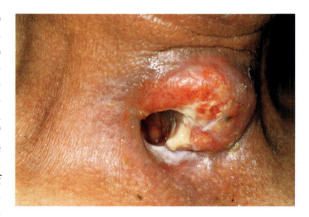

Figure 7.2

Recurrence at the tracheostoma

7.1.3.4 Peristomal Recurrence

The treatment of patients presenting with a so-called recurrence at the tracheostoma after previous laryngectomy (▶ Fig. 7.2) is still an oncologic challenge. Treatment choices are quite limited [48]. Recurrences at the tracheostoma can occur due to incomplete resection of the primary cancer, or lymphogenic metastatic spread to mediastinal lymph nodes [49]. However, the current view is that initial lymphogenic metastatic spread into lymph vessels of the cervical lymph nodes is the main cause for a recurrence at the tracheostoma. Continuity of the laryngotracheal lymph vessels in the area of the initial lymphatic system is the basis for this thought [50, 51].

Additional risk factors for the development of a recurrence at the tracheostoma are:

- tracheotomy prior to laryngectomy;
- extensive subglottic spread of the primary laryngeal cancer;
- the T-stage;
- the lymph node status; or
- previous ineffective surgical or radiochemotherapeutic treatment of the laryngeal carcinoma [52].

Due to the fact that approximately 8 % of patients suffering from peristomal recurrence initially had sub-

glottic tumor growth, the current opinion is that involvement of the subglottis is likely the most important pathogenic cause for the development of a recurrence at the tracheostoma [53–55].

The classification of recurrences at the tracheostoma elaborated by Sisson in 1989 [56], is still generally accepted. The author makes a distinction between four different types of recurrence:

- Type 1: localization above the stoma without involvement of the esophagus, trachea and/or corresponding vessels;
- Type 2: localization above the stoma with involvement of the esophagus, trachea and/or corresponding vessels;
- Type 3: localization below the tracheostoma with involvement of the esophagus and paratracheal skin; and
- Type 4: localization below the tracheostoma with involvement of structures other than the esophagus or paratracheal skin.

In order to determine the extent of the local findings and the resulting therapeutic options for patients with peristomal recurrence, an extensive pre-therapeutic diagnostic search for regional or distant metastases should be performed. This includes:

- biopsy in order to ascertain the histologic findings;
- tracheoscopy and esophagoscopy with biopsies; and
- CT scan or MRI of the neck and thorax.

Despite even extensive therapy, the prognosis for patients suffering from a recurrence at the tracheostoma is extraordinarily poor. Two-year survival rates after extended surgical resection with complex flap reconstruction is reported at 45% for Session type 1 and 2 and 9% for types 3 and 4 [57]. All patients treated by radiation alone had died by 24 months [58, 59]. Our experience suggests that the inclusion of new therapeutic approaches, such as locally applied cisplatin therapy, cannot improve the prognosis of patients suffering from a recurrence at the tracheostoma.

In view of this, the prevention of recurrences at the tracheostoma is critical. According to Rubin et al. [60] the following factors should be considered in the treatment of laryngeal and pharyngeal carcinomas in order to minimize the risk of a recurrence at the tracheostoma:

- no tracheotomy prior to planned laryngectomy (better: laser surgical debulking in the event of stridor);
- performance of hemithyroidectomy with laryngectomy (ipsilateral to the tumor);
- resection of the cervical trachea;
- resection of the paratracheal lymph nodes; and
- postoperative radiotherapy of the tracheal and paratracheal lymph nodes.

7.1.3.5 Retropharyngeal Lymph Nodes in Metastases from Head and Neck Cancers

One of the most common disease processes involving the retropharyngeal space is infectious pathology, such as deep neck abscess, which commonly originates in the retropharyngeal lymph nodes and may be bacterial or, on rare occasion, tubercular. Retropharyngeal lymph nodes are a group routinely not removed in classic radical, modified radical or selective neck dissection. However, several tumors of the upper aerodigestive tract mucous membranes metastasize to these lymph nodes. In particular, the retropharyngeal lymph nodes are important in carcinomas of the naso- and oropharynx, as well as in hypopharyngeal and cervical esophageal carcinomas, as depicted by Ferlito [61].

The retropharyngeal space is the most important route of communication between the neck and the mediastinum. Its nodes are divided into the lateral retropharyngeal nodes, also known as the Rouvière nodes, and the medial retropharyngeal nodes. The lateral retropharyngeal nodes are positioned posterolaterally to the nasopharynx and oropharynx from the C1 to the C3 vertebra. Normally, one to three lymph nodes on each side are present in infants, while in adults, retropharyngeal lymph nodes may be found on one side or the other [62]. The retropharyngeal lymph nodes decrease in diameter, measuring 10–15 mm in children, 5–8 mm in young adults and 3–5 mm in older individuals. The medial retropharyngeal lymph nodes can be found below the lateral retropharyngeal lymph nodes and are classified as upper and lower nodes [63].

Involvement of the retropharyngeal space poses significant diagnostic and therapeutic problems because the location of these lymph nodes is outside of the range of physical examination [61, 63, 64]. Image-guided fine-needle aspiration biopsy is the modality of choice in imaging this area. These methods are able to identify smaller nodes and to distinguish lymph nodes from a primary tumor of the adjacent nasopharynx; as a result, they have distinct advantages over CT in the assessment of retropharyngeal lymph nodes [65, 66]. Usually, the presence of necrosis or extracapsular spread, irrespective of lymph node size, is considered indicative of metastatic disease [63, 67].

Lam et al. [67] investigated the size of normal retropharyngeal lymph nodes and the incidence of retropharyngeal lymph node involvement in nasopharyngeal carcinoma in 44 cancer patients and 20 patients without cancer. Taking 4 mm as the upper limit of normal retropharyngeal lymph nodes, 89% of the patients with cancer had enlarged retropharyngeal lymph nodes. The number of nasopharyngeal walls involved and the maximum diameter of the primary tumor showed no statistical relationship with the involvement of retropharyngeal lymph nodes. There was a statistical association between retropharyngeal lymph nodes and level II node involvement. Despite the research of Lam et al., who, as indicated, considered 4 mm to be the largest diameter of normal lateral retropharyngeal lymph nodes, other investigators have felt any medial group node to be abnormal. King et al. [62] postulated that lateral retropharyngeal lymph nodes should be considered metastatically involved if the shortest axial diameter of the node was ≥5 mm. They agreed with Lam's group that any visible medial retropharyngeal lymph node should be classified as malignant.

A recent preliminary report from Miyashita et al. [68] on the value of percutaneous ultrasound with 3.5-MHz probes showed that retropharyngeal lymph nodes which are 1.5 cm or more in diameter can be demonstrated with percutaneous ultrasound using CT guidance. This technique may be utilized for the purpose of monitoring radiation therapy effect, but has no significance for the initial staging of disease.

Lymphogenic metastatic spread to retropharyngeal lymph nodes is a common finding in patients with nasopharyngeal carcinomas; it has a reported incidence of N+ neck disease between 85.7–93.9% [62, 69]. Based on MRI diagnosis and histological investigations, 8.6–14% of patients with carcinomas of the pyriform sinus or postcricoid area [69, 70], and 21.4–57.1% of patients suffering from carcinomas localized on the posterior pharyngeal wall, show metastatic involvement of retropharyngeal lymph nodes [69–71]. In 1995, McLaughlin et al. [69] reported on a large series of patients with squamous cell carcinomas of the oropharynx and supraglottis. The incidence of retropharyngeal adenopathy was 18.7% for carcinomas of the soft palate, 11.6% for carcinomas of the tonsillar region, 5.5% for carcinomas of the base of the tongue and 3.6% for carcinomas of the supraglottis. Based on histologic examination, Amatsu et al. [70] reported positive retropharyngeal lymph nodes in 19.5% of carcinomas of the cervical esophagus.

Although the treatment of retropharyngeal lymph nodes is controversial, there seems to be little doubt that the treatment of retropharyngeal nodes is indicated in cancer of the nasopharynx. Usually radiotherapy or chemoradiotherapy is used to treat the primary tumor and nodal metastases of this cancer [62]. Serious consideration should be given to the treatment of retropharyngeal lymph nodes in cases of advanced oropharyngeal, hypopharyngeal and cervical esophageal cancers [61, 70, 72]. As standard neck dissections (radical, modified radical and selective) do not address this area, consideration must be given to radiotherapy, or chemoirradiation, especially with newer IMRT approaches, for the treatment of oropharyngeal, hypopharyngeal or cervical esophageal cancers. Standard ablative primary site surgery – even with radical neck dissection – still leave the retropharyngeal nodes untreated. This may not be significant for necks ultimately shown to be pathologically negative, but, as indicated by studies referenced previously in this chapter, retropharyngeal nodes often can be involved by metastatic cancer. In contrast to radical primary site surgeries with major flap reconstruction and neck dissection, appropriately selected transoral resection, coupled with neck dissection in N+ patients and subsequent irradiation or chemoirradiation that includes the retropharyngeal nodes, may be a better approach. Additionally, in cases of lateralized hypopharyngeal or oropharyngeal cancers with N0 necks, transoral primary site resection, coupled with IMRT techniques that treats all appropriate ipsilateral nodal groups, including the retropharyngeal nodes, may confer control rates equal to or better than classical ablative approaches. A significant benefit is that patient morbidity in such a treatment scheme would be notably decreased.

So far, the evaluation and management of metastatic disease to the retropharyngeal nodes continue to be a diagnostic and therapeutic challenge in the treatment concept of head and neck squamous cell carcinomas. This area, however, should not be neglected in the evaluation and treatment of head and neck cancers.

7.2 Neck Dissection
for Lymphoepithelial Carcinomas

Lymphoepithelial carcinoma does not vary significantly from squamous cell carcinoma of the head and neck regarding its metastatic direction. Clearly, however, it metastasizes earlier and more frequently. While lymphoepithelial carcinoma can occur anywhere in Waldeyer's ring, it is most commonly observed in the area of the nasopharynx [34].

The tendency for lymphoepithelial carcinoma to infiltrate adjacent structures, and its frequent location in the area of the nasopharynx, makes it generally difficult to completely resect the primary tumor. Due to the fact that lymphoepithelial carcinoma is characterized by significantly higher radiotherapeutic sensitivity than squamous cell carcinomas, the treatment of choice in the area of the nasopharynx is radiotherapy, both for lymphoepithelial carcinoma and generally also for adjacent regions. Due to the high rate of occult lymph node metastases, the lymphatic drainage region – even retropharyngeal lymph nodes that would not normally be included in the surgical treatment of the lymphatic drainage region – must be included in the radiation field [32].

In spite of therapeutic and prophylactic radiation to the lymphatic drainage region, 9–12 % of patients develop recurrences in the area of cervical lymph nodes [30, 73]. Such recurrences are often associated with distant metastases and local recurrences. On the basis of pathologic examinations, which demonstrate a significantly higher-than-expected rate of tumorous lymph nodes and capsular extension after termination of radiotherapy, Wei and Sham [32] recommend a post-radiotherapy neck dissection, consisting of, generally, RND. This procedure seems reasonable based on their data, particularly in the case of initially extended lymphogenic metastatic spread with a high tumor volume in the lymph node metastases. We perform such neck dissections 6–8 weeks after termination of radiotherapy in order to wait for the lasting effect of the radiotherapy in patients who have clinically or radiologically persistent nodes.

7.3 Neck Dissection for Skin Malignancies

7.3.1 Squamous Cell Carcinomas

Squamous cell carcinomas of the facial, cervical or, in particular, auricular skin require a sonographic evaluation of the regional lymphatic drainage region, which should be performed prior to biopsy. With T1 carcinoma, sonographic study of the lymphatic drainage is indicated. Carcinomas staged T2 may require SND (especially in cases of primary cancer in the area of the cheek and the anterior aspect of the auricle). We treat the clinical N0 neck in advanced squamous cell carcinomas of the facial skin by means of SND (▶ Table 10.2).

7.3.2 Malignant Melanoma

While the influence of extracapsular lymph node growth of melanomas on the rate of regional metastases could not be proven [74], distant metastases of melanomas are detected in 81 % of patients. This number increases to 100 % in the event of multiple lymph node metastases with capsular rupture [75].

Selective Neck Dissection for Malignant Melanoma. The indication for performing SND for melanoma is controversial. Normally, SND is *not* indicated for the treatment of patients suffering from melanomas of lower tumor thickness (< 0.75 mm), and it is indicated only in exceptional cases (e.g., ulcerated tumor) for patients with a tumor size between 0.76–1.49 mm.

The value of SND for malignant melanoma of intermediate tumor size (1.5–3.99 mm) with a reported 7 % rate of lymph node metastases is controversial. Over the past 10 years, the so-called sentinel lymphadenectomy (see Chap. 7.6) as a minimally invasive and valid staging procedure has turned out to be appropriate for the detection of the lymphogenic metastatic spread of malignant melanomas. As such, it has replaced the routinely performed elective ND in many centers. The lymphogenic metastatic frequency of malignant melanomas with a tumor size of greater than 4.0 mm amounts to values up to 50 %. The performance of SND, however, is also disputed for this indication, due to the fact that the prognosis is not improved by this treatment measure and the staging function has been replaced by the introduction of sentinel lymphadenectomy [76].

Mucosal Melanomas. The treatment of mucosal melanomas of the upper aerodigestive tract does not include elective ND. Due to a primarily low occult lymphogenic metastatic spread, and a total rate of lymph node metastases between 20–25 %, surgical therapy should be limited to the N+ neck.

Regarding the extent of surgical intervention, it is important to note that in cases of mucosal melanomas localized in the area of the palate, the nasal cavity and the paranasal sinuses, the potential for metastases to the buccal lymph nodes and those adjacent to the skull base must be considered [77].

The use of radiotherapy for the treatment of malignant melanoma is described in Chap. 6.

7.3.3 Merkel Cell Carcinoma

Among the relatively rare, but highly aggressive, endocrine tumors of the skin, Merkel cell carcinoma must be mentioned, as it manifests in the head and in the neck region in 50 % of all cases. Merkel cell carcinomas are prone to early lymphogenic metastatic spread in regional cervical lymph nodes, and this always precedes distant metastatic spread. In 50–100 % of the cases, histologically proven micrometastases occur in clinically inconspicuous cervical lymph nodes. Due to the high rate of histologically detectable micrometastases in cases of the clinical N0 neck, the performance of elective ND is clearly indicated [78]. Based on the tumor location and the lymphatic drainage direction, SND may be indicated. Due to the high rate of lymphogenic metastatic spread of Merkel cell carcinomas, the extent of SND must not be limited. Potentially, sentinel node biopsy could gain importance as a preoperative staging procedure, just as it has with malignant melanoma [34, 79]. However, it must be pointed out that the therapeutic benefit of an elective ND in cases of Merkel cell carcinoma is currently not evident. Improvement in local control and reduction of the local recurrence rate has been demonstrated only for surgery with postoperative radiation (see Chap. 6) [80].

7.4 Neck Dissection for Carcinomas of the Salivary Glands

The first filter station for carcinomas of the salivary glands is localized intraglandularly (parotid gland) or in adjacent lymph nodes (submandibular gland); as a result, the lymphatic drainage must be included in the surgical treatment of carcinoma of the salivary glands. While intraglandular lymph nodes can usually be resected during surgery of carcinomas of the parotid gland, periglandular lymph nodes surrounding the submandibular gland must be removed. In addition, carcinomas of the major salivary glands must be resected in such a way that intraglandular and periglandular lymph nodes are resected during extirpation of the gland. The pathologist must pay attention to evaluating not only the primary cancer from a histological perspective, but also the associated lymph nodes [9].

The question of elective neck dissection in the event of carcinoma of the salivary glands has historically been determined by the histological type of cancer that is present, as ascertained either by fine needle aspiration biopsy before definitive surgery or by frozen section analysis at the time of surgery. It should be noted in this regard that both of these diagnostic procedures are not as definitive as the final, permanent pathological slide review. However, both fine needle aspiration biopsy and frozen section analysis can, at a minimum, strongly suggest the presence of cancer.

When surgery is approached with a presumption of malignancy, intraglandular lymph nodes are, of course, resected, with removal of the main salivary gland and periglandular lymph nodes as part of the approach to the actual gland resection. The issue of whether further neck dissection needs to be done must be evaluated on a case-by-case basis.

When malignancy is strongly suspected, we recommend that a SND be done at the time of the definitive cancer surgery. There are several reasons for this. By simply extending the cervical portion of a standard parotid incision medially, lymph node levels II and III are immediately in the surgical field. Resection in parotid cancers of levels II and III requires less than 30 additional minutes, and can be significant in cancer staging. Removal of level I lymph nodes in submandibular carcinomas should be included as part of the removal of the gland itself, for reasons already mentioned. Simple posterior extension of a typical submandibular gland incision allows access to lymph node levels II and III. These, again, can be resected with minimal additional time. In the presence of the resected salivary gland and associated lymph nodes (levels I, II or III, based on the primary cancer location), more definitive decisions must be made related to subsequent radiotherapy.

SND is not indicated in low-grade, mucoepidermoid cancers; nor (usually) is it indicated in acinic cell carcinoma. Additionally, most adenocarcinomas, including adenoid cystic carcinoma, have very low rates of regional metastatic spread. For this reason, many authors do not extend primary salivary gland excision to the adjacent nodes. In our opinion, however, the additional surgery is minimally morbid, requires little operative time and allows a better oncological staging if added to gland excision.

Patients with high-grade, mucoepidermoid carcinomas should be treated by SND. In the case of high-grade mucoepidermoid carcinoma of the parotid gland, the resection of lymph node levels II, III and IV can be coupled with the primary resection. Usually, lymph node level II B is included, as this is so easily accessed after parotidectomy. High-grade, mucoepidermoid carcinoma of the submandibular gland should also be treated by selective neck dissection of levels I–IV. If, on ultimate pathological review, these lymph node levels are free of cancer, then an interesting question develops concerning the extent to which the patient needs postoperative irradiation. While everyone would agree that the salivary gland bed needs irradiation, with current IMRT techniques it may be possible to spare the lower neck (lymph node level IV), which typically has been included in irradiation in the past.

Resection of minor salivary gland malignancies in the oral cavity, oropharynx or larynx present an interesting dilemma. Typically, SND is not done for these malignancies unless high-grade mucoepidermoid carcinoma is present. With the development of the sentinel lymph node concept, however, and the ability to perform this procedure even on deep-lying malignancies, this may ultimately prove to be a very effective modality in determining whether neck dissection is needed. In malignancies of minor salivary gland origin, sentinel node biopsies could be done to determine whether there is a need for neck dissection. If the sentinel nodes were negative, then most likely dissection would not be needed.

It should be noted that patients need preoperative imaging when fine needle aspiration biopsy suggests salivary gland malignancy. (Clearly, if the imaging suggests positive pathological nodes, then neck dissection is indicated.) It is usually the case, however, that such imaging will be negative.

It has been the author's observation that even parotid malignancies, which typically do not have regional metastatic spread, can, in fact, have intraglandular lymph node spread. In our experience, this has frequently been true of mucoepidermoid carcinoma, adenoid cystic carcinoma and acinic cell carcinomas. This is especially interesting in light of the fact that acinic cell carcinoma is usually not treated with selective neck dissection. The finding of such intraglandular lymph nodes in parotid malignancy lends further support to the contention that it is important to treat these tumor entities using SND.

A final comment must be made concerning the grading of mucoepidermoid carcinoma. Although everyone would agree that SND is not needed with low-grade mucoepidermoid cancers, and although there is a consensus that high-grade mucoepidermoid carcinoma patients need neck dissections, the issue of intermediate grade cancer requires discussion. In the author's experience, the actual metastatic potential of these lesions cannot be well predicted by histological analysis alone. For this reason, we feel that limited neck dissection at the time of parotidectomy is indicated for intermediate-grade mucoepidermoid carcinomas.

7.5 Neck Dissection for Carcinomas of the Thyroid Gland

Metastases is the first sign of cancer in up to 40 % of all cases of thyroid cancer. The metastatic frequency of papillary thyroid carcinomas has been reported to be approximately 50 %, with a range of 25–85 %. Occult metastases can occur in up to 60 % of patients. For follicular carcinoma of the thyroid gland, the metastatic frequency varies between 2–15 %; for medullary carcinoma it can be as high as 70 %; and for anaplastic carcinoma, the metastatic frequency is approximately 30 %. The actual rate of metastases in anaplastic cancer is probably much higher, but many patients die from local disease before regional or distant disease has manifested.

Surgical Therapy and Extent of Lymphadenectomy for Thyroid Cancer. Based on intraoperative findings, even without a clinical suggestion of lymphogenic metastatic spread, most differentiated carcinomas of the thyroid gland are treated by total thyroidectomy, with or without paratracheal node dissection, followed by radioactive iodine therapy [81, 82]. Because the paratracheal nodes are exposed with standard thyroidectomy techniques, this area must be carefully examined during surgery. Any abnormal mass should be evaluated by frozen section analysis, and paratracheal dissection should be done if the nodes have cancer spread.

In patients whose necks are difficult to examine (e.g., short necks, obese patients or muscular necks), preoperative MRI imaging is indicated. When patients have clinical or MRI-suggested regional cancer spread, preoperative FNA biopsy or intraoperative excisional biopsy, with frozen section analysis, must be done. Patients with demonstrated cancer should undergo SND (II, III, and IV) with paratracheal dissection, usually on the same side as the cancer in the thyroid, and contralaterally as needed, based on surgical findings.

Some papers report up to a 50 % incidence of occult spread in the contralateral neck in the presence of known ipsilateral disease. Whether contralateral selective neck dissection is indicated for such an No neck is controversial. Generally, these patients are treated with radioactive iodine therapy, followed by a determination of thyroglobulin levels and subsequent whole-body radioactive iodine scans. As not all patients take up radioactive iodine, MRI scans should be done in patients with initial neck disease or poor prognostic indicators in the primary cancer, e.g., large tumor size, extracapsular growth, etc.

Tumors with a diameter of more than 5 cm, and tumors that violate the thyroid capsule, have a significantly higher locoregional recurrence rate. For this reason, paratracheal dissection with ipsilateral neck dissection of levels II-IV is recommended concurrent with complete thyroidectomy [83].

Mediastinal lymph node spread is relatively rare, but can be observed in tumors with extrathyroidal extent (T4 tumors) [84]. In contrast, about one-third of the patients suffering from delayed primary site recurrences have mediastinal spread [85].

Indications for considering treatment of mediastinal lymph nodes include [81]:

- clinically detectable mediastinal lymph node metastases;
- histological proof of more than three lymph node metastases in the paratracheal area;
- detection of lymph node metastases in the cervico-lateral compartment (levels III or IV); and
- detection of lymph node metastases at the level of the right subclavian vein or the left brachiocephalic vein.

Patients with medullary cancers who are N+ should undergo MRND. Elective neck dissection for No patients is somewhat controversial. Generally, elective neck dissection is not recommended, but if patients have high calcitonin levels after total thyroidectomy, extensive imaging is indicated. Ipsilateral neck dissection (on the side of the initial thyroid lobe involvement) can be done for any suspicious lymph node indications as determined by scanning. In this setting, SND (levels II-IV) with paratracheal dissection can be done.

Neck dissection for anaplastic thyroid cancer is rarely done, as the primary site is so often inoperable. Where total thyroidectomy can be done with removal of all disease at that site, and with known operable neck spread, neck dissection (MRND or even RND) is indicated as a palliative measure. The goal of such dissection is to gain locoregional control, as most patients ultimately die of distant metastases or local failure in spite of surgery and postoperative irradiation.

Technique of Lymphadenectomy. Cervical access for resection of the thyroid gland, the paratracheal area and the lower neck is obtained via a Kocher's incision extended in cranio-lateral direction (collar incision). The thyroid gland is first mobilized, and then the dissection of the paratracheal and the neck levels is performed. Neck levels III and IV are easily accessed by extending the typical thyroid collar incision more laterally, and by detaching the sternal head of the sternocleidomastoidal muscle. Level II can be reached through a wide "collar-type" incision, or by placing a parallel incision in the upper neck within a natural crease. This "MacFee-type" incision allows excellent access, and is cosmetically pleasing.

If mediastinal resection must be performed, it is generally done transsternally. The thymus must be mobilized and prepared to the edge of the mediastinal pleura as well as the azygos vein. En-bloc resection of the mediastinal lymph nodes is done subsequent to the resection of the lymph nodes of the upper paratracheal area compartment [81]. Full sternotomy is rarely needed. If anterior mediastinal nodes cannot be safely removed through the neck incision, a partial sternotomy usually provides adequate access.

According to the Division of American Head and Neck surgeons [86], a radical or modified radical neck dissection is performed only in extraordinary cases, except, as previously noted, for medullary carcinoma of the thyroid gland. The surgical therapy of the lymphatic drainage in differentiated carcinomas of the thyroid gland usually consists of SND (II-IV± V). Subsequent to such therapy, special attention must be paid to possible recurrences in the area of the retro- and parapharyngeal lymph nodes.

7.6 Sentinel Node Biopsy

The so-called sentinel node concept was first described in 1977 by Cabanas [87] for squamous cell carcinoma of the penis. It is based on the assumption that the lymphogenic metastatic spread of a malignant process occurs via a first-draining lymph node situated in the drainage region of the primary tumor, the so-called *sentinel node* (SN), and that from there further lymphogenic metastatic spread occurs.

The presence of a first draining lymph node in the drainage region of the primary tumor is based on the assumption that in an early stage of lymphogenic metastatic spread, the first metastasis arises in this lymph node (▶ Fig. 7.3).

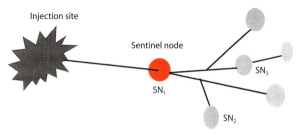

Figure 7.3

The sentinel node concept is based on the assumption that the first metastasis of a primary tumor can be found in the first draining lymph node of the primary tumor. This lymph node is called the sentinel lymph node and can be identified by intra- or peritumoral injection of radioactive tracer by means of a gamma probe

7.6.1 Marking of the Sentinel Node

A description of the SN is obtained by means of blue dye injection alone, the application of a radiopharmaceutical alone (e.g., ^{99m}technetium nanocolloid, where its intraoperative accumulation can be detected via a gamma probe) or by a combination of both procedures.

The most frequently applied dyes for lymphography [88] are

- Patent blue and
- Evans blue (used more rarely).

Substitute dyes are

- Methylene blue, and
- Indigo carmine.

Radionuclides. Garzom et al. were the first (1965) to report on the successful application of a colloidal [99m]technetium radionuclide for lymphoscintigraphy [89]. [99m]Technetium (^{99m}Tc) has a very short half-life of only 6 hours and an energy output of 140 keV. Low cost is another reason for the wide distribution of radiopharmaceuticals associated with [99m]technetium.

The biokinetics of the identification of the sentinel node, as indicated by measuring intranodal activity accumulation, largely depends on the size of the particles of the applied radiopharmaceutical [90].

The larger the particle size, the lower the absorption rate into the lymphatic system, and the better the accumulation in the sentinel node.

For lymphoscintigraphy, a multitude of different radiopharmaceuticals can be used. One radiopharmaceutical frequently applied in the USA is the filtered ^{99m}Tc sulfur colloid, which has a mean particle size of 38 nm (about 90 % of the particles are smaller than 50 nm). It is drained from the injection point with a half-life of 10.5 hours.

The radiopharmaceutical most frequently used in Europe is ^{99m}Tc nanocolloid. It is drained with a half-life of 4 hours from healthy tissue [90]. Another radiopharmaceutical is ^{99m}Tc human albumin. This radiopharmaceutical has a molecular weight of 60,000 Daltons and is transported in the lymphatic system at a velocity of about 10 cm per minute. It reaches the sentinel node after 1–12 minutes [91, 92].

Concerning the question of which radiopharmaceutical is best, representative evaluations comparing large patient populations are missing. Only a few studies on the above-mentioned radiopharmaceuticals exist, and their results are somewhat contradictory. While some studies report a quicker transport of ^{99m}Tc nanocolloid, compared with filtered ^{99m}Tc sulfur colloid, other studies show no relevant difference between filtered ^{99m}Tc sulfur colloid and ^{99m}Tc human albumin [90, 93]. The size of the single particles and the slow transport of filtered ^{99m}Tc sulfur colloid carries the risk of not identifying the SN. The quick intra-lymphatic drainage time of ^{99m}Tc human albumin allows passage to the first draining SN. We prefer to use ^{99m}Tc nanocolloid, which combines a quick intralymphatic transport with a longer storage period in the SN. This allows a successful sentinel lymphadenectomy to be performed even 24 hours after injection.

Radiotracer and/or Blue Dye. The groups reporting on the value of sentinel lymphadenectomy mostly do not apply blue dye in addition to the radionuclide. In agreement with earlier communications by Pitman and co-workers [94], a recent study [95] indicates that the false negative rate is not reduced significantly by additional color lymphography. Radioactive marking of the sentinel lymph node is the basis for sentinel lymphadenectomy in the head and neck region. The high sensitivity of the results obtained by means of radiotracer marking makes the additional application of blue dye, as well as the various complications associated with the use of dyes, unnecessary. Accidental trauma to the lymph collector draining the dye could lead to an extravasation of the dye, with a resulting reduction of intraoperative information [96]. The probability of this happening is especially high in the area of cervical soft tissues, with their multitude of neural and vascular structures. Furthermore, already in 1985, Longnecker, et al. reported on anaphylaxis after subcutaneous injection of blue dye [96]. In the current literature, up to 2 % of the examined patients have anaphylaxis [97]. Results of the clinical application and benefit of [99m]radiotracers coupled with methylene blue for sentinel lymphadenectomy requires further investigation [98].

Dose and Quantity. Regarding the minimal dose of radionuclides, no comparable evaluations exist. Due to an unphysiologic increase in interstitial pressure, the application of abnormally high volumes leads not only to additional drainage in a secondary drainage region adjacent to the main drainage region, but also to the accumulation of the radionuclide in multiple lymph nodes that are not representative of the first-draining lymph node station. With regard to the classic rule of lymphology according to Mascagni, fluid from the first-draining lymph node station passes an average of eight lymph nodes before being re-transported into the venous blood system. In view of this, it is important to reduce the number of lymph nodes accumulating the radionuclide to 1–3 representative first-order nodes (SN1–3) [99].

In our experience, the application of a dose of 1.2 mCi ^{99m}Tc nanocolloid, dissolved in 0.2–0.35 ml physiologic saline, is sufficient to successfully identify the SN up to 24 hours after injection [99–103].

With carcinomas of the anterior oral cavity and oropharynx, 1.2 mCi ^{99m}Tc nanocolloid, dissolved in 0.3 ml physiologic saline, is placed in an insulin syringe (PlastiPak, Becton Dickinson, Madrid, Spain) and injected by means of a 24-gauge needle 25 mm long (Microlance3, Becton Dickinson, Drogheda, Ireland). This is done in separate 0.05 ml injections into four positions of the lateral tumor wall.

With carcinomas of the supraglottis and glottis, 1.2 mCi ^{99m}Tc nanocolloid, dissolved in 0.4 ml physiologic saline, is placed into an insulin syringe (Plasti-Pak, Becton Dickinson, Madrid, Spain) and injected by means of a 23-gauge needle 80 mm long (Sterican, B. Braun, Melsungen, Germany) in four 0.05 ml injections around the lateral tumor wall.

7.6.2 Intraoperative Detection of Activity

The detection of intranodal activity is accomplished intraoperatively by means of a gamma probe.

Injection Technique. The radiopharmaceutical and/or dye can be applied to the aerodigestive tract via:

- 4–6 peritumoral injections, i.e., in the lateral wall of the carcinoma; or
- via one intratumoral injection.
- For other carcinomas (e.g., breast cancer), a subdermal injection has been described.

Because critically needed evaluations comparing the various injection techniques are missing, we prefer peritumoral injection in the lateral wall of the tumor. This assumes that the absorption of the radiopharmaceutical is probably in the initial lymph vessels in this area of highly active tumor growth. With intratumoral injection, one might postulate that, in the cen-

ter of the tumor, growth is accompanied by a destruction of the draining lymph vessels. This is an element of uncertainty that needs to be considered regarding the transport of the radiopharmaceutical.

The classic procedure, e.g., in cases of melanoma and breast cancer, is to inject a radiopharmaceutical intra- or peritumoral on the day prior to surgery and to describe the lymphatic drainage by means of lymphoscintigraphy. On the following day, the localization of the SN is identified via a gamma probe and the SN is directly resected through a small skin incision.

In the event of a tumor-free SN in the frozen section diagnosis, a sufficiently experienced surgeon can decide not to perform an extended lymph node dissection. Initial results with regard to melanomas and breast cancer seem to favor this procedure [87, 104–107], which not only allows a reduction in the surgery-related morbidity and an accompanying increase in quality of life, but also reduces costs.

Pretherapeutic dynamic lymphoscintigraphy of the head and neck can detect preoperatively an adequate functional capacity of lymphatic drainage of the primary tumor, as well as the main direction of lymphatic drainage (ipsi- or contralateral). This is due to the intranodal accumulation of a sufficient amount of the radionuclide (▶ Fig. 7.4). Other communications [108, 109], however, have found the procedure to be unreliable in identifying the SN in the area of the lymphatic drainage of grossly enlarged jugular lymph nodes of neck levels II–IV.

When SN biopsy is used as a purely intraoperative detection procedure, our own results with SN biopsy performed in a surgically opened neck seem to be promising with regard to the detection of metastatic spread not identified preoperatively, and also with regard to identifying spread in early squamous cell carcinomas of the upper aerodigestive tract [100, 101, 110, 111].

Procedure. At the beginning of the surgical intervention (tumor resection and neck dissection), the peritumoral tracer application is performed. The intraoperative identification of the SN by means of a gamma probe with a 14 mm collimator aperture (Navigator Gamma Guidance System, Auto Suture, Toenisvorst, Germany) is performed identically in all patients. In

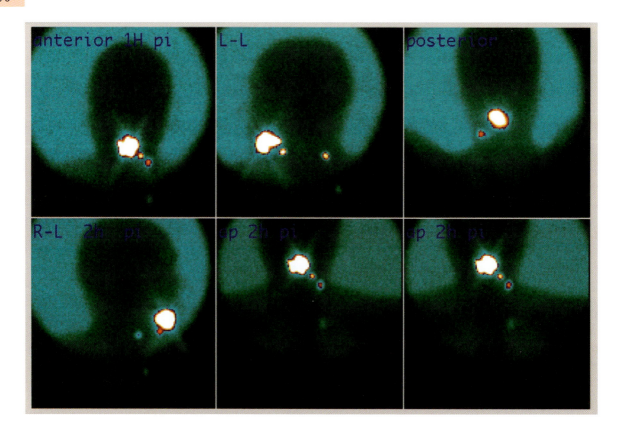

Figure 7.4

Description of the cervical lymphatic drainage by planar scintigraphs under the double detector camera with description of the body silhouette by a phantom placed behind the head, which is injected with ^{99m}technetium

order to reduce the dispersion of radiation, resection 15–20 minutes after injection of the primary tumor is optimal [112]. This procedure is justified by our findings on dynamic lymphoscintigraphy of the head and neck. Lymphatic drainage can be detected immediately after injection in 75 % of the cases, which allow a clear description of the first draining lymph node stations after 30 minutes [101, 103].

Intraoperative lymphatic mapping is taken after complete raising of the skin flap, while the dissection of the vascular sheath occurs during mobilization of the ND specimen (▶ Fig. 7.5). Following the intraoperative identification, marking or resection of the SN, as well as other lymph nodes accumulating in the radionuclide, further dissection is performed until

the value of the SN biopsy of the head and neck is clarified. The residual neck is then dissected according to the original indication for ND. After removal of the ND specimen, an intracervical control is performed in order to clarify possible residual activity, and this is followed by an extracorporeal re-measurement of the neck dissection specimen.

Although studies published by various groups [95, 109, 114–123] are inconclusive regarding the value of sentinel lymphadenectomy in squamous cell carcinomas of the upper aerodigestive tract, early results with easy-to-expose carcinomas of the anterior oral cavity confirm the significance of this new diagnostic concept. Additionally, our evaluations appear to show value for this procedure in pharyngeal and laryngeal

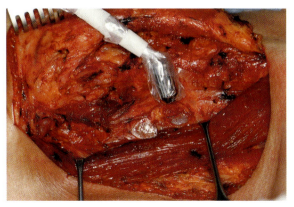

Figure 7.5

Intraoperative measurement of the activity by means of a gamma probe

T1 and T2 carcinomas, as well as in T3 glottic carcinomas exposable during general anesthesia [98–101, 110, 111]. In contrast, our results show that an advanced intranodal tumor growth with extracapsular metastatic spread leads to a significant reduction in the absorption of the radionuclide or no accumulation at all, due to total loss of the nodal storage capacity. Because of this, the identification of a histologically non-representative SN cannot be excluded reliably. Therefore, ipsilateral SN biopsy should not be performed in cases of clinically advanced lymphogenic metastatic spread. However, the intraoperative SN biopsy may be important for the contralateral clinical N0 neck.

7.6.3 Limits and Sources of Errors

A limitation of the SN concept in carcinomas of the upper aerodigestive tract is the technical difficulty in clearly identifying radioactively-marked lymph nodes, which may be disturbed by the dispersion of radiation at the primary injection point.

Dispersion of Radiation. Tumors of the upper aerodigestive tract present anatomical peculiarities in the head and neck region. Given the close proximity of the primary tumor and first-draining lymph node

station, the undisturbed measurement of radiation in a single lymph node is not always reliable. This is because of the accumulation of radiation from the primary injection point. Misrepresentation of the intranodal activity measured by means of a gamma probe cannot be excluded in all cases due to this problem [101]. For reasons already explained, the identification of very small, first-draining lymph nodes adjacent to the primary tumor is often only possible after mobilization of the ND specimen from the operation site away from the primary site.

For this reason, some authors recommend the intraoperative placement of a lead plate to insulate against radiation at the primary injection point [112, 124]. In our experience, misrepresentations cannot be avoided reliably even with the use of this tool. Consequently, we recommend resection of the primary site 15–20 minutes after injection, when there is a reduction in the effect of the dispersion of radiation [111].

Extracorporal determination of the activity of the lymph nodes accumulating the radionuclide can increase significantly the reliability of SN biopsy [110]. Further examinations are needed to determine whether the gamma probe can be substituted by a less expensive and less interference-prone instrument for sentinel lymphadenectomy in cases of squamous cell carcinomas of the head and neck.

Injection Related to the Lymphatic Drainage Region. Detailed examinations have revealed differences of density in the regional distribution pattern of the initial lymph vessels of the head and neck [51, 98, 125, 126], which has a direct effect on the identification of the first-draining lymph node. Due to the close proximity of the different lymphatic drainage regions in the head and neck, the injection technique bears the risk of injecting into a drainage region adjacent to the main drainage area. Hence, the quality of the examination is directly related to the quality of injection and, as a result, also to the experience of the examiner. The use of intraoperative injection can contribute significantly to the reliability of the injection due to a better general view and the lack of movement of the patient [99–103].

There is also the question of an optimal volume of the tracer substance to be injected. Because of an unphysiologic increase in the interstitial pressure, the application of a large quantity of radionuclide not only leads to additional drainage in a secondary drainage region adjacent to the main drainage region, but also to the accumulation of the radionuclide in multiple lymph nodes that are no longer representative of the first draining lymph node station. With regard to the classic rule of lymphology as stated by Mascagni – namely, that the lymph fluid passes an average of 8 lymph nodes before being re-transported into the venous blood system, it is important to reduce the number of lymph nodes accumulating the radionuclide to 1–3 representative first-draining lymph nodes (SN1–3) [99]. The general description and resection of the most highly accumulating lymph node (SN1) does not seem to be sufficiently representative when considering the distribution pattern of collateral formations of initial lymph vessels of the head and neck [51, 98, 125, 126]. The primary tumor can drain into two adjacent lymphatic drainage regions due to its location and thus have more than one draining lymph node. For this reason, i.e., based on the dense lymph node system of the head and neck, we believe that the identification of two or at most three lymph nodes (SN1, SN2, SN3) accumulating the radiopharmaceutical is helpful in reducing the risk of false negative results in cases of the N0 neck.

7.7 Conclusion

In the context of elaborating a standardized diagnostic and therapeutic approach for the lymphatic drainage of carcinomas of the upper aerodigestive tract, there is a great deal of interest in sentinel lymphadenectomy, which is also used in the treatment other tumor entities (especially breast cancer and melanomas). A critical and careful evaluation of the validity of this method as it applies to carcinomas of the head and neck remains to be done. An uncritical transfer cannot be recommended, due to the possibility of tumor cells escaping the first-draining lymph node and metastasizing to other lymph nodes (skip metastases), which is well documented for head and neck carcinomas [127]. Furthermore, in the node-negative neck, intraoperative assessment does not

seem to improve the accuracy of staging [128]. Last, but not least, accurate pathologic staging of the neck has revealed that a third of the metastatic nodes are 3 mm or less in diameter [129]. This also underscores the need for critical evaluation of the SN concept in future studies.

Another important task will be to clarify (1) whether the intraoperative lymphatic mapping is useful in reducing the extent of SND in cases of suspected N0 neck, and (2) whether this method can avoid neck dissection in cases of a histologically proven tumor-free sentinel node. Opponents of this line of thought argue that SND is already minimally morbid. Supporters of intraoperative lymphatic mapping desire to protect the intact, i.e., metastatically unaffected, cervical lymph node system, as well as to reduce the extent of neck surgery. Scar contracture, disturbed sensation and persisting partial lymph edema might all be reduced by a circumscribed extirpation of the sentinel lymph node(s). These benefits warrant intense future investigation of intraoperative lymphatic mapping as it applies to N0 neck staging of mucosal carcinomas of the head and neck.

References

1. Bataini JP (1993) Radiotherapy in N0 head and neck cancer patients. Eur Arch Otorhinolaryngol 250:442–445
2. Rabuzzi DD, Chung CT, Saagerman RH (1980) Prophylactic neck irradiation. Arch Otolaryngol Head Neck Surg 106: 454–455
3. Steiner W (1984) Surgical treatment of the cervical lymph node system in laryngeal carcinoma. In: Wigand ME, Steiner W, Stell PM (eds) Functional partial laryngectomy. Springer, Berlin, 253–264
4. Ambrosch P, Kron M, Pradier O, Steiner W (2001) Efficacy of selective Neck dissection: A review of 503 cases of elective and therapeutic treatment of the neck in squamous cell carcinoma of the upper aerodigestive tract. Otolaryngol Head Neck Surg 124:180–187
5. Vandenbrouck C, Sancho-Garnier H, Chassagne D, Saravane D, Cachin Y, Micheau C (1980) Elective versus therapeutic radical Neck dissection in epidermoid carcinoma of the oral cavity. Results of a randomized clinical trial. Cancer 46:386–390
6. Rodrigo JP, Suarez C, Ferlito A, Devaney KO, Petruzzelli GJ,

Rinaldo A (2003) Potential molecular prognostic markers for lymph node metastasis in head and neck squamous cell carcinoma. Acta Otolaryngol 123:100–105

7. Maula SM, Luukkaa M, Grenman R, Jackson D, Jalkanen S, Ristmäki R (2003) Intratumoral lymphatics are essential for the metastatic spread and prognosis in squamous cell carcinomas of the head and neck region. Cancer Res 63: 1920–1926

8. Werner JA, Dünne AA, Lippert BM (2002) Indikationen zur Halsexploration bei nicht nachweisbaren Lymphknotenmetastasen. Teil I HNO 50:253–262

9. Werner JA, Dünne AA, Lippert BM (2002) Indikationen zur Halsexploration bei nicht nachweisbaren Lymphknotenmetastasen. Teil II HNO 50:370–378

10. Lippert BM, Werner JA (2001) Metastases in head and neck cancer. Tectum, Marburg

11. Kaneko S, Yoshimura T, Ikemura K, Shirasuna K, Kusukawa J, Ohishi M, Shiba R, Sunakawa H, Tominaga K, Sugihara K, Shinohara M, Katsuki T, Yanagisawa S, Kurokawa H, Mimura T, Ikeda H, Yamabe S, Ozeki S (2002) Primary neck management among patients with cancer of the oral cavity without clinical nodal metastases: A decision and sensitivity analysis. Head Neck 24:582–590

12. Gavilán C, Gavilán J (1989) Five-year results of functional Neck dissection for cancer of the larynx. Arch Otolaryngol Head Neck Surg 115:1193–1196

13. van den Brekel MW, van der Waal I, Meijer CJ, Freeman JL, Castelijns JA, Snow GB (1996) The incidence of micrometastases in Neck dissection specimens obtained from elective Neck dissections. Laryngoscope 106:987–991

14. Hosal AS, Carrau RL, Johnson JT, Myers EN (2000) Selective Neck dissection in the management of the clinically node-negative neck. Laryngoscope 110:2037–2040

15. Ambrosch P, Freudenberg L, Kron M, Steiner W (1996) Selective Neck dissection in the management of squamous cell carcinoma of the upper digestive tract. Eur Arch Otorhinolaryngol 253:329–335

16. Barrera JE, Miller ME, Said S, Jafek BW, Campana JP, Shroyer KR (2003) Detection of occult cervical micrometastases in patients with head and neck squamous cell cancer. Laryngoscope 113:892–896

17. Rhee D, Wenig BM, Smith RV (2002) The significance of immunohistochemically demonstrated nodal micrometastases in patients with squamous cell carcinoma of the head and neck. Laryngoscope 112:1970–1974

18. Wirtschafter A, Benninger MS, Moss TJ, Umiel T, Blazoff K, Worsham MJ (2002) Micrometastatic tumor detection in patients with head and neck cancer: a preliminary report. Arch Otolaryngol Head Neck Surg 128:40–43

19. DeSanto LW, Magrina C, O'Fallon WM (1990) The "second" side of the neck in supraglottic cancer. Otolaryngol Head Neck Surg 102:351–361

20. Gavilán J, Gavilán C, Herranz J (1994) The neck in supraglottic cancer. In: Smee R, Bridger GP (eds) Laryngeal cancer Elsevier, Amsterdam, 576–581

21. Teicher BA, Holden SA, Kelley MJ, Shea TC, Cucchi CA, Rosowsky A, Henner WD, Frei E 3d (1987) Characterization of a human squamous carcinoma cell line resistant to cis-diamminedichloroplatinum(II). Cancer Res 47:388–93

22. Fakih AR, Rao RS, Borges AM, Patel AR (1989) Elective versus therapeutic Neck dissection in early carcinoma of the oral tongue. Am J Surg 158:309–313

23. Vartanian JG, Pontes E, Agra IM, Campos OD, Goncalves-Filho J, Carvalho AL, Kowalski LP (2003) Distribution of metastatic lymph nodes in oropharyngeal carcinoma and its implications for the elective treatment of the neck. Arch Otolaryngol Head Neck Surg 129:729–732

24. Ferlito A, Kowalski LP, Byers RM, Pellitteri PK, Bradley PJ, Rinaldo A, Silver CE, Wei WI, Shaha AR, Medina JE (2002) Is the standard radical neck dissection no longer standard? Acta Otolaryngol 122:792–795

25. dos Santos CR, Goncalves Filho J, Magrin J, Johnson LF, Ferlito A, Kowalski LP (2001) Involvement of level I neck lymph nodes in advanced squamous carcinoma of the larynx. Ann Otol Rhinol Laryngol 110:982–984

26. Ferito A, Kowalski LP, Silver CE, Shaha AR, Rinaldo A, Byers RM (2002) The use and misuse of level Ia dissection for head and neck cancer. Acta Otolaryngol 122:553–555

27. Silverman DA, El-Hajj M, Strome S. Esclamado RM (2003) Prevalence of nodal metastases in the submuscular recess (level IIb) during selective neck dissection. Arch Otolaryngol Head Neck Surg 129:724–728

28. Talmi YP, Horowitz Z, Wolf M, Bedrin L, Peleg M, Yahalom R, Kronenberg J (2001) Upper jugular lymph nodes (submuscular recess) in non-squamous-cell cancer of the head and neck: surgical considerations. J Laryngol Otol 115:808–811

29. Hamoir M, Desuter G, Gregoire V, Reychler H, Rombaux P, Lengele B (2002) A proposal for redefining the boundaries of level V in the neck: is dissection of the apex of level V necessary in mucosal squamous carcinoma of the head and neck? Arch Otolaryngol Head Neck Surg 128:1381–1383

30. Ho CM, Lam KH, Wei WI (1992) Occult lymph node metastasis in small oral tongue cancers. Head Neck 14:359–363

31. Cunningham MJ, Johnson JT, Myers EN (1986) Cervical lymph node metastasis after local excision of early squamous cell carcinoma of the oral cavity. Am J Surg 152:361–366

32. Wei WI, Sham JS (1996) Cancer of the Nasopharynx. In: Myers EN, Suen JY. Cancer of the head and neck. Philadelphia, Saunders

33. Batsakis JQ (1979) Squamous cell carcinomas of the oral cavity and the oropharynx. In: Batsakis JG (ed) Tumors of the Head and Neck: Clinical and Pathological Considerations. 2nd ed. Baltimore, Williams & Wilkins, 144–176

34. Choe W, Housini I, Mello AM (1995) Lymphoscintigraphy in a case of Merkel cell tumor. Clin Nucl Med 20:922–924

35. Redaelli de Zinis LO, Nicolai P, Tomenzoli D, Ghizzardi D, Trimarchi M, Cappiello J, Peretti G, Antonelli AR (2002) The distribution of lymph node metastases in supraglottic

squamous cell carcinoma: therapeutic implications. Head Neck 24:913–920

36. Pinilla M, Gonzalez FM, Lopez-Cortijo C, Arellano B, Herrero J, Trinidad A, Vergara J (2003) Management of N0 neck in laryngeal carcinoma. Impact on patient's survival. J Laryngol Otol 117:63–66

37. Ganzer U, Meyer-Breiting E, Ebbers J, Vosteen KH (1982) Der Einfluss von Tumorgrösse, Lympknotenbefall und Behandlungsart auf die Prognose des Hypopharynxkarzinoms. Laryngorhinootologie 61:622–628

38. Weissler MC (1994) Technique of radical Neck dissection. In: Shockley WW, Pillsbury III HC (eds) The neck. Diagnosis and Surgery. Mosby, St. Louis, 573–588

39. Muzaffar K (2003) Therapeutic selective neck dissection: a 25-year review. Laryngoscope 113:1460–1465

40. Ferlito A, Robbins KT, Shaha AR, Pellitteri PK, Kowalski LP, Gavilan J, Silver CE, Rinaldo A, Medina JE, Pitman KT, Byers RM (2002) Current considerations in neck dissection. Acta Otolaryngol 122:323–329

41. Konno A, Togawa K, Iizuka K (1981) Analysis of factors affecting complication of carotid ligation. Ann Otol Rhinol Laryngol 90:222–226

42. Schobel G, Hollmann K, Millesi W (1992) Über das Risiko der Mitresektion der Arteria carotis communis bzw. interna bei der Exstirpation von Tumoren im maxillo-facialen Bereich. In: Vinzenz K, Waclawiczek HW (eds) Chirurgische Therapie von Kopf-Hals-Karzinomen. Springer, Wien, 269–282

43. Boysen M, Lovdal O, Natvig K, Tausjo J, Jacobsen AB, Evensen JF (1992) Combined radiotherapy and surgery in the treatment of neck node metastases from squamous cell carcinoma of the head and neck. Acta Oncol 31:455–460

44. Somerset JD, Mendenhall WM, Amdur RJ, Villaret DB, Stringer SP (2001) Planned postradiotherapy bilateral neck dissection for head and neck cancer. Am J Otolaryngol 22:383–386

45. Mendenhall WM, Villaret DB, Amdur RJ, Hinerman RW, Mancuso AA (2002) Planned neck dissection after definitive radiotherapy for squamous cell carcinoma of the head and neck. Head Neck 24:1012–1018

46. Roy S, Tibesar RJ, Daly K, Pambucian S, Lee HK, Gapany M, Adams GL (2002) Role of planned neck dissection for advanced metastatic disease in tongue base or tonsil squamous cell carcinoma treated with radiotherapy. Head Neck 24:474–481

47. McHam SA, Adelstein DJ, Rybicki LA, Lavertu P, Esclamado RM, Wood BG, Strome M, Carroll MA (2003) Who merits a neck dissection after definitive chemoradiotherapy for N2-N3 squamous cell head and neck cancer? Head Neck 25:791–798

48. Ferlito A, Silver CE, Rinaldo A, Kim H, Shaha AR (2002) Parastomal recurrence: a therapeutic challenge. Acta Otolaryngol 122:222–229

49. Kowalski LP, Rinaldo A, Robbins KT, Pellitteri PK, Shaha AR, Weber RS, Ferlito A (2003) Stomal recurrence: pathophysiology, treatment and prevention. Acta Otolaryngol 123:421–432

50. Duenne AA, Werner JA (2000) Functional anatomy of lymphatic vessels under the aspect of tumor invasion. Recent Results Cancer Res 157:82–89

51. Werner JA, Schünke M, Rudert H, Tillmann B (1990) Description and clinical importance of the lymphatics of the vocal fold. Otolaryngol Head Neck Surg 102:13–19

52. Eckel HE (2001) Peristomal recurrences of laryngeal and hypopharyngeal carcinoma. In: Lippert BM, Werner JA (eds) Metastases in head and neck cancer. Tectum, Marburg, 389–394

53. Leon X, Quer M, Burgues J, Abello P, Vega M, de Andres L (1996) Prevention of stomal recurrence. Head Neck 18:54–59

54. Yotakis J, Davris S, Kontozoglou T, Adamopoulos G (1996) Evaluation of risk factors for stomal recurrence after total laryngectomy. Clin Otolaryngol 21:135–138

55. Zbaren P, Greiner R, Kengelbacher M (1996) Stoma recurrence after laryngectomy: an analysis of risk factors. Otolaryngol Head Neck Surg 114:569–575

56. Sisson GA (1989) Ogura memorial lecture: mediastinal dissection. Laryngoscope 99:1262–1266

57. Gluckman JL, Hamaker RC, Schuller DE, Weissler MC, Charles GA (1987) Surgical salvage for stomal recurrence: a multi-institutional experience. Laryngoscope 97:1025–1029

58. Mantravadi R, Katz AM, Skolnik EM, Becker S, Freehling DJ, Friedman M (1981) Stomal recurrence. A critical analysis of risk factors. Arch Otolaryngol 107:735–738

59. Rockley TJ, Powell J, Robin PE, Reid AP (1991) Post-laryngectomy stomal recurrence: tumour implantation or paratracheal lymphatic metastasis? Clin Otolaryngol 16:43–47

60. Rubin J, Johnson JT, Myers EN (1990) Stomal recurrence after laryngectomy: interrelated risk factor study. Otolaryngol Head Neck Surg 103:805–812

61. Ferlito A, Shaha AR, Rinaldo A (2002) Retropharyngeal lymph node metastasis from cancer of the head and neck. Acta Otolaryngol 122:556–560

62. King AD, Ahuja AT, Leung SF, Lam WW, Teo P, Chan YL, Metreweli C (2000) Neck node metastases from nasopharyngeal carcinoma: MR imaging of patterns of disease. Head Neck 22:275–281

63. Mancuso AA, Harnsberger HR, Muraki AS, Stevens MH (1983) Computed tomography of cervical and retropharyngeal lymph nodes: normal anatomy, variants of normal, and applications in staging head and neck cancer. Part I: normal anatomy. Radiology 148:709–714

64. Pfreundner L, Pahnke J, Willner J (2000) Systematics in lymphatic tumor spread of carcinomas of the upper aerodigestive tract – a clinical study based on embryologic data. Eur Arch Otorhinolaryngol 257:561–569

65. Watanabe H, Komiyama S, Soh N, Kudoh S. Metastases to the Rouviere nodes and headache. Auris Nasus Larynx 1985; 12:53–56

66. Maghami EG, Bonyadlou S, Larian B, Borges A, Abemayor E, Lufkin RB (2001) Magnetic resonance imaging-guided fine-needle aspiration biopsies of retropharyngeal lesions. Laryngoscope 111:2218–2224

67. Lam WW, Chan YL, Leung SF, Metreweli C (1997) Retropharyngeal lymphadenopathy in nasopharyngeal carcinoma. Head Neck 19:176–181

68. Miyashita T, Tateno A, Ablimit I, Nakamizo M, Kumazaki T, Yagi T (2003) Ultrasonographic demonstration of retropharyngeal lymph nodes: Preliminary report. Ultrasound Med Biol 29:633–636

69. McLaughlin MP, Mendenhall WM, Mancuso AA, Parsons JT, McCarty PJ, Cassisi NJ, Stringer SP, Tart RP, Mukherji SK, Million RR (1995) Retropharyngeal adenopathy as a predictor of outcome in squamous cell carcinoma of the head and neck. Head Neck 17:190–198

70. Amatsu M, Mohri M, Kinishi M (2001) Significance of retropharyngeal node dissection at radical surgery for carcinoma of the hypopharynx and cervical esophagus. Laryngoscope 111:1099–1103

71. Ballantyne AJ (1964) Significance of retropharyngeal nodes in cancer of the head and neck. Am J Surg 108:500–504

72. Hasegawa Y, Matsuura H (1994) Retropharyngeal node dissection in cancer of the oropharynx and hypopharynx. Head Neck 16:173–180

73. Chen WZ, Zhou DL, Luo KS (1989) Long-term observation after radiotherapy for nasopharyngeal carcinoma (NPC). Int Radiat Oncol Biol Phys 16:311–314

74. O'Brien CJ, Petersen-Schaefer K, Ruark D, Coates AS, Menzie SJ, Harrison RI (1995) Radical, modified, and selective Neck dissection for cutaneous malignant melanoma. Head Neck 17:232–241

75. Singletary SE, Byers RM, Shallenberger R, McBride CM, Guinee UF (1986) Prognostic factors in patients with regional cervical nodal metastases from cutaneous malignant melanoma. Am Surg 152:371–375

76. Hauschild A, Lischner S, Christophers E (2000) Surgical and adjuvant drug therapy in head and neck cutaneous melanoma. Laryngorhinootologie 79:428–433

77. Scherer H (1984) Behandlungsmöglichkeiten des malignen Melanoms des Gaumens, der Nasenhöhle und der Nasennebenhöhlen. Laryngorhinootologie 63:9–10

78. Victor NS, Blaine M, Smith JW (1996) Merkel cell cancer: is prophylactic lymph node dissection indicated? Am Surg 62:879–882

79. Sian KU, Wagner JDW, Sood R, Park HM, Havlik R, Coleman JJ (1999) Lymphoscitigraphy with sentinel lymph node biopsy in cutaneous merkel cell carcinoma. Ann Plast Surg 42:679–68

80. Morrison WH, Peters LJ, Silva EG, Wendt CD, Ang KK, Goepfert H (1990) The essential role of radiation therapy in securing locoregional control of Merkel cell carcinoma. Int J Radiat Oncol Biol Phys 19:583–591

81. Goretzki P, Dotzenrath C (2000) Differenziertes Schilddrüsenkarzinom. In: Rothmund, M. (ed) Endokrine Chirurgie. Springer, Berlin

82. Röher HD, Simon D, Sitte J, Goretzki P (1994) Principals of limited or radical surgery for differentiated thyroid cancer. Thyroidology 5:93

83. Goretzki P, Simon D, Frilling A (1993) Surgical reintervention for differentiated thyroid cancer. Br J Surg 80:1009

84. Gimm O, Ukkat J, Dralle H (1998) Determinative factors of biochemical cure after primary and reoperative surgery for sporadic medullary thyroid carcinoma. World J Surg 22:562–567

85. Gimm O, Dralle H (1997) Reoperation in metastasizing medullary thyroid carcinoma: is tumor stage-oriented approach justified? Surgery 122:1124–1130

86. Robbins KT, Woodson GE (1985) Thyroid carcinoma presenting as a parapharyngeal mass. Head Neck Surg 7:434–436

87. Cabanas RM (1977) An approach for the treatment of penile carcinoma. Cancer 39:456–466

88. Barke R (1983) Farbstoffe. In: Wiljasalo M, Weissleder H (eds) Lymphographie bei malignen Tumoren. Thieme, Stuttgart, 32–33

89. Garzom OL, Palcos MC, Radicella R (1965) Technetium-99m labelled colloid. Int J Appl Radiat Isotopes 16:613

90. Borgstein PJ, Pijpers R, Comans EF, van Diest PJ, Boom RP, Meijer S (1998) Sentinel lymph node biopsy in breast cancer: Guidelines and pitfalls of lymphoscintigraphy and gamma probe detection. J Am Coll Surg 186:275–283

91. Nathanson SD, Nelson L, Karvelis KC (1996) Rates of flow of technetium-99m-labeled human serum from peripheral injection sites to sentinel lymph nodes. Ann Surg Oncol 3:329–335

92. Offodile R, Hoh C, Barsky SH, Nelson SD, Elashoff FR, Eilber FR (1998) Minimally invasive breast carcinoma staging using lymphatic mapping with radiolabeled dextran. Cancer 82:1704–1708

93. Glass EC, Essner R, Guilano A, Morton DL (1995) Comparative efficacy of three lymphoscintigraphic agents. J Nucl Med 36:199

94. Pitman KT, Johnson JT, Edington H, Barnes L, Day R, Wagner RL, Myers EN (1998) Lymphatic mapping with isosulfan blue dye in squamous cell carcinoma of the head and neck. Arch Otolaryngol Head Neck Surg 124:790–793

95. Ross GL, Soutar DS, Shoaib T, Camilleri IG, MacDonald DG, Robertson AG, Bessent RG, Gray HW (2002) The ability of lymphoscintigraphy to direct sentinel node biopsy in the clinically N0 neck for patients with head and neck squamous cell carcinoma. Br J Radiol 75:950–958

96. Longnecker SM, Guzzardo MM, Van Voris LP (1985) Life-threatening anaphylaxis following subcutaneous administration of isosulfan blue 1%. Clin Pharm 4:219–221

97. Plut EM, Hinkle GH, Guo W, Lee RJ (2002) Kit formulation for the preparation of radioactive blue liposomes for sentinel node lymphoscintigraphy. J Pharm Sci 91: 1717–1732

98. Werner JA (1995) Morphologie und Histochemie von Lymphgefässen der oberen Luft- und Speisewege: Eine klinisch orientierte Untersuchung. Laryngorhinootologie 74: 568–576

99. Werner JA, Dünne AA, Ramaswamy A, Folz BJ, Brandt D, Külkens C, Moll R, Lippert BM (2002) Number and location

of radiolabeled, intraoperatively identified Sentinel Nodes in 48 head and neck cancer patients with clinically staged N0 and N1 neck. Eur Arch Oto Rhino Laryngol 259:91–96

100. Dünne AA, Külkens C, Ramaswamy A, Folz BJ, Brandt D, Lippert BM, Behr T, Moll R, Werner JA (2001) Value of sentinel lymphadenectomy in head and neck cancer patients without evidence of lymphogenic metastatic disease. Auris Nasus Larynx 28:339–344

101. Werner JA, Dünne AA, Brandt D, Ramaswamy A, Külkens C, Lippert BM, Folz BJ, Joseph K, Moll R (1999) Untersuchungen zum Stellenwert der Sentinel Lymphonodektomie bei Karzinomen des Pharynx und Larynx. Laryngorhinootologie 78:663–670

102. Werner JA, Dünne AA, Brandt D (2001) Sentinel Lymphonodektomie bei Plattenepithelkarzinomen im Kopf-Hals-Bereich. In: Schlag PM (ed) Sentinel Lymphknoten Biopsie. Ecomed, Landsberg, 129–139

103. Werner JA, Dünne AA, Ramaswamy A, Brandt D, Külkens C, Moll R, Lippert BM (2002) Das Sentinel Node Konzept bei Plattenepithelkarzinomen der oberen Luft- und Speisewege – eine kritische Analyse an 100 Patienten. Laryngorhinootologie 81:31–39

104. Czerniecki BJ, Scheff AM, Callans LS, Spitz FR, Bedrosian I, Conant EF (1999) Immunohistochemistry with pancytokeratins improves the sensitivity of sentinel lymph node biopsy in patients with breast carcinoma. Cancer 85:1098–1103

105. Jansen L Koops HS, Nieweg OE, Doting E, Kapteijn AE, Balm AJM (2000) Sentinel node biopsy for melanoma in the head and neck region. Head Neck 22:272–33

106. Veronesi U, Paganelli G, Viale G, Galimberti V, Luini A, Zurrida S (1999) Sentinel lymph node biopsy and axillary dissection in breast cancer: results in large series. J Natl Cancer Inst 91:368–373

107. Yu LL, Flotte TJ, Tanabe KK, Gadd MA, Cosimi AB, Sober AJ (1999) Detection of microscopic melanoma metastases in sentinel lymph nodes. Cancer 86:617–627

108. Colnot, DR, Nieuwenhuis EJC, Castelijns JA, Pijpers R, Brakenhoff RH, Snow GB (1999) Ultrasound guided aspiration of sentinel nodes for improved staging of head and neck cancer patients. Eur J Nucl Med 26:70

109. van den Brekel MW, Reitsma LC, Quak JJ, Smeele LE, van der Linden JC, Snow GB, Castelijns JA (1999) Sonographically guided aspiration cytology of neck nodes for selection of treatment and follow-up in patients with N0 head and neck cancer. Am J Neuroradiol 20:1727–1731

110. Dünne AA, Jungclas H, Werner JA (2001) Intraoperative sentinel node biopsy in patients with squamous cell carcinomas of the head and neck-experiences using a well-type NaI detector for gamma ray spectroscopy. Otolaryngol Pol 55:127–134

111. Werner JA, Dünne AA, Ramaswamy A, Folz BJ, Lippert BM, Moll R, Behr T (2002) Sentinel node detection in N0 cancer of the pharynx and larynx. Br J Cancer 87:711–715

112. Shdanov DA (1932) Röntgenologische Untersuchungsmethoden des Lymphgefässsystems des Menschen und der Tiere. Fortschr. Röntgenstr. 46:680

113. Alex JC, Sasaki CT, Krag DN, Wenig B, Pyle PB (2000) Sentinel lymph node radiolocalization in head and neck squamous cell carcinoma. Laryngoscope 110:198–203

114. Barzan L, Sulfaro S, Albert F, Politi D, Marus W, Pin M, Savignano MG (2002) Gamma probe accuracy in detecting the sentinel lymph node in clinically N0 squamous cell carcinoma of the head and neck. Ann Otol Rhinol Laryngol 111:794–798

115. Bilde A, von Buchwald C, Dreyer M, Eigtved AI (2002) Sentinel node biopsy in head and neck cancer. Is there an indication for use of this new surgical technique in the treatment of head and neck cancer? Ugeskr Laeger 164:4276–4280

116. Chiesa F, Mauri S, Grana C, Tradati N, Calabrese L, Ansarin M, Mazzarol G, Paganelli G (2000) Is there a role for sentinel node biopsy in early N0 tongue tumors? Surgery 128:16–21

117. Civantos FJ, Gomez C, Duque C, Pedroso F, Goodwin WJ, Weed DT, Arnold D, Moffat F (2003) Sentinel node biopsy in oral cavity cancer: Correlation with PET scan and immunohistochemistry. Head Neck 25:1–9

118. Hyde N, Prvulovich E (2002) Is there a role for lymphoscintigraphy and sentinel node biopsy in the management of the regional lymphatics in mucosal squamous cell carcinoma of the head and neck? Eur J Nucl Med 29:579–584

119. Ionna F, Chiesa F, Longo F, Manola M, Villano S, Calabrese L, Lastoria S, Mozzillo N (2002) Prognostic value of sentinel node in oral cancer. Tumori 88:S18–19

120. Nieuwenhuis EJ, Castelijns JA, Pijpers R, van den Brekel MW, Brakenhoff RH, van der Waal I, Snow GB, Leemans CR (2002) Wait-and-see policy for the N0 neck in early-stage oral and oropharyngeal squamous cell carcinoma using ultrasonography-guided cytology: is there a role for identification of the sentinel node? Head Neck 24:282–289

121. Ross G, Shoaib T, Soutar DS, Camilleri IG, Gray HW, Bessent RG, Robertson AG, MacDonald DG (2002) The use of sentinel node biopsy to upstage the clinically N0 neck in head and neck cancer. Arch Otolaryngol Head Neck Surg 128:1287–1291

122. Von Buchwald C, Bilde A, Shoaib T, Ross G (2002) Sentinel node biopsy: the technique and the feasibility in head and neck cancer. ORL J Otorhinolaryngol Relat Spec 64:268–274

123. Zitsch RP 3rd, Todd DW, Renner GJ, Singh A (2000) Intraoperative radiolymphoscintigraphy for detection of occult nodal metastasis in patients with head and neck squamous cell carcinoma. Otolaryngol Head Neck Surg 122:662–666

124. Shoaib T, Soutar DS, Prossar JE, Dunaway DJ, Gray HW, McCurrach GM (1999) A suggested method for sentinel node Biopsie in squamous cell carcinoma of the head and neck. Head Neck 21:728–733

125. Hosemann W, Kühnel T, Burchard AK, Werner JA (1998) Histochemical detection of drainage pathways in the middle nasal meatus. Rhinology 36:50–54
126. Werner JA (1995) Untersuchungen zum Lymphgefässsystem von Mundhöhle und Rachen. Laryngorhinootologie 74:622–628
127. Ferlito A, Shaha AR, Rinaldo A, Pellitteri PK, Mondin V, Byers RM (2002) "Skip metastases" from head and neck cancers. Acta Otolaryngol 122:788–791
128. Finn S, Toner M, Timon C (2002) The node-negative neck: accuracy of clinical intraoperative lymph node assessment for metastatic disease in head and neck cancer. Laryngoscope 112:630–633
129. Jose J, Coatesworth AP, MacLennan K (2003) Cervical metastases in upper aerodigestive tract squamous cell carcinoma: histopathologic analysis and reporting. Head Neck 25:194–197

Complications

8.1 Surgical Complications

8.1.1 General Considerations

In about 1% of the cases, radical neck dissection (RND) leads to a fatal outcome [1]. The mortality for simultaneous bilateral RND amounts to 17%, which is reduced to 3.2% in cases of RND performed in two sessions. When two sessions are used, bilateral RND is also associated with fewer complications [2–4]. After ND, there is a peak in the mortality rate during the first 3 days. The exact mechanism of this sudden incidence of death remains unclear [5].

Prevention. In order to reduce the surgery-associated complications of ND, several precautions should be taken. Undoubtedly, the complication rate is directly related to the indication. It is well known that previous radiotherapy leads to increased risk of postoperative wound healing impairment. This knowledge is the reason for special attention to careful wound control and early care for probable wound dehiscence. Not only exogenous but also endogenous factors, such as existing diabetes mellitus, are related to an increased risk of postoperative wound healing impairment. A thorough knowledge of possible complications must be included in the planning of the treatment. Although problems cannot be totally avoided, their extent can be reduced. Finally, clear preoperative communication between the surgeon and patient leads to appropriate informed consent and a healthy relationship in spite of probable morbidity.

    Beyond the general considerations involved in any surgical procedure, there are certain special considerations unique to ND which must be mentioned and which can often avoid unintentional damage to anatomic structures. These include the careful identification of the spinal accessory nerve, which frequently runs superficially, and the avoidance of exaggerated retraction of this nerve when dissecting on or through the sternocleidomastoid muscle in its middle and upper segments. Also, the marginal branch of the facial nerve must be protected from damage during dissection of region I, the neural supply of the levator muscle of the scapula must be conserved and the branches reaching into the skin of the cervical plexus must be ligated or coagulated in order to reduce the risk of developing a neuroma. Finally, the sympathetic trunk and the superior laryngeal nerve must be preserved in dissection behind the carotid artery. When levels IV and V are dissected, it is important to clamp the fatty tissue containing lymph nodes before dividing this tissue, and then to place suture ligatures in order to avoid chylus fistulae. When the oral cavity or pharynx is opened to the neck, skin sutures should not be continuous.

For quality control, optimized postoperative control and early rehabilitation, a special documentation sheet that the surgeon must fill out at the end of the neck dissection is very appropriate.

8.1.2 Preoperative Informed Consent

Possible complications should be discussed in an open and extensive preoperative consultation with the patient. The patient must be informed about the probability of both minor and serious complications and provided with information on the possibilities of their control. Clearly, the consultation for any neck dissection procedure is best performed by experienced surgeons.

8.1.3 Wound Healing Impairment

Incidence. For all extended surgical interventions of the neck, the danger of developing a fistula amounts to about 13% [6]. With preoperative radiotherapy, the risk of wound healing impairment increases consid-

erably [7, 8]. Specific risks include increased vulnerability of the vessels during dissection, slowed hemostasis due to reduced vascular contraction and a higher risk of local infections and wound dehiscences. Because of these factors, postoperative radiation is generally recommended instead of preoperative radiotherapy.

When RND is done alone, the incidence of oropharyngo-cutaneous fistulae is very low. With the simultaneous resection of oral carcinomas, this rate increases to 6%, and in cases of simultaneous laryngectomy, it can be as high as 40% [9].

8.1.4 Vascular System

Two significant vascular complications that require special attention are thrombosis of the internal jugular vein and postoperative rupture of the carotid artery.

Non-elective ligation of the carotid artery results in a 50% incidence of stroke and a mortality rate of about 38%. Elective ligation of the carotid artery is associated with a 23% risk of stroke and a 17% mortality rate [10, 11]. When the carotid artery is ligated, low-dose heparin should be started at the forty-eighth hour postoperatively (▶ Table 8.1). In this way, an embolism originating from a distally localized thrombus can be avoided [12].

Intraoperative Damage of Major Vessels. Damage to larger veins can lead to an air embolism [13]. Negative pressure, allowing penetration of air into a cervical vein, causes the air embolism. In the event of accidental opening of a large vein, the open area should be compressed immediately and the patient brought into the Trendelenburg position. Additionally, ventilation with increased pressure must be applied until the perforation can be identified and definitively treated. In any case of inadvertent opening of a large vein, the anesthesiologist must be informed immediately. For treatment of intravascular air, the patient can be rotated to the left so that the air reaches the right atrium. The air can then be removed via a central venous catheter [1]. There are also reports of venous air embolisms occurring after the removal of

Table 8.1. Treatment of intraoperatively occurring complications during performance of neck dissection

Complication	Recommended action
Threatened complication	
Damage to sympathetic trunk	Avoidance of preparation posterior to carotid artery
Damage to brachial plexus	Identification of deep neck fascia
Chylus fistula	Wide resection of lymph-node-containing fatty tissue of regions IV and V
Actual complication	
Injury of subclavian vein	Resection of medial third of clavicle
Resection of carotid artery	Postoperative low-dose heparin
Opening of a major vein	Immediate compression
	Trendelenburg position
	Positive-pressure ventilation
Injury of accessory nerve	Conservation of motor fibers C_2–C_4

the axillary nodes. In order to avoid such events, a tourniquet can be placed on the respective area for 24 hours after removing these lymphatics [14]. In the event of damage to the subclavian vein or other vessels situated below the clavicle, the surgeon should not hesitate to resect the medial third of the clavicle in order to have better access. It is important to mention that not all operating rooms are necessarily equipped with the potentially necessary rib scissors (N. Bethune 340mm, Aesculap FB 878R, Tuttlingen, Germany) that allow for rapid resection of the medial third of the clavicle.

Thrombus of the Internal Jugular Vein. The risk of developing a thrombus of the internal jugular vein can be reduced by avoiding, as much as possible, mechanical damage to the intima of the vessel. Another potential complication results from the ligation of vascular branches, which can lead to sacculations, where blood clots can develop. Surgical removal of the adventitia results in the devascularization of the vascular wall with an increased risk of transmural vascular damage. Finally, care must be taken to avoid dissection of the venous surface during the operation process [15]. Following SND, long-term internal jugular vein occlusion has to be considered an exceedingly rare event [16].

Postoperative Rupture of the Carotid Artery or Internal Jugular Vein. Patients who have a complete circumferential dissection of the internal jugular vein low in the neck and go on to have fistulas develop may be more prone to internal jugular vein rupture [17]. Postoperative rupture of the carotid artery occurs in about 3–7 % of all patients who undergo RND in connection with resection of laryngeal, pharyngeal or oral cavity carcinoma [14, 18–20]. This dramatic event can occur as a result of thrombosis of the vasa vasorum caused by surgical removal of the surrounding tissue, desiccation or salivary drainage on the vessel, or by radiotherapy. Ruptures of the carotid artery occur very rarely without preceding wound healing impairment. In the event of overlying flap necrosis with exposure of the carotid artery, it is necessary to cover this area with a myocutaneous flap as soon as possible [21]. This condition has been described in an analysis by Maran et al. [8]. Carotid artery rupture occurred in 17 of 394 patients treated with RND and led to a fatal outcome in all cases. Fifteen of these seventeen patients had wound infections (82.2 %), compared with a wound infection rate of only 10.3 % in patients without rupture of the carotid artery. This difference is of statistical significance. Fourteen of 17 patients were treated preoperatively with radiotherapy, and seven of the 17 patients had a lymph node recurrence at the time of artery rupture. In the event of a perceived danger of impending postoperative rupture of the carotid artery, vessel ligation must evaluated.

8.1.5 Neural Impairment

Neural damage leading to functional impairment is the most frequent complication of ND. The nerves at risk are discussed below.

Accessory Nerve. The transection of the spinal accessory nerve often leads to the so-called shoulder syndrome first described by Nahum [22] (▶ Fig. 8.1). This occurs in up to 70 % of the patients treated with ND [23, 24]. In a follow-up study of 46 patients who had undergone RND, Shone and Yardley showed that 46 % of these patients had to resign from their jobs because of severe shoulder problems, whereas 30 % suffered from moderate to severe pain in this area [25]. In order to compensate for or to prevent these problems, several techniques have been recommended, including the transplantation of the levator muscle of the scapula and fixation of the scapula via a fascial loop [26], as well as the basic procedure for re-anastomosing check the neural stumps via free neural transplantation [27]. Weitz and co-workers [28] described a technique for conserving the function of the trapezius muscle in the event of RND. The technique takes into consideration the double innervation of the mentioned muscle from the accessory nerve and from motor fibers from C_2–C_4.

The most important measure, however, seems to be intensive physical therapy [6]. When resection or conservation of the accessory nerve is considered, it must be realized that conservation of the nerve cannot always guarantee undisturbed postoperative function of the shoulder [23]. In spite of careful protection during dissection to preserve the accessory nerve, up to 60 % of the patients develop shoulder symptoms [29, 30]. Preservation of the nerve nonetheless results in significantly greater muscle strength, compared with transection of the nerve [31]. Concerning the intraoperative neuromonitoring of the facial nerve in lateral parotidectomies or extirpation of the submandibular gland, various groups

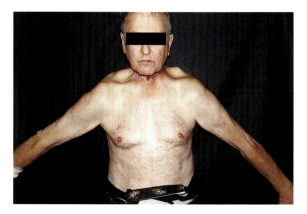

Figure 8.1

Shoulder arm syndrome with inability to lift the arm beyond 90° as a consequence of a bilateral neck dissection (radical and modified radical neck dissection)

are working on the development of intraoperative electromyography for the accessory nerve [32, 33]. The physical basis for the stimulation and dissipation procedure must be defined, and the intraoperative electromyography procedure must be performed with a view of lessening the otherwise probable outcome of postoperative paralysis [32]. Further steps to lessen accessory nerve injury include location of the nerve in the upper neck as it exits the sternocleidomastoid muscle, versus in the lower posterior neck, and the avoidance of paralysis during surgery.

Hypoglossal Nerve. Very seldom has bilateral transection of the hypoglossal nerve been observed. This terrible complication nearly always necessitates placement of a PEG (percutaneous endoscopic gastrostomy) tube, and even laryngectomy in cases of chronic aspiration [14].

Brachial Plexus. The performance of ND can also lead to damage of the brachial plexus. In order to avoid this complication, the level of the deep cervical fascia that overlays the brachial plexus must be identified before clamping the supraclavicular fatty tissue.

Sympathetic Trunk and Superior Laryngeal Nerve. The risk of damaging the sympathetic trunk, and the resulting development of a Horner's syndrome, increases for dissections performed behind the carotid artery. The classic Horner's syndrome includes ptosis, miosis and enophthalmos. Additionally, similar deep dissection behind the carotid artery can lead to damage to the superior laryngeal nerve and the resultant loss of ipsilateral cricothyroid muscle function and superior laryngeal sensation.

Phrenic Nerve. Iatrogenic injury to the phrenic nerve occurs in about 8 % of ND [34]. Bilateral injury to this nerve would lead to severe respiratory problems. In order to avoid damage to the phrenic nerve or to the motor branches of the levator scapula muscle, these nerves should be dissected and the sensory branches transected at a distance of at least 1cm from where they emerge from between the anterior and middle scalene muscle. In light of the potential risk of injury to the mentioned nerves, the recommendation of Awengen and Donald [35] should be considered. In their opinion, every patient undergoing ND should receive a postoperative chest x-ray to rule out paralysis of the phrenic nerve, as evidenced by diaphragm elevation, and to also rule out pneumothorax or atelectasis. To lessen radiation exposure and cost, in our opinion, a clinical examination performing auscultation and percussion after ND should be performed to diagnose these potential complications before ordering radiologic tests.

8.1.6 Vasovagal Response

Manipulation of the pressure receptors situated in the wall of the carotid bulb can elicit bradycardia, hypotension and/or cardiac arrhythmia. Babin and Panje determined that the incidence of the vasovagal response in 76 cases of RND was about 10 % [36]. The topical application of 2 % lidocaine solution is not adequate prophylaxis to avoid vasovagal response during RND. Manipulations of the pressure receptors of the carotid bulb has been reported to result in patient deaths during neck dissection [37].

8.1.7 Chylus Fistula and Chylothorax

Chylus Fistula. The anatomy of the terminal part of the thoracic duct reveals a large variability. According to Greenfield and Gottlieb [38], the thoracic duct drains in about 50 % of the cases as a single channel at the lateral side of the venous angle between the internal jugular and subclavian veins into the venous system. In about one-third of the cases, however, it drains directly into the subclavian vein. Kinnaert [7] indicated that, in only 13 % of the cases, an isolated lymphatic channel exists, whereas, in 66 % of the cases, multiple lymphatic channels can be found that drain into a common terminal vessel joining the venous system and, in 21 % of the cases, multiple lymphatic channels drain separately into the venous system.

The thoracic duct emerges from the upper mediastinum behind the common carotid artery and the left subclavian artery into the deep inferior neck. This cervical duct describes an arc (▶ Fig. 8.2), in which it is situated between the anterior scalene muscle and the internal jugular vein on the deep cervical fascia below the phrenic nerve. The duct courses in front of the thyrocervical trunk in an arcuate line in the direction of the left venous angle [39, 40]. As a rule of thumb, it can be said that the thoracic duct emerges about 2cm above the venous angle into the venous system. Accordingly, the mentioned arcuate line of the duct can be expected 3–5cm above the clavicle [40].

The risk of developing a chylus fistula after RND amounts to about 1–2.5 % of all cases. This occurs on the left side 75–92 % of the time [41]. Preoperative radiotherapy increases the risk of developing a chylus fistula [42]. The accumulation of chyle can lead to a lifting of the neck flaps, often with an intense erythematous reaction and occasionally orocutaneous fistulae, as well as exposure of the carotid artery to the risk of postoperative rupture [40].

During dissection of the neck regions IV and V, it is recommended that the fatty tissue containing lymph nodes be generously ligated in order to avoid the development of a chyle fistula [12]. Ligation is also required when lymph channels are unintentional-

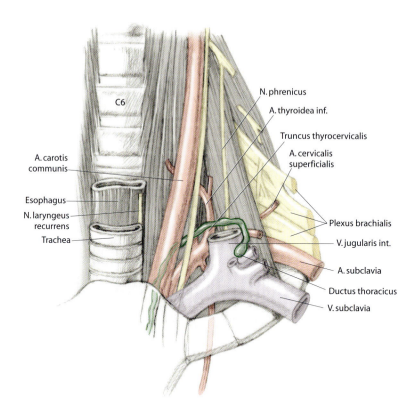

A. carotis communis

Esophagus

N. laryngeus recurrens

Trachea

C6

N. phrenicus

A. thyroidea inf.

Truncus thyrocervicalis

A. cervicalis superficialis

Plexus brachialis

V. jugularis int.

A. subclavia

Ductus thoracicus

V. subclavia

Figure 8.2

Schematized description of the cervical direction of the thoracic duct

ly divided during surgery. Bipolar or monopolar cautery of lymph vessels is discouraged. Great attention must be given to the identification and control of all lymphatic channels. After deep dissection, the neck must be carefully examined for leaks during and at the end of dissection. Use of the Valsalva maneuver by anesthesia is helpful in identifying some leaks. Final neck closure should not be done until careful observation and use of these techniques is complete.

Despite great caution, there are cases where chyle leaks are not recognized or where the chyle fistula can only be identified postoperatively. Since 1875, when the first description of accidental injury to the thoracic duct was reported, the optimal treatment concept for a chyle fistula is still controversial [43]. Whereas many surgeons thought at the beginning of the 19th century that ligature of the thoracic duct was potentially life-threatening, Stuart [44] concluded in a follow-up description of 14 patients, who nevertheless had undergone treatment of a chyle fistula by ligation of the thoracic duct, that ligature should be performed when a chyle fistula could not be controlled by initial compression. In the following years, several studies were able to demonstrate that after ligation of the thoracic duct, a contralateral vascular formation occurs that assures the re-circulation of lymph fluid into the venous system [40]. Up until the 1970s, various authors recommended operative ligature of the thoracic duct accompanied by rotation of a flap taken from the anterior scalene muscle as the therapy of choice in the treatment of postoperative chylus fistulae [45, 46]. Only in later years have other authors indicated that operative intervention should only be performed in cases where conservative compression measures could not achieve a spontaneous closure of the chylus fistula [40, 47].

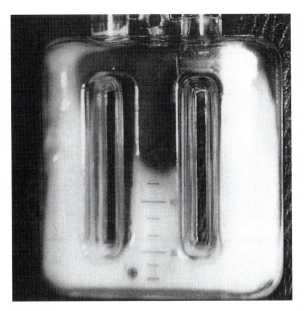

Figure 8.3

Drainage bottle with typical milky chyle

Currently, specific conservative therapy can be used in most of the cases to successfully treat a postoperative chylus fistula. Exact monitoring of the chyle quantity (▶ Fig. 8.3) and hematocrit, radiographic studies of the thorax, urinalysis and evaluation of liver function tests, electrolytes and serum proteins, including serum albumin, are necessary. Small fistulae can be treated conservatively by reducing chyle production through the nutritional use of middle chain triglycerides. Parenteral hyperalimentation does not seem reasonable because of the cost. Conservative treatment measures for chylus fistulae should be limited to a maximum of 30 days in order to start scheduled postoperative radiotherapy in a timely manner. Patients with therapy-resistant hypoalbuminemia, or patients who suffer from a chylus fistula that produces more than 600 ml in 24 hours, should undergo surgical revision [41].

Finally, for the sake of completeness, it should be mentioned that another alternative to surgical exploration, sclerotherapy with tetracycline, has been performed successfully in the therapy of a postoperative chylus fistula. This method takes advantage of the fact that a local inflammatory process leads to a sclerosis of the open thoracic duct with the surrounding tissue and, thus, to closure of the chylus fistula. Due to possible paralytic irritations of neighboring neural structures, e.g., the phrenic nerve, this treatment concept is very controversial. This concept may, on rare occasion, be considered where exposure of the thoracic duct is extremely difficult [40].

Chylothorax. Division of the right thoracic duct can lead to the development of a bilateral chylothorax [14]. The right accessory thoracic duct is intrathoracic and inferior to the subclavian artery, which generally protects it from injury during RND. Chylothorax is a serious complication which produces both cardio-respiratory and metabolic effects.

The *cardio-respiratory effect* can be explained by a mechanic alteration. The accumulation of liquids leads to lung compression, with a resulting reduction of vital capacity and displacement of the mediastinum with a so-called kinking of the great vessels. The *metabolic effect* consists in a loss of lymph fluid, together with a loss of electrolytes, including calcium, in addition to proteins, fat, liposoluble vitamins and circulating lymphocytes [48].

The therapy for a bilateral chylothorax consists of repeated thoracocentesis, a fat-depleted diet and, usually, intravenous liquids and electrolytes. Ligature of the thoracic duct should be performed only in cases where conservative therapy fails [49].

8.1.8 Increased Intracranial Pressure

Increased intracranial pressure is a well-documented complication of bilateral RND, which – although it is most commonly seen in cases of simultaneous bilateral operations – can also occur with RND performed in two sessions [50], as well as with unilateral ND [51].

Bilateral ligation of the internal jugular vein leads to a direct and drastic increase of venous flow through the vertebral plexus, which is not able to drain such a quantity immediately. The inner part of the vertebral plexus fills the space between the dura and bony spinal canal, and the outer part of the venous plexus is situated deeply in the area of the muscles of the neck and the back, communicating with the thoracic and abdominal veins. In addition to the direct communication between the inner and outer parts of the vertebral plexus, the intracranial and extracranial vascular systems are connected via the emissary veins and the diploic veins. In addition, the veins of the orbit and the veins situated in the region of the foramina of the skull base allow some cerebral egress.

Intracranial pressure achieves its maximum level about 30 minutes after internal jugular vein ligation is performed at the level of the clavicle [50]. The increase of flow-in resistance of the cerebral arteries in the context of a reduced venous drainage can explain the postoperative neurological symptoms in patients who already have an exhausted perfusion reserve [19]. Jackson and Stell indicate that the occurrence of symptoms that increase intracranial pressure, such as rising blood pressure and decreasing heart rate, justifies the intravenous use of mannitol [52].

In cases of postoperatively persisting headaches and nausea, even after unilaterally performed RND, increased intracranial pressure must be considered. Development of tinnitus can also indicate an increase in intracranial pressure [53].

At least nine cases of intracranial increase in pressure after unilateral ND have been described [29]. Eight of these nine patients had undergone surgery on the right side. In this context, it is interesting to note that anatomic studies have shown that in the majority of cases the right jugular foramen and right sigmoid sinus are larger than on the left side [54].

8.1.9 Visual Loss and Blindness

Vision reduction after RND is a rare but very serious complication that occurs mostly after bilateral RND. This unusual complication of bilateral cortical blindness has been reported following unilateral ND [55]. In a review of the literature, Marks et al. [21] found that four patients out of 935 suffered from blindness after bilateral RND. Two of these cases occurred after simultaneous RND and two cases after staged RNDs. Intraoperative hypotension, with the resulting risk of

infarction of the occipital lobe, must be mentioned as a risk for visual loss [21]. The ophthalmic veins are considered to be an important component of the collateral circulation. That these veins are certainly involved is evidenced by the fact that patients generally develop serious facial edema and cyanosis. Due to the increased pressure, the ophthalmic arteries can be poorly perfused.

A vision reduction after RND is not necessarily permanent. Jackson and Stell [52] reported on a patient who underwent staged RND. This patient suffered from severe postoperative lymphedema and an almost complete visual loss after the second surgery. However, vision returned to normal in two weeks.

In the event of vision reduction that does not result from macular edema, surgical decompression of the optic nerve should be performed [56]. If there is an increase in intracranial pressure and vision loss after unilateral RND, a subtemporal decompression may lead to a partial vision recovery.

Finally, a case of papilledema without visual loss must be mentioned. In a 51-year-old man treated by staged bilateral RND (nine months between the two surgeries), the papilledema disappeared completely within three and a half months [51].

8.1.10 Lymphedema

Lymphedema is a consequence of insufficiency of the lymphatic system. A primary and secondary form can be differentiated.

- *Primary* lymphedema develops in the context of lymphatic malformations, such as aplasia (either hypo- or hyperplasia) [57].
- *Secondary* lymphedema occurs after mechanical impact or trauma, and from disease states such as inflammatory processes and tumor infiltration.

The extent of lymphedema in the head and neck region is mainly determined by the conserved venous collateral circulation. In the head and neck region, numerous vascular collaterals between the valveless, low-pressure systems can be found that allow reflux [53].

The well-documented lymphedemas that occur postoperatively after ND develop due to lymphatic interruptions or to lymphatic stasis that occurs after lymph node resections. Those lymphedemas are made worse by additional radiotherapy because the lymph vessels have to undergo the strain of increased resorption and transport. Furthermore, more cellular debris and cells elicited from cell aggregation must be transported. Additionally, the lymphatic drainage must be intensified because of the increased interstitial level of liquids and proteins occurring after damage to the blood capillaries. Surpassing the lymphogenic transportation capacity leads to the development of an interstitial edema. During radiotherapy, some of the bracing filaments that are important for inter-endothelial junctions are lost [13], which significantly disturbs the interaction between the vascular wall and surrounding tissue, which is necessary to decompress the increased interstitial pressure. This may result in the development of secondary lymphedema.

Frequently, facial edema (▶ Fig. 8.4) is at its maximum after 72 to 96 hours, [13] and it regresses after 7–10 days. The lymphedemas of the pharynx or supraglottis observed after simultaneous bilateral ND [10] may lead to a respiratory obstruction that, in some cases, requires a temporary tracheotomy. This can even occur with staged neck dissections. Therefore, for simultaneous bilateral RND with resection of both internal jugular veins, a protective tracheotomy is recommended [50, 58]. The advent of endolaryngeal CO_2 laser surgery has provided a method that can be used to avoid tracheotomy, in very select cases, by excising voluminous mucosal tissues.

Reconstruction of the internal jugular vein can reduce complications accompanying simultaneous bilateral RND with resection of both internal jugular veins [59]. Depending on the localization of the lymph node metastases, as well as on the full venous system, three different types of reconstruction of the internal jugular vein are possible. The so-called type A is applied in the event of lymph node metastasis localized cranially and medio-jugularly, provided a sufficiently long external jugular vein is available. The external jugular vein is removed in the region of the parotid gland and anastomosed directly end-to-end

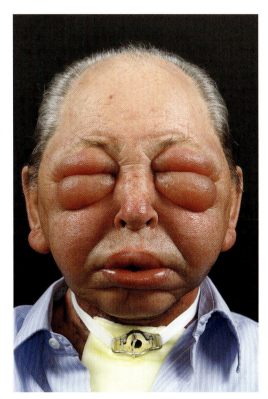

Figure 8.4

Severe lymphedema after bilateral neck dissection and postoperative radiochemotherapy

with the cranial stub of the internal jugular vein. If the external jugular vein is not available, then a type B reconstruction is performed. This involves interposing the great saphenous vein between the upper and lower stubs of the internal jugular vein. In the event of inferior jugular lymph node metastasis, a type C reconstruction is performed. In this situation, the great saphenous vein is directly anastomosed end-to-end with the cranial stub of the internal jugular vein and the caudal stub of the external jugular vein. In each of the three reconstruction types, systemic heparinization is started prior to vascular anastomosis in order to avoid thrombosis. The patency of the venous interposition should be verified postoperatively by duplex sonography.

8.1.11 Clavicular Fracture

After RND, sternoclavicular abnormalities may occur [60] that can be described, in many cases, as subluxations in different directions up to a torsion-like rotation of the clavicle. When the sternocleidomastoid muscle is absent, the cranially directed tension is missing. This leads to an imbalanced caudal tension in the subclavius muscle, the greater pectoral muscle and the deltoid muscle [61]. The resulting transformed biomechanical situation is mainly responsible for the complications already mentioned in the sternoclavicular region.

Postoperative spontaneous clavicular fractures (▶ Fig. 8.5), which may even require claviculectomy, can be caused by radiation therapy damage to capillary vessels [62] or by a surgical devascularization of the clavicle, with resulting aseptic bone necrosis [63]. Developing scar tissue can appear as a pseudotumor. Bizarre exostoses of the clavicle are also known to occur. In some cases, after clavicular fracture in the presence of severe scarring, extended contractions in the region of the shoulder occur and result in significant functional impairment. The scarring and contractions after ND (▶ Fig. 8.6) cause problems esthetically as well as functionally. Incisions performed according to the skin tension line can frequently avoid such scarring.

Finally, the development of myositis ossificans as a consequence of RND must be mentioned. A surgical correction should be performed after six months at the earliest to give this process enough time for "maturing."

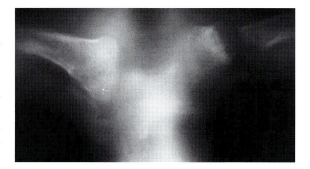

Figure 8.5

Spontaneous clavicular fracture after neck dissection and postoperative radiochemotherapy

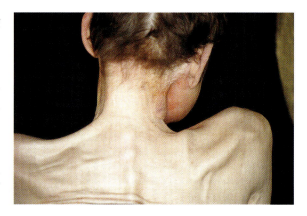

Figure 8.6

Severe shoulder contraction after clavicular fracture and development of massive scars as a consequence of radical neck dissection

8.1.12 Postoperative Care

The postoperative follow-up of patients having undergone uni- or bilateral neck dissection is basically the same as for more extended tumor surgical interventions. However, there are clinical indications of possible complications that must be recognized as early as possible. Among these is postoperative hypertension with simultaneous decreased heart rate as a possible hint of cerebral edema. Nausea and headache can also be signs of increased intracranial pressure. Indications of the so-called vasovagal reflex can include a reduced heart rate, cardiac arrhythmia and hypotension. Additionally, postoperative bleeding may occur and lead to swelling or even cyanosis of cervical soft tissue, not to mention pain, pressure sensations and increased collateral blood flow. Hypotension and tachycardia occur in cases of more severe bleeding and requires immediate surgical revision and possible transfusion. Swelling of neck flaps can accompany the development of a postoperative chyle fistula and also cause pain and pressure, but without hypotension or tachycardia.

8.2 Complications from Radiation Therapy

The effects from radiation therapy on normal tissues can be divided into two major categories: early effects which occur during and immediately after a course of radiotherapy; and late effects which may occur months to many years after radiation. Early effects tend to be treatable and for the most part reversible, while late effects are often progressive and irreversible. The pathologic changes that occur in normal tissues have been well described by Fajardo [64] and Mettler [65]. Acute injury is often due to parenchymal cell loss and injury, while late effects are more commonly due to injury of the vasculoconnective tissue [66].

Damage to normal tissues is related to the total dose of radiation, the daily fractionation (or hyperfractionation) and the volume irradiated, as well as to the differing normal tissue tolerances. Empirically, the daily dose of radiation is decreased if the volume irradiated is large, and it may be increased if the volume is very small. In general, the early and late effects from radiation occur from directly or indirectly killing target cells, although this is a highly complex process involving cellular signaling cascades, radiation-inducible gene expression and compensatory proliferative responses and apoptosis, as well as necrosis and clonogenic death [67].

8.2.1 Clinically Evident Acute Toxicities

Acute toxicities are related to the volume and organs irradiated, the daily fractionation and the total dose. Acute toxicity is intensified both in frequency and severity by the addition of concomitant chemotherapy [68–72] and with hyperfractionated radiation [73]. The addition of a brachytherapy boost may also increase local toxicity.

With irradiation of large volumes of tissue in the head and neck, a number of acute toxicities occur. The skin will develop erythema and can progress to moist desquamation especially around the pinna of the ear (if treated). Hair (or beard) loss will occur in the irradiated field after 2–3 weeks of treatment. Mucositis and dysphagia can lead to significant weight loss and require dietary changes (a soft bland diet) or even support by enteral feedings (either naso-duodenal or via gastrostomy tube). Acute pain from these conditions can usually be managed by narcotic analgesics or topical anesthetics. Saliva will become thick and ropy with markedly decreased fluidity. Taste bud function will be altered (in part by decreased salivary function). Often all foods take on a bland or flavorless taste. Both bacterial and more commonly fungal infections can occur, making good oral hygiene critical for the patient undergoing radiation to the head and neck area. The addition of concomitant chemotherapy has been associated with neutropenia and even the rare acute neutropenic death (3 % in the RTOG-5).

Patients undergoing either radiotherapy or chemoradiation (post-operatively or as primary treatment) for head and neck cancer are often already debilitated and have significant preexisting comorbidities. This results in an increased need for acute management during radiation. Nutritional support is extremely important throughout treatment, as these patients have often lost significant weight either because of the cancer or surgery before radiation is initiated.

If radiotherapy is needed, it should be initiated as early as possible in the treatment course. Liberal use of narcotic and non-narcotic analgesics may be used, as indicated above, for pain management. Pre-radiation dental and periodontal evaluations and institution of oral hygiene and dental prophylaxis will reduce the severity of oral complications.

8.2.2 Delayed Radiation Effects

Perhaps the most common and symptomatically bothersome result of radiation to the oral cavity and head and neck region is xerostomia. Virtually all patients will have some degree of xerostomia if the parotid glands are included in the radiation field. A dose of less than 52 Gy will result in chronic xerostomia in 50 % of patients, while doses less than 33 Gy will result in subacute xerostomia, with half the of the patients recovering in the first 6 months [74]. Symptomatically, xerostomia itself leads to a number of other long term complaints, including changes in taste (75 % of patients), dysphagia (63%), altered speech (51%), difficulty using dentures (49%) and dental decay (31%) [75].

The use of intensity-modulated radiotherapy (IMRT) in the treatment of head and neck cancers can potentially lessen the dose to the parotid glands. Mean dose thresholds needed to reduce stimulated and unstimulated salivary flow to less than 25% of pretreatment baseline are 26Gy and 24Gy, respectively [76]. Chao et al. have also demonstrated a reduction in stimulated saliva flow by less than 25% if both parotid glands receive a mean dose of 32Gy or less [77].

Pilocarpine, a parasympathomimetic drug, has been approved by the FDA as a sialogogue. Typical dosing begins at 5mg three times per day and can be titrated according to symptom relief. Studies by Johnson et al. [78] and LeVeque et al. [79] have demonstrated some symptomatic relief in approximately 50% of patients experiencing radiation-induced xerostomia. Conversely, it has not been shown to be beneficial in patients whose parotid glands were irradiated to tumoricidal doses [80]. Because pilocarpine stimulates the parts of the salivary glands that are not fully irradiated, it may be most beneficial in patients who have some salivary gland sparing in their radiation ports.

Amifostine is a free radical scavenger and radioprotectant which shows promise in reducing acute mucositis and long term xerostomia. Brizel and colleagues conducted a randomized study of conventional radiotherapy with and without amifostine [81]. The incidence of grade 2 or higher xerostomia (using RTOG criteria) was reduced from 78% to 51% (p < 0.001). The local regional control does not appear to have been compromised in this relatively small study.

Amifostine is FDA approved for the prevention of xerostomia and off-label use to decrease acute mucositis.

Subcutaneous and oropharyngeal fibrosis, usually associated with mucosal atrophy, can occur, especially at doses exceeding 70Gy. Soft tissue necrosis occurs in 5–10% of patients receiving doses in excess of 70Gy [82]. Fortunately, the majority of these will heal spontaneously or with conservative management.

More severe cases may benefit from hyperbaric oxygen treatment by increasing the oxygenation of the injured tissues. One must exercise particular caution with IMRT, as significant "hot spots" may occur which can lead to a higher risk of soft tissue injury.

Osteoradionecrosis is most commonly felt to be a complication of interstitial implants of either the tongue or, more commonly, the floor of mouth. Mazeron and colleagues [83] noted a 3% risk of grade 2 osteonecrosis (requiring antibiotics and steroids) and a 7% incidence of grade 3 osteonecrosis (requiring surgery or leading to substantial disability) in 95 patients undergoing brachytherapy for T1 and T2 floor of mouth cancers. Osteonecrosis occurs at a rate of approximately 5–10% in conventionally irradiated patients (2Gy per day to 60–70Gy; 20, 21). The rate increases with increasing dose to as high as 22% reported by Niewald in patients treated with 1.2–82.8Gy fractions twice per day [84].

In a series by Stenson et al., radiation given prior to surgical neck dissection lead to wound healing complications in approximately 10% of patients [85]. They reported a series of 69 patients receiving accelerated radiation with concomitant chemotherapy followed by neck dissection. Six percent of those patients ultimately required surgical intervention for closure.

In summary, in patients undergoing radiation therapy for head and neck cancers, extreme care must be exercised when planning the volume of normal and "at risk" tissue to be irradiated, the dose fractionation and the overall dose. Special attention must be paid to normal-tissue tolerance doses. This is especially true for patients undergoing IMRT where dose gradients are very steep, unconventional treatment angles are used and very high doses can occur, albeit to small volumes, either within tumor tissue or normal tissue. Patients undergoing radiation to the head and neck area require attentive care during treatment to manage the acute side effects. Close follow-up by both the surgeon and the radiation oncologist is critical in order to recognize and treat tumor recurrence and also late complications.

References

1. Ogura JH, Piller HF, Wette R (1971) Elective Neck dissection for pharyngeal and laryngeal cancers: An evaluation. Ann Otol Rhinol Laryngol 80:646–651
2. Million RR, Cassisi NJ (1994) Management of head and neck cancer. Lippincott, Philadelphia, 130
3. Razack MS, Baffi R, Sako K (1981) Bilateral radical Neck dissection. Cancer 47:197–199
4. Genden EM, Ferltio A, Shaha AR, Talmi YP, Robbins KT, Rhys-Evans H, Rinaldo A (2003) Complications of neck dissection. Act Otolaryngol 123:795–801
5. Gueret G, Cosset MF, McGee K, Luboinski FB, Bourgain JL (2002) Sudden death after neck dissection for cancer. Ann Otol Rhinol Laryngol 111:115–119
6. Brown H, Burns S, Kaiser CW (1988) The spinal accessory nerve plexus, the trapezius muscle, and shoulder stabilization after radical neck cancer surgery. Ann Surg 208:654–661
7. Kinnaert P (1973) Anatomical variations of the cervical portion of the thoracic duct in man. J Anat 1973:45–52
8. Maran AGD, Amin M, Wilson JA (1989) Radical Neck dissection: A 19-year experience. J Laryngol Otol 103:760–764
9. Lavelle RJ, Maw RA (1972) The aetiology of postlaryngectomy pharyngocutaneous fistulae. J Laryngol Otol 86:785–793
10. Lore JM (1988) An atlas of head and neck surgery. Saunders, Philadelphia
11. Gavilan J, Ferlito A, Silver CE, Shaha AR, Martin L, Rinaldo A (2002) Status of carotid resection in head and neck cancer. Acta Otolaryngol 122:453–455
12. Medina JE (1996) Radical Neck dissection. Supraomohyoid Neck dissection. Modified radical Neck dissection. Posterolateral Neck dissection. In: Bailey BJ, Calhoun KH, Coffey AR, Neely JG (eds) Atlas of head and neck surgery – otolaryngology. Lippincott, Philadelphia, 140–153, 162–163
13. Mann W, Beck C, Freudenberg N, Leupe M (1981) Der Bestrahlungseffekt auf die Lymphkapillaren des Kehlkopfes. HNO 29:381–387
14. Prim MP, de Diego JI, Fernandez-Zubillaga A, Garcia-Raya P, Madero R, Gavilan J (2000) Patency and flow of the internal jugular vein after functional Neck dissection. Laryngoscope 110:47–50
15. Fisher CB, Mattox DE, Zinreich JS (1988) Patency of the internal jugular vein after functional Neck dissection. Laryngoscope 98:923–927
16. Cappiello J, Piazza C, Berlucchi M, Peretti G, De Zinis LO, Maroldi R, Nicolai P (2002) Internal jugular vein patency after lateral neck dissection: a prospective study. Eur Arch Otorhinolaryngol 259:409–412
17. Cleland-Zamudio SS, Wax MK, Smith JD, Cohen JI (2003) Ruptured internal jugular vein: a postoperative complication of modified/selected neck dissection. Head Neck 25:357–360
18. Docherty JG, Carter R, Sheldon CD, Falconer JS, Bainbridge LC, Robertson AG, Soutar DS (1993) Relative effect of surgery and radiotherapy on the internal jugular vein following functional Neck dissection. Head Neck 15:553–556
19. Werner C, Pau HW, Kessler G, Koch U (1990) Veränderungen der Blutfluss-geschwindigkeit in den basalen Hirnarterien nach Neck dissection. Laryngorhinootologie 69:538–542
20. Witz M, Korzets Z, Shnaker A, Lehmann JM, Ophir D (2002) Delayed carotid artery rupture in advanced cervical cancer – a dilemma in emergency management. Eur Arch Otorhinolaryngol 259:37–39
21. Marks SC, Jaques DA, Hirata RM, Saunders JR (1990) Blindness following bilateral radical Neck dissection. Head Neck 12:342–345
22. Nahum AM, Mullall YW, Marmor L (1961) A syndrome resulting from radical Neck dissection. Arch Otolaryngol Head Neck Surg 74:424–428
23. Leipzig B, Suen JY, English JL, Barnes J, Hooper H (1983) Functional evaluation of the spinal accessory nerve after Neck dissection. Am J Surg 146:526–530
24. Dijkstra PU, van Wilgen PC, Buijs RP, Brendeke W, de Goede JT, Kerst A, Koostra M, Marinus J, Schoppink EM, Stuiver MM, van de Velde CF, Roodenburg JLN (2001) Incidence of shoulder pain after neck dissection: a clinical explorative study for risk factors. Head Neck 23:947–953
25. Shone GR, Yardley MPJ (1991) An audit into the incidence of handicaps after unilateral radical Neck dissection. J Laryngol Otol 105:760–762
26. Dewar FP, Harris RI (1960) Restoration of function of the shoulder following paralysis of the trapezius by fascial sling fixation and transplantation of the levator scapulae. Ann Surg 132:1111
27. Harris RI, Dickey JR (1965) Nerve grafting to restore function of trapezius muscle after radical Neck dissection. Ann Otol Rhinol Laryngol 74:880
28. Weitz JW, Weitz SL, McElhinney AJ (1982) A technique for preservation of spinal accessory nerve function in radical Neck dissection. Head Neck Surg 5:75–78
29. Blessing R, Mann W, Beck C (1986) Wie sinnvoll ist der Erhalt des Nervus accessorius bei der Halsausräumung? Laryngorhinootologie 65:403–405
30. Mann W, Wolfensberger M, Fhller U, Beck C (1991) Radikale versus modifizierte Halsausräumung. Kanzerologische und funktionelle Gesichtspunkte. Laryngo-rhinootol 70:32–35
31. Berghaus A, Holtmann S, von Scheel J, Tausch-Treml R, Herter M (1988) Zur Frage der Schonung des Nervus accessorius bei der Neck dissection. HNO 36:68–73
32. Fuchs M, Mehnert S, Stumpf R, Keiner S, Bootz F (2001) Intraoperative monitoring of spinal accessory nerve in neck surgery. In: Lippert BM, Werner JA (eds) Metastases in head and neck cancer. Tectum, Marburg, 307–312
33. Romstock J, Strauss C, Fahlbusch R (2000) Continuous electomyography monitoring of motor cranial nerves during cerebellopontine angle surgery. J Neurosurg 93:586–593

34. de Jong AA, Mann JJ (1991) Phrenic nerve paralysis following Neck dissection. Eur Arch Otorhinolaryngol 248:132–134

35. Àwengen DF, Donald PJ (1994) Complications of radical Neck dissection. In: Shockley WW, Pillsbury III HC (eds) The neck. Diagnosis and Surgery. Mosby, St. Louis, 483–509

36. Babin RW, Panje WR (1980) The incidence of vasovagal reflex activity during radical Neck dissection. Laryngoscope 90:1321–1323

37. Harlowe HD (1942) Carotid sinus syndrome and sudden death during surgical procedure of the neck. Dis Eye Ear Nose Throat 2:188–190

38. Greenfield J, Gottlieb MI (1956) Variation in the terminal portion of the human thoracic duct. Arch Surg 73:955–959

39. Gregor RT (2000) Management of chyle fistulization in association with neck dissection. Otolaryngol Head Neck Surg 122:434–439

40. Nussenbaum B, Liu JH, Sinard RJ (2000) Systemic management of chyle fistula: The southwestern experience and review of the literature. Otolaryngol Head Neck Surg 122:31–38

41. de Gier HHW, Balm AJM, Bruning PF, Gregor RT, Hilgers FJM (1996) Systematic approach to the treatment of chylous leakage after Neck dissection. Head Neck 18:347–351

42. Kassel RN, Havas TE, Gullane PJ (1987) The use of topical tetracycline in the management of persistent chylous fistulae. J Otolaryngol 16:174–178

43. Allen DP, Briggs CE (1901) Wounds of the thoracic duct occurring in the neck: report of 2 cases. Resume of 17 cases. Am Med 14:401–404

44. Stuart WJ (1907) Operative injury of the thoracic duct in the neck. Edinburgh Med J 22:301–317

45. Fitz-Hugh GS, Cowgill R (1970) Chylous fistula – complication of neck dissection. Arch Otolaryngol 91:543–547

46. Myers EN, Dinerman WS (1975) Management of chylous fistulas. Laryngoscope 85:835–840

47. Crumley RL, Smith JD (1976) Postoperative chylous fistula prevention and management. Laryngoscope 86:804–813

48. Har-El G, Segal K, Sidi J (1985) Bilateral chylothorax complicating radical Neck dissection: report of a case with no current external chylus leakage. Head Neck Surg 7:2252–230

49. Bocca E, Pignataro O, Oldini C, Cappa C (1984) Functional Neck dissection: an evaluation and review of 843 cases. Laryngoscope 94:942–45

50. Weiss KL, Wax MK, Haydon RC, Kaufman HH, Hurst MK (1993) Intracranial pressure changes during bilateral radical Neck dissections. Head Neck 15:546–552

51. De Vries WAEJ, Balm AJM, Tiwari RM (1986) Intracranial hypertension following Neck dissection. J Laryngol Otol 100:1427–1431

52. Jackson SR, Stell PM (1991) Second radical Neck dissection. Clin Otolaryngol 16:52–58

53. Lindberg R (1972) Distribution of cervical lymph node metastasis from squamous cell carcinoma of the upper respiratory and digestive tracts. Cancer 29:1446–1449

54. Lefebvre JL, Coche-Dequeant B, Van JT, Buisset E, Adenis A (1990) Cervical lymph nodes from an unknown primary tumor in 190 patients. Am J Surg 160:443–446

55. Raj P, Moore PL, Henderson J, Macnamara M (2002) Bilateral cortical blindness: an unusual complication following unilateral neck dissection. J Laryngol Otol 116:227–229

56. Corbett JJ, Thompson S (1989) The rational management of idiopathic intracranial hypertension. Arch Neurol 46:1049–1051

57. Regnault F (1887) Die malignen Tumoren der Gefässscheide. Arch Klin Chir 35:50

58. McGuirt WF, McCabe BF (1980) Bilateral radical Neck dissections. Arch Otolaryngol Head Neck Surg 106:427–429

59. Katsuno S, Ishiyama T, Nezu K, Usami S (2000) Three types of internal jugular vein reconstruction in bilateral radical neck dissection. Laryngoscope 110:1578–1580

60. Gorman JB, Stone RT, Keats TE (1971) Changes in the sternoclavicular joint following radical Neck dissection. Am J Roentgenol 3:584–587

61. Cummings CW, First R (1975) Stress facture of clavicle after a radical Neck dissection. Plast Reconstruct Surg 55:366–367

62. Suárez O (1963) El problema de las metástasis linfáticas y alejadas del cáncer de laringe e hipofaringe. Rev Otorrhinolaryngol 23:83–99

63. Temesvari A, Vandor F (1945) Über die Komplikationen nach cervikalen Dissectionoperationen. Chirurg 25:437–442

64. Fajardo L (1982) Pathology of Radiation Injury. New York, Masson Publishing.

65. Mettler F, Upton A (1995) Medical Effects of Ionizing Radiation, 2nd Ed. Philadelphia, WB Saunders Company.

66. Casarett GW (1964) Similarities and Contrasts between Radiation and Tissue Pathology. In Strehler B, ed. Advances in Gerontological Research. New York, Academic, 109–163

67. Coleman CN, Stevenson MA, et al. (2000) "Molecular and Cellular Biology" in Gunderson LL, Tepper JE eds. Clinical Radiation Oncology. New York, Churchill Livingstone, 42– 63

68. Cooper JS, Scott CB, Laramore GE, et al. (2002) Patterns of Failure for Resected Advanced Head and Neck Cancer Treated by Concurrent Chemotherapy and Radiation Therapy: An Analysis of RTOG 95–01/Intergroup Phase III Trial. Int J Radiat Oncol Biol Phys 54 (Suppl.):2

69. Bernier J, Domenge C, Eschwege F, et al. (2001) Chemo-Radiotherapy as Compared to Radiotherapy Alone Significantly Increases Disease-Free and Overall Survival in Head and Neck Cancer Patients after Surgery: Results of EORTC Phase III Trial 22931. Int J Radiat Oncol Biol Phys 1 (Suppl.):1

70. Calais G, Alfonsi M, Bardet E, et al. (1999) Randomized Trial of Radiation Therapy Versus Concomitant Chemotherapy and Radiation Therapy for Advanced-Stage Oropharynx Carcinoma. J Natl Cancer Inst 91:2081–2086

71. Brizel DM, Albers ME, Fisher SR, et al. (1998) Hyperfractionated Irradiation With or Without Concurrent Chemotherapy for Locally Advanced Head and Neck Cancer. New Eng J Med 338:1788–180

72. Wendt TG, Grabenbauer GG, Rodel CM, et al. (1998) Simultaneous Radiochemotherapy versus Radiotherapy Alone in Advanced Head and Neck Cancer: A Randomized Multicenter Study. J Clin Oncol 16:1318–1324

73. Fu K, Pajak T, Trotti A, et al. (2000) A Radiation Therapy Oncology Group (RTOG) Phase III Randomized Study to Compare Hyperfractionated and Two Variants of Accelerated Fractionated to Standard Fractionated Radiotherapy for Head and Neck Squamous Cell Carcinoma: First Report of RTOG 90–03. Int J Radiat Oncol Biol Phys 48:7–16

74. Kareko M, Shirato H, et al. (1998) Scintigraphic Evaluation of Long Term Salivary Function after Bilateral Whole Parotid Gland Irradiation in Radiotherapy for Head and Neck Tumour. Oral Oncol 34:140–146

75. Epstein JB, Emerton S, et al. (1999) Quality of Life and Oral Function Following Radiotherapy for Head and Neck Cancer. Head Neck 21:1–11

76. Eisbruch A, Ten-Haken RK, et al. (1999) Dose, Volume and Function Relationships in Parotid Salivary Glands Following Conformal and Intensity-Modulated Irradiation of Head and Neck Cancer. Int J Radiat Oncol Biol Phys 45:577–587

77. Chao KSC, Deasy JL, et al. (2001) A Prospective Study of Salivary Function Sparing in Patients with Head and Neck Cancer Receiving Intensity-Modulated or Three-Dimensional Radiation Therapy: Initial Results. Int J Radiat Oncol Biol Phys 49:907–916

78. Johnson JT, Ferret GA, et al. (1993) Oral Pilocarpine for Post Irradiation Xerostomia in patients with Head and Neck Cancer. N Engl J Med 329:390–395

79. LeVeque FG, Montgomery, et al. (1993) A Multicenter Randomized Double-Blind Placebo-Controlled, Dose Titration Study of Pilocarpine for Treatment of Radiation-Induced Xerostomia in Head and Neck Cancer Patients. J Clin Oncol 7:535–541

80. Valdez IH, Wolff A, et al. (1993) Use of Pilocarpine during Head and neck Radiation Therapy to Reduce Xerostomia and Salivary Dysfunction. Cancer 71:1848–1851

81. Brizel DM, Wasserman TH, et al. (2000) Phase III Randomized Trial of Amifostine as a Radioprotector in Head and Neck Cancer. J Clin Oncol 18:3339–3345

82. Perez, CA (1997) Tonsillar Fossa and Faucial Arch. In: Perez CA, Brady LW eds. Principles and Practice of Radiation Oncology. 3d Edition. Philadelphia, Lippincott-Raven 897–939

83. Mazeron JJ, Grimard L, et al. (1990) Iridium-192 Curietherapy for T1 and T2 Epidermoid Carcinomas of the Floor of Mouth. Int J Radiat Oncol Biol Phys 18:1299–1306

84. Niewald M, Barbie O, et al. (1996) Risk Factors and Dose-effect Relationship for Osteoradionecrosis after Hyperfractionated and Conventionally Fractionated Radiotherapy for Oral Cancer. Br J Radiol 69:847–851

85. Stenson KM, Haraf DJ, et al. (2000) The Role of Cervical Lymphadenectomy after Aggressive Concomitant Chemoradiotherapy. Arch Otolaryngol Head Neck Surg 126:950–956

Cancer of Unknown Primary Sites

9.1 General Considerations

The so-called CUP syndrome (cancer of unknown primary) is defined as one or more histologically proven metastases of a malignant tumor for which the localization cannot be determined in spite of intensive diagnostic measures [1].

Epidemiology. About 3–5% of newly diagnosed malignant diseases in the head and neck region are cervical lymph node metastases of an unknown primary tumor [2, 3]. In former times, the incidence amounted to about 10% [4] or even more. The current ability to detect histologically similar malignant entities by means of immunohistochemical procedures may explain the decrease in frequency of the CUP syndrome. Additionally, improved imaging techniques allow optimized diagnosis.

About 37% of metastases of a CUP syndrome manifest first in the lymph node stations of the body. Metastases to lymph nodes in the head and neck account for 84% of these. Sites of metastases outside the lymph nodes in unknown primary cancer are, with decreasing frequency, the liver, bones and lungs.

Seventy percent of cervical lymph node metastases in CUP are squamous cell carcinomas [4] and 9–16% are adenocarcinomas [5–7]. The incidence of lymph node metastases from an occult malignant melanoma ranges between 1–14%, when considering all body regions [8]. In the head and neck region, fewer than 10% of lymph node metastases in unknown primary cancer are due to malignant melanoma [9, 10].

Age and Sex Distribution. Men are affected by the CUP syndrome about twice as often as women [11, 12]. The mean age of diagnosis is 60 years [4, 13].

Hypothesis for Genesis. In the CUP syndrome, the primary tumor often reveals unspecific characteristics regarding its localization and growth behavior [14]. The following mechanisms in unknown primary cancers will be discussed:

- A small primary tumor can induce multiple metastases that can be identified by a rapid growth earlier than the primary.
- The regression of the primary tumor can be explained by changes in the tumor phenotype and genotype [15].
- The growth rate of the primary tumor can decrease due to local immunologic influences [16].
- Generally, malignant tumors metastasize lymphogenously into the regional lymph nodes or hematogenously into the first subsequent capillary system. The first station can be skipped in CUP syndrome [17].

The development of lymph node metastases in occult malignant melanoma allows further discussion of more-or-less specific mechanisms for this tumor entity, which include:

- Overlooking the primary tumor due to its small size or location (e.g., a hairy head);
- Complete regression of the primary cancer; a process that is repeatedly documented for malignant melanoma [18];
- Localization of the primary tumor in the region of the mucosa of the upper aerodigestive tract or the visceral organs [19].
- De novo development of a malignant melanoma within a nevocellular nevus [20];
- Unwitting destruction of the unknown primary tumor by accidental trauma [21].

9.2 Topography of Lymph Node Metastases in Cancer of Unknown Primary

Density differences in the distribution pattern of initial lymph vessels have a direct influence on tumor cell dissemination and also on the localization of possible lymph node metastases in the head and neck [12, 22]. The localization of cervical lymph node metastases allows conclusions on the possible primary tumor site that should be considered when looking for the primary cancer (▶ Table 9.1). The following general observations must be taken into consideration:

- More than 70 % of the patients suffering from cervical lymph node metastases of the upper and mid-deep jugular lymph nodes (levels I–III [23]) have unknown primary squamous cell carcinomas in the area of the tonsils, the base of the tongue and the nasopharynx.
- Lymph node metastases localized in the lower third of the vascular sheath (level IV and medial aspect of level V [23]) frequently originate from an unknown squamous cell carcinoma of the hypopharynx or the bronchial system [24].
- In cases of metastases to the supraclavicular triangle, the primary tumor may be from the area of the ovary, the breast, the ventricle or the prostate gland.
- In cases of supraclavicular lymph node swellings in young men, there is also the possibility of a metastasizing testicular carcinoma [25].
- The origin of a cervical lymph node metastasis can also be an occult malignant melanoma [26]; this can be the case for all lymph node levels of the head and neck.

Table 9.1. Typical metastatic pattern of squamous cell carcinomas in certain cervical lymph node levels depending on probable primary tumor site location.

Level	Probable primary tumor site
I	Lower lip Floor of the mouth Ventral area of the mucosa of the cheek Mobile part of the tongue Gingival, alveolar ridge Nasal cavity and paranasal sinuses
II	Oropharynx including soft palate, tonsil, base of tongue Glossotonsilar vallecula, glossoepiglottic vallecula Supraglottis, glottis **More rarely:** facial skin, concha, all regions of level I and nasopharynx
III	Larynx, especially glottis, also supra- and subglottis Hypopharynx Caudal part of the base of tongue **More rarely:** other regions of the oropharynx
IV	Hypopharynx Subglottis Cranial part of trachea Thyroid gland
V	Epipharynx Scalp (especially dorsal part), partly also concha Gastrointestinal (especially stomach in case of left-sided metastatic spread)
VI	Thyroid gland Subglottis (so-called Delphian lymph nodes) Caudal part of trachea

9.3 Diagnostics

Preoperative Diagnosis. By definition, prior to the diagnosis of the CUP syndrome an intensive search for the primary tumor must be performed [27].

To make a diagnosis of CUP syndrome in the cervical region the workup should at the very least include:

- A careful history directed toward examination of the skin;
- Endoscopy of the nose and nasopharynx;
- Inspection and palpation of the oral cavity;
- Endoscopy of the base of the tongue (including palpation), as well the hypopharynx, the larynx, the tracheo-bronchial system and the esophagus.

Furthermore, the following procedures are indicated:

- B-mode sonography of the cervical soft tissue with fine needle aspiration cytology;
- B-mode sonography of the abdomen (especially if adenocarcinoma is suspected);
- Computed tomography and/or magnetic resonance imaging of the head and neck region [4, 24]. The significance of positron emission tomography (PET) as a diagnostic tool is not yet clear. Recent results, however, seem very promising (see Chap. 4.6).

In cases of lymph node metastases in the lower part of the neck, a CT scan of the thorax should be performed, given that up to 32 % of the occult primary tumors with cervical lymph node metastases occur in the lung [26].

If a cervically localized *lymph node metastasis of an unknown adenocarcinoma* is suspected, the following should be performed in addition to the previously mentioned diagnostic steps:

- Careful examination of the breast, the prostate, the rectum and the other pelvic viscera by colleagues of the respective specialties;
- Additional imaging, to include:
  - A CT of the abdomen, skull and pelvis;
  - As well as mammography in female patients;
- Additional tests include:
  - Urinalysis;
  - An extensive serologic examination that includes thyroid function parameters (calcitonin and thyroglobulin) and thyroid function levels, plus serum calcium;
  - Determination of the carcinoembryonic antigen, ss-human chorionic gonadotropin and alpha-fetoprotein [15].

Invasive Diagnosis. Based on clinical experience of the most frequent sites of unknown primary squamous cell carcinoma or undifferentiated carcinoma, panendoscopy in combination with ipsilateral palatine tonsillectomy is recommended [28], as well as an extended excision of epipharyngeal specimens and excision of tissue from the base of the tongue. The latter can be accomplished with an extended laser resection of the lingual tonsil, unilaterally or bilaterally. This procedure allows a significantly higher identification rate of occult carcinomas than blind biopsy of the base of the tongue.

Autofluorescence and ALA-Induced Fluorescence. Diagnosis in the upper aerodigestive tract has been optimized by means of fluorescence techniques. The application of autofluorescence has increased intraoperative identification rates from 15.4 to 38.5 % [29].

Salivary Gland and Thyroid Gland Scintigraphy. In cases of unclear cytological findings in lymph node metastases, the presence of primary thyroid gland or salivary gland carcinomas must be considered. Knothe and Fritsch [30] have reported on scintigraphy of the salivary glands and the thyroid gland in their search for the primary tumor in the CUP syndrome. In our experience, the major salivary glands must be included in the sonographic examination in the CUP syndrome. The necessity for regularly performing scintigraphic examinations of the salivary glands needs to be verified, ideally, by several independent studies.

18FDG Positron Emission Tomography. Generally, high metabolic activity can be observed in malignant tumors. It is based on a predominance of intracellular hexokinase in glucose metabolism. Fluoro-deoxyglucose (^{18}FDG) is metabolized by hexokinase to ^{18}FDG-6-phosphate. This is not further changed in glucose metabolism and is enhanced in cells with superior hexokinase activity (neurons, malignant cells, etc.) [31]. Because of this, ^{18}FDG positron emission tomography can selectively detect malignancies and their soft tissue metastases in addition to describing the metabolic processes in the brain and heart. This method is highly sensitive and allows a relatively exact detection and localization of malignancies in comparison to other imaging procedures. The drawback is that ^{18}FDG positron emission tomography is not specific. Inflammatory processes with tissue acidosis and mainly anaerobic metabolism can cause false positive results [32, 33].

A final assessment of the significance of ^{18}FDG positron emission tomography is not yet possible, although reports exist which show a significantly increased rate of tumor detections in up to 50 % of the cases [34–38]. A detailed description regarding PET can be found in Chap. 4.6.

Special Serologic Diagnosis. In cases of a suspected CUP syndrome, the determination of the EBV antibody titer seems to be reasonable, especially the IgA antiviral capsid antigen (VCA). This titer is increased in approximately 70 % of the patients with an EBV-associated nasopharyngeal carcinoma, provided a lympho-epithelial carcinoma cannot be excluded. In this context, it must be mentioned that titer control is particularly important for the follow-up of epipharyngeal carcinomas, especially lympho-epithelial carcinomas [39].

9.4 Prognosis in Patients with Cancer of Unknown Primary Site

Prognosis for patients and treatment strategies are dependent on the histology of the lymph node metastasis.

9.4.1 Metastases in Squamous Cell Carcinoma of Unknown Primary

About one-third of patients with cervical metastases from an unknown primary survive more than 5 years. In more than half of these patients, the primary tumor may never be detected [40]. The prognosis for metastases of squamous cell carcinomas of unknown primary site is better than for other histological types [15]. It is critical in diagnosis to determine the location and number of metastases.

Localization of Lymph Node Metastases. Location of the lymph node metastases plays an important role in relation to long-time survival rate. Tumor-specific 5-year-survival rates are:

- 63% in cases of high cervical lymph node metastases and 47% in the cases of total survival.
- In cases of deep cervical location, the 5-year-survival rate is reported to be $9 \pm 6\%$ and the total survival $9.2 \pm 9\%$. This is due to the high rate of distant metastases, which is 67% in cases of deep cervical localization, in contrast to 12% in cases of high cervical position [39].

In the context of a CUP syndrome, the survival rate is directly proportional to the *number* and *location* of lymph node metastases, as well as to the identification of *perinodal tumor growth* (extracapsular extension) [4, 41–45].

9.4.2 Metastases in Adenocarcinoma of Unknown Primary

In comparison to lymph node metastases from unknown squamous cell carcinoma, the detection of lymph node metastases from unknown site adenocarcinoma generally reflects an already-advanced stage of tumor dissemination. This knowledge influences the treatment concept of lymph node metastases of an unknown site adenocarcinoma. The prognosis in these patients is significantly poorer than the prognosis in patients suffering from an unknown squamous cell carcinoma.

Earlier publications, such as the study performed by Snyder et al. [46], report a mean survival of 2 months in 49 patients with a lymph node metastasis of an unknown adenocarcinoma. Another study showed a mean survival of 9 weeks in patients older than 57 years and only 2 weeks in patients who were younger than 57 years [47]. Actual examinations report a mean survival of 8 months, with a 2-year-survival rate of 20% and a 5-year-survival rate of 9% [48].

In light of previously mentioned factors, the necessity of finding the primary tumor must be weighed against three factors:

- From the time of diagnosis, the remaining survival time is often very short due to the generally advanced-stage disease.
- There is little chance of finding the primary location of an adenocarcinoma in the lifetime of the patient. In a representative study, in only 22 out of 266 patients (8%) could the primary cancer be diagnosed. This identification rate was increased to 48% by post mortem examination [49]. The low identification rate has been confirmed by further examinations [47].
- Although research of every possible location can eventually lead to identification of the primary tumor, this is not in time to initiate effective therapy.

Lymph Node Localization. Location of metastasis in adenocarcinoma has an influence on mean survival. Lee et al. [48] were able to detect a significantly higher survival rate in patients who had lymph node metastases cranio- and medio-jugularly to the parotid gland, as well as suboccipitally, compared with patients with caudo-jugular lymph node metastases.

9.4.3 Metastases in Malignant Melanoma of Unknown Primary

Considering biologic behavior, the prognosis in patients with cervical lymph node metastases of an occult malignant melanoma is similar, or perhaps even better, than in patients with a known primary site malignant melanoma of stage II. In the literature, the 5-year-survival rate is reported to be 11–48 % and the 10-year-survival rate 32 % [9, 10, 50].

Generally, the prognosis in patients with the CUP syndrome or a cervical lymph node metastasis of a known squamous cell carcinoma is determined directly by the number of metastatic lymph nodes. In contrast, the number of cervical lymph node metastases, or the identification of an extracapsular metastatic growth, does not seem to be relevant for the prognosis of occult malignant melanoma [51, 52].

Cervical lymph node metastases from an occult malignant melanoma are most frequently localized:

- In level V, dorsal to the sternocleidomastoid muscle; or
- In the superior-jugular level II, as well as
- In the parotid gland.
- However, cervical lymph node metastases of an occult malignant melanoma must be expected in all levels.

This pattern of metastasis reflects the lymphogenic metastatic spread of cutaneous malignant melanomas of the face, the haired scalp, the ears and the upper aerodigestive tract.

9.5 Treatment Concepts of Lymph Node Metastases in Squamous Cell Carcinoma of Unknown Primary Site

The identification of one or even several lymph node metastases of an unknown squamous cell carcinoma of course does not allow classical treatment of the primary tumor. In reference to cervical lymph node stage, however, diagnostic and therapeutic approaches equivalent to the classic approach could be used as if the primary site were known.

9.5.1 Primary Radio(chemo)therapy

Radiotherapy. Radiotherapy plays a central role in the treatment of the CUP syndrome because it includes the lymphatic drainage and the probable primary tumor location in the treatment field.

The medical literature reports that a total dose of 60–70 Gy is required for curative intent for the devitalization of macroscopic metastases of squamous cell carcinoma, adenocarcinoma or an undifferentiated carcinoma.

The mean survival of patients who undergo radiation only to possible primary tumor regions corresponding to metastatic cervical lymph node levels is generally similar to the survival of patients who undergo radiation to all known primary tumor locations [53].

Based on current imaging techniques, which screen the nasopharynx with great accuracy, and based on knowledge originating from prospective studies showing that most unknown primary squamous cell carcinomas ultimately manifest in the region of the tonsils and the base of the tongue, a question arises concerning the possibility of reducing the inevitable side effects of radiotherapy by *not* irradiating the nasopharynx, larynx and pharynx, as is generally recommended using dosages up to 70 Gy [4]. The downside to this approach is that the occurrence of a nasopharyngeal carcinoma after completed therapy is more difficult to treat. In the past, such treatment of the nasopharyngeal the primary cancer was felt not to be curative. With newer concepts of IMRT (irradiation), or even re-irradiation with or without chemotherapy, this risk is not as great.

Glynne-Jones et al. [54], report that radiation of the nasopharynx should be performed when:

- Cervical lymph node metastases of an unknown primary are situated dorsally to the sternocleido-mastoid muscle;
- The patient is younger than 30 years;
- An increased EBV capsid titer is present;
- Epstein–Barr virus is identified in the biopsy material; or
- A genetic predisposition exists for developing a nasopharyngeal carcinoma (as is the case, e.g., in patients of Asiatic origin).

In current clinical practice, the so-called shrinking field technique in regional irradiation has proven to be useful. This means that:

- The whole cervical lymphatic drainage region receives a dose of 45–50 Gy;
- The oropharynx and hypopharynx are radiated up to at least 50 Gy;
- the ipsilateral cervical lymphatic drainage is irradiated up to 56–60 Gy; and
- The affected lymph nodes are radiated with a boost of rapid electrons to a total dose of 70 Gy. In this manner, the spinal cord and pharynx are spared.
- In contrast, when nasopharyngeal cancer is suspected, the nasopharynx should receive 70 Gy.

Radiochemotherapy. A non-randomized study revealed that in comparison to patients who underwent only radiotherapy, patients suffering from metastases of squamous cell carcinomas who had been treated with concurrent chemotherapy and irradiation had an increased 5-year-survival rate, as well as an improved local response rate [11]. A recent study, however, shows improved local control during combined therapy with cisplatin and 5-fluorouracil (5-FU) without a significant increase in survival [5].

At this time, it is not possible to provide a definitive statement on the significance of chemotherapy in cases of the CUP syndrome. Based on the above-mentioned results, however, concurrent chemotherapy and irradiation in the treatment of lymph node metastases of unknown squamous cell carcinoma seems reasonable. It is also probable that irradiation of the nasopharynx can be avoided in unknown primary squamous cell cancers without the risk factors already mentioned.

9.5.2 Combined Radiotherapy and Surgery

Locoregional Control and Survival Rate. Radiotherapy alone is felt to be inferior to combined therapy with surgery and postoperative irradiation or chemo-irradiation. As a general rule, patients with positive cervical lymph nodes greater than 2 cm who undergo surgical intervention of the lymphatic drainage, in addition to postoperative radiotherapy, are described in the literature as having a significantly higher survival than patients treated exclusively with radiotherapy.

According to an examination performed by Dunst et al. [55], patients who had undergone radical neck dissection and subsequent radiotherapy had a locoregional tumor control rate of 83%, in contrast to only 20% in the group treated exclusively by radiotherapy. None of the patients treated exclusively with radiotherapy survived longer than 4 years.

Kirschner et al. [39] reported similarly good results with a complete remission rate of 95% (46/48) in patients who had neck dissection of the ipsilateral neck according to their N status, followed postoperatively by radiotherapy. After 5 years, they had a locoregional control rate of 76% and a tumor-specific survival rate of 67%. In contrast to this, all patients (p < 0.0001) who were not surgically treated died within 4 years (mean: 9.2 months). The complete remission in this last group amounted to only 37.5% with locoregional control, and, after three years, to only 27.9% (p < 0.0001).

Reports of significantly higher local control of the ipsilateral neck are another indication of the importance of the surgical treatment of cervical lymphatic drainage, independent of the type of radiotherapy (ipsilateral or bilateral), when compared to excisional

ated with a significantly higher rate of complications. These include cervical tissue necrosis, chylous fistulae, recurrent nerve paresis, suture dehiscence and postoperative bleeding. Furthermore, after such "rescue surgery" local recurrences have been shown to occur in more than 60 % of the cases during the first year and in over 90 % of the cases by the third postoperative year.

Due to the obstacles already discussed, the possibility of surgical salvage in cases of squamous cell carcinoma of the upper aerodigestive tract cannot be assured. Hence, in the context of the CUP syndrome, it seems reasonable that the initial therapy should aim at achieving local control [65] and that the treatment of the CUP syndrome N1 neck should include a combination of surgery and postoperative radiotherapy.

Combined Therapy Depending on the Number of Histologically Detected Lymph Node Metastases. It is important to mention a study by that Leemans et al. [63], in which they investigated a group of patients with known primary cancer who were treated *only* with MRND (i.e., without postsurgical radiotherapy). After pathological review, these patients revealed only one or two lymph node metastases without extracapsular growth, and the local recurrence rate did not differ from the local recurrence rate of patients treated radiotherapeutically after surgery. Based on this observation, Friedman et al. [66] recommended a therapeutic concept in cases of known primary cancer that requires radiotherapy only in cases of *three* histologically proven cervical lymph node metastases. Transferring this knowledge to the CUP syndrome, the approach assumes the excision of a sufficiently extended ND specimen and subsequent histopathology that accurately assesses cervical lymph node status. In the case of SND, the cervical lymph node tissue removed in the respective cervical lymph node regions would have to equal the tissue removed from this region with MRND in cases of known primary cancer [42].

Actually, this treatment strategy of the N1 neck in the cases of CUP syndrome cannot be totally supported given that current results, not related solely to the N1 neck, require a combination of surgery and ra-

diotherapy. Prospective randomized studies would be necessary for further assessment.

9.5.4 Treatment Concept of the Contralateral Neck Side (N0)

Most authors answer the question of whether uni- or bilateral neck dissection must be performed in the case of the CUP syndrome based on the sonographic and aspiration cytology findings [4, 15, 26, 67].

To determine the need for contralateral ND in patients with upper and deeper cervical lymph node metastases, the prognostic factors, as already mentioned, must be considered. In cases of advanced metastatic growth in levels I–II, a contralateral neck dissection with curative intention is justified.

In the cases of advanced metastatic growth in levels IV–V (caudal), however, an extended contralateral neck dissection should be avoided. This is because in most cases treatment is a palliative therapeutic measure and, as such, does not justify any resulting impairment to the quality of life. This refers also to the results obtained by Fu, who, in a literature review of the significance of surgery with and without radiotherapy, showed that there were no important differences between the occurrence of contralateral lymph node recurrences in contralateral radiotherapy, versus surgical treatment (or a combination of surgical treatment and radiotherapy) to the lymphatic drainage region [43].

9.6 Treatment Concepts of Lymph Node Metastases in Adenocarcinoma

The detection of a cervical lymph node metastasis of an unknown adenocarcinoma is a therapeutic dilemma because generally it is a sign of an advanced stage of disease. Metastasis from an unknown adenocarcinoma of the salivary glands, however, must be excluded from this generalization. In this case, the possibility of upper lymph node metastases must always be taken into consideration, and if present, requires surgical treatment of the cervical lymphatic drainage region and postoperative radiotherapy [68].

In spite of the generally poor prognosis in adenocarcinoma, there are groups that recommend the performance of a MRND or RND combined with postoperative radiotherapy [48]. Most surgeons, however, avoid an extended cervical lymph node dissection in cases of deeply located cervical lymph node metastases with adenocarcinoma, preferring instead a palliative therapeutic approach that avoids the accompanying impairment to the quality of life [68, 69]. Due to the disseminated tumor state, Stiernberg and Mostert [68] recommend systemic chemotherapy, possibly combined with palliative radiotherapy of the cervical regions, or a ND performed with palliative purposes.

The results of controlled studies of chemotherapy given for cervical metastases of adenocarcinomas of unknown primaries, however, are discouraging. A response rate of 27% and a median survival rate of 10 months after therapy with cisplatin, tamoxifen and 5-FU have been reported [70]. A treatment regimen with doxorubicin and cyclophosphamide, as well as etoposide and carboplatin, achieved a median survival of 8 months. More aggressive regimes with Taxol and cisplatin or Taxol and carboplatin have also been examined, but in a recent phase II study, these agents extended the median survival only to one year [71].

In summary, due to the extremely poor prognosis, the therapeutic approach should be planned individually in cases of a cervical lymph node metastasis of an unknown adenocarcinoma.

9.7 Treatment Concepts of Lymph Node Metastases in Occult Malignant Melanoma

The literature reveals a local recurrence rate of 68% in patients treated only by lymph node extirpation [72]. This high local failure rate could indicate that ND is a reasonable surgical approach for the treatment of cervical metastases from melanomas. Given this situation, Jonk et al. [19] recommend radical neck dissection. Other authors favor a MRND on the ipsilateral neck side, as this would also be performed in cases of a known malignant melanoma in order to avoid the functional impairments that are more likely to be seen after RND [50, 73].

O'Brien et al., in cases of known malignant melanoma, recommend dissection of levels I–V, anteriorly to an imagined line through the acoustic meatus, usually in combination with parotidectomy [52]. In cases of localization of the melanoma posterior to this arbitrary level, these authors recommend dissection of levels II–V. According to their results, MRND is highly effective in gaining local control of a metastasizing melanoma. As the discussion relates to unknown primary melanomas, the use of sentinel node techniques is not relevant.

The cervical lymph node metastasis of an occult malignant melanoma can be treated by modified radical neck dissection. This is because the biologic behavior of a cervical lymph node metastasis of an occult malignant melanoma corresponds very closely to that of a known malignant melanoma of stage II [9, 10, 50].

9.8 Value of Post-Therapeutic Appearance of the Primary Cancer

In 6–58% of the patients suffering from CUP syndrome, the carcinoma appears post therapeutically [2, 4, 41, 44, 55, 64]. However, it must be taken into consideration that in about 5% of these cases, it is a second primary carcinoma [74].

The appearance of the primary tumor in the further course of the disease is assessed in the literature by other means. Geyer and Wisser [44] compared the survival rates of patients with primary tumors that remained occult with the survival rates of those where the primary appeared in the further course of the disease. Their results showed that the prognosis was similarly poor for both groups. This supported by other authors [15, 26], who confirm that there is no difference in the 5-year-survival rate of both patient populations.

The results of numerous other groups, however, indicate a significant deterioration in survival where the primary tumor appears after completed therapy [4, 6, 15, 44, 47, 55, 64]. A final assessment of the question can actually not be given.

9.9 Branchiogenic Carcinoma

The finding of a branchiogenic carcinoma again and again leads to confusion. Usually the removal of the tumorous mass is performed under the suspicion of a lateral cervical cyst. The postoperatively diagnosed branchiogenic carcinoma must then be considered as development of a carcinoma in a lateral cervical cyst. The difficulty of diagnosing this rare disease is explained below.

The malignant degeneration of a lateral cervical cyst was described first by von Volkmann, in 1882, who coined the term of "deep branchiogenic cervical carcinoma" [75]. Squamous cell carcinoma cells within a cystic mass have engendered much controversy since first described by von Volkmann. The diagnosis of a malignant lateral cervical cyst (so-called "branchiogenic carcinoma") must be differentiated from centrally fused-in, necrotic, and thus, cystically imposing lymph nodes [76].

In 1950, Martin et al. [77] defined the histologic and clinical criteria that are still used today as a measure for justifying the diagnosis of the so-called *branchiogenic carcinoma*:

1. Location of a cystic mass in the area of the carotid triangle;
2. Histomorphologic tissue structures that appear in branchiogenic residues;
3. Absence of a primary tumor of a cystic cervical lymph node metastasis in the first five years after diagnosis; and

4. Histologic detection of carcinoma cells in the wall of an epithelial- lined cyst.

The retrospective analysis of the published 250 case reports performed by Martin et al. [77] revealed that only three of the patients fulfilled the abovementioned criteria. In following years, ten more patients were described, who, this time, fulfilled all four criteria [78, 79].

Clinically, an isolated mass is usually identified at the anterior edge of the sternocleidomastoid muscle in the area of the carotid triangle. It is characterized by a firm elasticity with fluctuation. Sonographically, it appears in image as a cyst. Other otolaryngologic examinations and imaging diagnostics do not reveal the presence of a tumor in any other area of the upper aerodigestive tract.

The theory of a branchiogenic carcinoma originating from relics of embryonic development was already in 1893 called "pure fiction" by Sutton [80]. In addition to its strict diagnostic criteria [82, 83], the differential diagnosis of a cystic cervical lymph node metastasis of an unknown primary tumor has created a great deal of skepticism regarding the existence of this disease [80, 81].

In many cases, isolated lymph node metastases are located in the area of the upper venous angle. As already mentioned, Lindberg [84] demonstrated in an extended study that the primary tumors which metastasize in the area of the carotid triangle are often situated in the region of the tonsils. Small carcinomas localized in the submucosa can then be the reason for a large isolated cervical lymph node metastasis. Such small carcinomas located in the region of the Waldeyer's tonsillar ring are usually accompanied by cystic cervical lymph node metastases. Having said this, it is important to point out that many authors consider cervical masses (branchiogenic carcinomas) as misinterpreted cystic cervical lymph node metastases of an occult squamous cell carcinoma in the area of Waldeyer's tonsillar ring [85–95].

In lymph node metastases of squamous cell carcinomas, partially cystic formations and collagen connective tissue reactions are known. The detection of a cystic metastasis on the base of residing lymph node tissue is possible as long as the cystic degeneration processes are not completely finished. The differentially diagnostic way to find a "branchiogenic carcinoma" begins when the carcinoma cells have displaced lymph node tissue and start to imitate the cystic wall. The additional occurrence of a distinct capsular connective tissue reaction leads to the image of a "malignant lateral cervical cyst" [88].

The unsolved oncologic problem of the "branchiogenic carcinoma" was extensively discussed by Hamperl in 1939 from a formal, pathologic point of view [96]. Hamperl argued that only masses should be called branchiogenic tumors, at least according to the definition that such tumors develop from tissue that is already present during the development of the branchial arcs, which implies that they are innate. Thus, the tissue malformation can be *branchiogenic*, i. e., as originating from the branchial arch system. However, this is not the case with respect to the autonomous carcinomatous development of a tumor. According to Hamperl, the connection between branchiogenic and malignant cannot be made from a formally pathological point of view. The missing detection of a primary tumor as well is no proof for a neoplasia from embryonic branchial arch residues.

Finally, the criteria elaborated by Martin et al. [77], with mainly differentially diagnostic value is questionable in relation to the difference between the existence and non-existence of a "branchiogenic carcinoma" [82, 97]. This is especially true for the third criterion (five-year limit regarding a later development of a primary tumor). Here, the objection can be made that occult primary tumors are often treated by the frequently performed postoperative radiotherapy and do not manifest clinically. The non-appearance of a primary cannot be considered certain proof for the non-existence of a primary tumor, especially given the fact that a regression of occult tumors is also known without radiotherapy [98]. As a result this situation, two other criteria have been postulated [82]:

- Missing evidence of a primary tumor after careful diagnosis (endoscopy, biopsies, CT scan); and
- Histologic evidence of a cystic mass with parts of squamous cell carcinoma cells.

However, even these differential diagnostic criteria seem insufficient for a clear-cut diagnosis of a "branchiogenic carcinoma." The difficulty defining useful criteria resides partly in the fact that even now there is no agreement on the pathogenesis of a simple lateral cervical cyst. The purported origin of the lateral cervical cyst as "dispersed residues of the second branchial pouch [or the branchial cleft]" conflicts with the idea that the cyst developed out of heterotropic epithelial inclusions in the cervical lymph nodes as "tonsilogenic lymph node disease" [99, 100].

Many authors believe that squamous cell carcinoma cells in a cervical cystic mass are caused by an occult squamous cell carcinoma [85–95]. In the treatment of such a case, a sufficiently radical oncologic treatment concept, which is accompanied by a relatively low morbidity, must be chosen. Up to 95 % of the metastases of a tonsillar carcinoma or of an unknown primary in the head and neck are localized in the cranio-jugular lymph nodes [89, 97, 101]. The occurrence of an isolated cervical lymph node metastasis outside this region indicates the location of the primary tumor outside Waldeyer's tonsillar ring [95]. In this context, it must be mentioned that occult papillary thyroid carcinomas can cause cystic cervical lymph node metastases [102–104].

If there is cytologic suspicion of a cystic mass associated with carcinoma cells, the treatment concept should be the same as for the CUP syndrome. Regarding the "branchiogenic carcinoma", more often situations occur when the suspected disease (lateral cervical cyst) suddenly and drastically turns out to be malignant after pathologic/anatomic preparation. In such a situation, the diagnosis should be continued as follows:

- Palpation of the oral cavity and oropharynx;
- Endoscopy of the upper aerodigestive tract, completed by the excision of specimens in the event of suspicious findings;
- Tonsillectomy;
- Possible lingual tonsillectomy, done by transoral laser surgery; and
- So-called blind specimen excisions from the nasopharynx – this is necessary because carcinomas localized in this area sometimes metastasize into level II.

If the "branchiogenic carcinoma" is diagnosed in another cervical region, the abovementioned steps must be extended to include screening other suspected locations for the primary cancer (CT scan of the lung, sonography and, possibly, cytology of the thyroid gland).

Finally, the uncertainty surrounding the differential diagnosis of a "branchiogenic carcinoma" should be reduced by performing neck dissection – if not MRND, then at least SND (I–III or I–IV).

In summary, even though the pathomorphologic and clinical lines between cystic cervical lymph node metastases and "branchiogenic carcinoma" and are blurred, the latter disease cannot be totally ignored. The question remains whether the disease of the malignant lateral cervical cyst and the disease of the cystic cervical lymph node metastasis of an unknown squamous cell carcinoma exist in parallel with varying frequency. According to the literature, the "branchiogenic carcinoma is assumed to occur with an incidence of 0.3% among all malignant supraclavicularly localized neoplasms [105]. However, there is no doubt that most of the published case reports of "branchiogenic carcinomas" have been cystic cervical lymph node metastases.

References

1. Fischer DS (1975) Management of cancer of unknown primary. Conn Med 39:205–208
2. Coker DD, Casterline PF, Chambers RG, Jaques DA (1977) Metastases of the lymph nodes of the head and neck from the unknown primary site. Am J Surg 134:517–522
3. Lefebvre JL, Coche-Dequeant B, Ton Van J, Buisset E, Adenis A (1990) Cervical lymph nodes from an unknown primary tumor in 190 patients. Am J Surg 160:443–446
4. Jungehülsing M, Eckel HE, Ebeling O (1997) Diagnostik und Therapie des okkulten Primärtumors mit Lymphknotenmetastasen. HNO 45:573–583
5. Barrie JR, Knapper WH, Strong EW (1970) Cervical nodal metastases of unknown origin. Am J Surg 120:466–470
6. Jesse RH, Neif LE (1966) Metastatic carcinoma in cervical nodes with an unknown primary lesion. Am J Surg 112:547–553
7. Winegar LK, Griffin W (1973) The occult primary tumor. Arch Otolaryngol 98:159–163
8. Mastrangelo MJ, Baker AR, Katz HR (1983) cancer principles and practice of oncology. Cutaneous melanoma. In: De Vita VY, Hellman S, Rosenberg SA (eds) Lippincott; Philadelphia, 1371–1422
9. Balm AJM, Kroon BBR, Hilgers FJM, Jonk A, Mooi WJ (1994) Lymph node metastases in the neck and parotid gland from an unknown primary melanoma. Clin Otolaryngol 19:161–165
10. Jonk A, Kroon BBR, Rumke P, Mooi WJ, Hart AAM, van Dongen JA (1990) Lymph node metastasis from melanoma with unknown primary site. Br J Surg 77:665–668
11. de Braud F, Heilbrun LK, Ahmed K (1989) Metastatic squamous cell carcinoma of an unknown primary localized to the neck. Advantages of an aggressive treatment. Cancer 64:510–515
12. Werner JA, Schünke M, Lippert BM, Koeleman-Schmidt H, Gottschlich S, Tillmann B (1995) Das laryngeale Lymphgefässsystem des Menschen. Eine morphologische und lymphographische Untersuchung unter klinischen Gesichtspunkten. HNO 35:525–531
13. Abrahms HL, Spiro R, Goldstein N (1950) Metastases in carcinoma. Analysis of 1000 autopsied cases. Cancer 3:74–85
14. Altman E, Cadman E (1986) An analysis of 1539 patients with cancer of unknown primary site. Cancer 57:120–124
15. Abbruzzese JL, Raber MN, Frost P (1988) An effective strategy for the evaluation of unknown primary tumors. Cancer Bull 41:157–161
16. Frost P (1985) Unknown primary tumors: an example of accelerated (type2) tumor progression. In Sudilovski O (ed.) Boundaries between promotion and regression during carcinogenesis. Cancer 55:1163–1166
17. Scanlon EF (1985) The process of metastasis. Cancer 55:1163–1166
18. McGovern VJ (1975) Spontaneous regression of melanoma. Pathology 7:91–99
19. Jonk A, Kroon BBR, Rümke Ph, van der Esch EP, Hart AAM (1988) Results of radical dissection of the groin in patients with stage II melanoma and histologically proved metastases of the iliac or obturator lymph nodes, or both. Surg Gynecol Obstet 167:28–32
20. Shenoy BV, Fort III L, Benjamin SP (1987) Malignant melanoma primary in lymph node. Am Surg Pathol 11:140–146
21. Milton GW, Lane Brown MM, Gilder M (1967) Malignant melanoma with an occult primary lesion. Br J Surg 54:651–658
22. Werner JA (1995) Untersuchungen zum Lymphgefässsystem von Mundhöhle und Rachen. Laryngorhinootologie 74:622–628
23. Medina JE (1989) A rational classification of Neck dissections. Otolaryngol Head Neck Surg 100:169–176
24. Werner JA (1997) Aktueller Stand der Versorgung des Lymphabflusses maligner Kopf-Hals-Tumoren. Eur Arch Otorhinolaryngol Suppl I 47–85
25. Zeph RD, Weisberger EC, Einhorn LH, Williams SD, Lingeman RE (1985) Modified Neck dissection for metastatic testicular carcinoma. Arch Otolaryngol Head Neck Surg 111:667–672

26. Wang RC, Goepfert H, Barber AE, Wolf P (1990) Unknown primary squamous cell carcinoma metastatic to the neck. Arch Otolaryngol Head Neck Surg 116:1388–1393

27. Haas I, Hoffmann TK, Engers R, Ganzer U (2002) Diagnostic strategies in cervical carcinoma of an unknown primary (CUP). Arch Otorhinolaryngol 259:325–333

28. Randall DA, Johnstone PA, Foss RD, Martin PJ (2000) Tonsillectomy in diagnosis of the unknown primary tumor of the head and neck. Otolaryngol Head Neck Surg 122:52–55

29. Kulapaditharom B, Boonkittichareon V, Kunachak S (1999) Flourescence-guided biopsy in the diagnosis of an unknown primary cancer in patients with metastatic cervical lymph nodes. Ann Otol Rhinol Laryngol 108:700–704

30. Knothe J, Fritsche F (1980) Zur Halslymphknotenmetastasierung bei unbekanntem Primärtumor. Laryng Rhinol Otol 59:221–226

31. Wilson CBJH (1992) Pet scanning in oncology. Eur J Cancer 28:508–510

32. Bailet JW, Abermayour E, Jabour BA, Hawkins RA, HoC War PH (1992) Positron emission tomography: a new, precise imaging modality for detection of primary head and neck tumors and assessment of cervical adenopathy. Laryngoscope 102:281–288

33. Jungehülsing RM, Scheidhauer K (1994) FDG-PET im Vergleich mit CT, MRT und Sonographie zum Staging von Kopf-Halskarzinomen. Eur Arch Otol Rhinol Laryngol Suppl II, 171–172

34. Bohuslavizki KH, Klutmann S, Sonnemann U, Thomas J, Kroger S, Werner JA, Mester J, Clausen M (1999) F-18-FDG for detecting occult primary tumors in patients with lymph node metastases in the neck. Laryngorhinootologie 78:445–449

35. Bohuslavizki KH, Klutmann S, Kröger,S, Sonnemann U, Buchert R, Werner JA, Mester J, Clausen M (2000) Impact of positron emission tomography using 18F-FDG for detection of unknown primary tumors. J Nucl Med 41:816–820

36. Mendenhall WM, Mancuso AA, Parsons JT, Stringer SP, Cassisi NJ (1998) Diagnostic evaluation of squamous cell carcinoma metastatic to cervical lymph nodes from an unknown head and neck primary site. Head Neck 20:739–744

37. Safa AA, Tran LM, Rege S, Brown CV, Mandelkern MA, Wang MB, Sadeghi A, Juillard G (1999) The role of positron emission tomography in occult primary head and neck cancers. Cancer J Sci Am 5:214–218

38. Stokkel MP, Terhaard CH, Hordijk GJ, van Rijk PP (1999) The detection of unknown primary tumours in patients with cervical metastases by dual-head positron emission tomography. Oral Oncol 5:390–394

39. Kirschner MJ, Fietkau R, Waldfahrer F, Iro H, Sauer R (1997) Zur Therapie von zervikalen Lymphknotenmetastasen ohne bekannten Primärtumor. Strahlenther Oncol 173:362–368

40. Koivunen P, Laranne J, Virtaniemi J, Bäck L, Mäkitie A, Pulkkinen J, Grenman R (2002) Cervical metastases of un-

known origin: a series of 72 patients. Acta Otolaryngol 122:569–574

41. Boysen M, Lövdal O, Natvig K, Tausjö J, Jacobsen AB, Evensen JF (1992) Combined radiotherapy and surgery in the treatment of neck node metastases from squamous cell carcinoma of the head and neck. Acta Oncologica 31:455–460

42. Busaba NY, Fabian LR (199) Extent of lymphadenectomy achieved by various modifications of Neck dissection: a pathologic analysis. Laryngoscope 109:212–215

43. Fu KK (1994) Neck node metastases from unknown primary. Controversies in management. Front Radiat Ther Oncol 28:66–78

44. Geyer G, Wisser G (1983) Die Bedeutung der Panendoskopie bei der Primärtumorsuche cervikaler Metastasen. Laryngorhinootologie 62:359–362

45. Maulard C, Housset M, Brunel P, Rozec C, Ucla L, Delanian S, Baillet F (1992) Primary cervical lymph node of epidermoid type. Results of a series of 123 patients treated by the association surgery-radiotherapy or irradiation alone. Ann Otolaryngol Chir Cervicofac 109:6–13

46. Snyder RD, Mavligit GM, Valdivieso M (1979) Adenocarcinoma of unknown primary site: A clinico-pathological study. Med Pediatr Oncol 6:289–294

47. Stewart JF, Tattersall MHN, Woods RL (1979) Unknown primary adenocarcinoma: incidence of over investigation and natural history. Br Med J 1:1530–1533

48. Lee NK, Byers RM, Abbruzzese JL, Wolf P (1991) Metastatic adenocarcinoma to the neck from an unknown primary source. Am J Surg 162:306–309

49. Nystrom JS, Weiner JM, Wolf RM (1979) Identifying the primary site in metastatic cancer of unknown primary origin. JAMA 241:381–383

50. Wong JH, Cagle LA, Morton DL (1987) Surgical treatment of lymph nodes with metastatic melanoma from unknown primary site. Arch Surg 122:1380–1383

51. Andersson A, Gottlieb J, Drzewiecki KT, Hou-Jensen K, Sondergaard K (1992) Skin melanoma of the head and neck. Prognostic factors and recurrence free survival in 512 patients. Cancer 69:1153–1156

52. O'Brien CJ, Petersen-Schäfer K, Ruark D, Coates AS, Menzie SJ, Harrison RI (1995) Radical, modified and selective Neck dissection for cutaneous malignant melanoma. Head Neck 17:232–241

53. Subramianan R, Chilla R (1995) Halslymphknotenmetastasen bei unbekanntem Primärtumor. Verlaufsbeobachtung an 58 Patienten. HNO 43:299–303

54. Glynne-Jones RGT, Anand A, Young TE, Berry RJ (1990) Cervical metastatic squamous cell carcinoma of unknown or occult primary source. Head Neck 12:440–443

55. Dunst J, Sauer R, Weidenbecher M (1998) Halslymphknotenmetastasen bei unbekanntem Primärtumor. Strahlenther Oncol 164:129–135

56. Reddy SP, Marks MD, Marks JE (1997) Metastatic carcinoma in the cervical lymph nodes from an unknown primary site:

results of bilateral neck plus mucosal irradiation vs. ispilateral neck irradiation. Int J Radiat Oncol 37:797–802

57. Kuntz AL, Weymuller EA (1999) Impact of Neck dissection on quality of life. Laryngoscope 109:1334–1338
58. Köybasioglu A, Tokcear AB, Uslu SS, Ileri F, Beder L, Özbilen S (2000) Accessory nerve function after modified radical and lateral Neck dissection. Laryngoscope 110:73–77
59. Brazilian Head and Neck Cancer Study Group (1999) End results of a prospective Trial on elective lateral Neck dissection vs. type III modified radical Neck dissection in the management of supraglottic and transglottic carcinomas. Head Neck 21:694–702
60. Prim MP, de Diego JI, Fernandez-Zubillaga A, Garcia-Raya P, Madero R, Gavilan J (2000) Patency and flow of the internal jugular vein after functional Neck dissection. Laryngoscope 110:47–50
61. Byers RM, Clayman GL, McGill D, Andrews T, Kare RP, Roberts DB, Goepfert H (1999) Selective Neck dissections for squamous carcinoma of the upper aerodigestive tract: patterns of regional failure. Head Neck 21:499–505
62. Carvalho AL, Kowalski LP, Borges JALB, Aguiar S, Magrin J (2000) Ipsilateral neck cancer recurrences after elective supraomohyoid Neck dissection. Arch Otolaryngol Head Neck Surg 126:410–412
63. Leemans CR, Tiwari R, van der Waal I, Karim ABMF, Nauta JJP, Snow GB (1990) The efficacy of comprehensive Neck dissection with or without postoperative radiotherapy in nodal metastases of squamous cell carcinoma of the upper respiratory and digestive tracts. Laryngoscope 100:1194–1198
64. Smith PE, Krementz ET, Chapman W (1967) Metastatic cancer without a detectable primary site. Am J Surg 113:633–637
65. Mabanta SR, Mendenhall WM, Stringer SP, Cassissi NJ (1999) Salvage treatment for neck recurrence after irradiation alone for head and neck squamous cell carcinoma with clinically positive neck nodes. Head Neck 21:591–594
66. Friedman M, Lim JW, Dickey W, Tanyeri H, Kirshenbaum GL, Phadke DM, Calarelli D (1999) Quantification of lymph nodes in selective neck dissection. Laryngoscope 109:368–370
67. Coster JR, Foote RL, Olsen KD, Jack SM, Schaid DJ, DeSanto LW (1992) Cervical nodal metastasis of squamous cell carcinoma of unknown origin: indications for withholding radiation therapy. Int J Radiat Oncol Biol Phys 23:743–749
68. Stiernberg CM, Mostert JF (1994) Unknown primary lesion. In: WW Shockley, HC Pillsbury III (eds) The neck. Diagnosis and Surgery. Mosby; St. Louis, 431–437
69. Templer J, Perry MC, Davis WE (1981) Metastatic cervical adenocarcinoma from unknown primary tumor. Arch Otolaryngol 107:45–47
70. Culine S, Fabro M, Ychou M, Romieu G, Cupissol D, Pujol H (1999) Chemotherapy in carcinomas of unknown primary site: a high-dose intensity policy. Ann Oncol 10:569–575

71. Greco FA, Erland JB, Morrissey LH, Burris HA 3rd, Hermann RC, Steis R, Thompson D, Gray J, Hainsworth JD (2000) Carcinoma of unknown primary site: phase II trials with docetaxol plus cisplatin or carboplatin. Ann Oncol 11:211–215
72. Kane M, McClary E, Ballet RE (1987) Frequency of occult residual melanoma after excision of a clinically positive regional lymph node. Ann Surg 205:88–89
73. Leipzig B, Winter ML, Hokanson JA (1981) Cervical nodal metastases of unknown primary origin. Laryngoscope 91:593–598
74. Vikram B (1980) Changing patterns of failure in advanced head and neck cancer. Arch Otolaryngol 110:11–17
75. von Volkmann R (1882) Das tiefe branchiogene Halskarzinom. Zbl Chir 9:49
76. Knöbber D, Lobeck H, Steinkamp HJ (1995) Gibt es die malignisierte laterale Halszyste doch? HNO 43:104–107
77. Martin H, Morfit HM, Ehrlich H (1950) The case for branchiogenic cancer (malignant branchioma). Ann Surg 132: 867
78. Park SS, Karmody CS (1992) The first branchial cleft carcinoma. Arch Otolaryngol 118:969–971
79. Singh B, Balwally AN, Sundaram K, Har-El G, Krgin B (1998) Branchial cleft cyst carcinoma: Myth or reality? Ann Otol Rhino Laryngol 107:519–524
80. Sutton JB (1983) Tumors – Innocent and Malignant. London: Cassel
81. Willis RA (1934) The spread of tumors in the human body. London: J&A Churchill
82. Khafif RA, Prichep R, Minkowitz S (1989) Primary branchiogenic carcinoma. Head Neck 11:153–163
83. Robinson AC, Powell CR, Kenyon GS, East JM (1987) Branchiogenic carcinoma: A review of diagnostic criteria. J Laryngol Otol 101:399–403
84. Lindberg R (1929) Distribution of cervical lymph node metastases from squamous cell carcinoma of the upper respiratory and digestive tracts. Cancer 29:1446–1449
85. Carbone A, Micheau C (1982) Pitfalls in microscopic diagnosis of undifferentiated carcinoma of nasopharyngeal type (lymphoepithelioma). Cancer 50:1344–1351
86. Charlton G, Singh B, Landers G (1996) Metastatic carcinoma in the neck from occult primary lesion. South Afr J Surg 34:37–39
87. Compagno J, Hyams VJ, Safacian M (1976) Does branchiogenic carcinoma really exist? Arch Pathol Lab Med 100: 311–314
88. Delank KW, Freytag G, Stoll W (1992) Klinische Relevanz der malignen lateralen Halszysten. Laryngorhinootologie 71:611–617
89. Flanagan PM, Roland NJ, Jonas AS (1994) Cervical node metastases presenting with features of brachial cysts. J Laryngol Otol 108:1068–1071
90. Foss RD, Warnock GR, Clark WB, Graham SJ, Morton AL, Yunan ES (1991) Malignant cyst of the lateral aspect of the neck: branchial cleft carcinoma or metastasis? Oral Surg Oral Med Oral Pathol 71:214–217

91. Hassmann-Poznanska E, Musiatowicz B (1995) Branchiogenic carcinoma: cystic metastases from oropharyngeal primary. Otolaryngol Pol 49:364–370

92. Micheau C, Cachin Y, Caillou B (1974) Cystic metastases in the neck revealing occult carcinoma of the tonsil: a report of six cases. Cancer 33:228–233

93. Swoboda H, Braun O (1989) The branchiogenic cyst in an oncologic context. Laryngorhinootologie 68:337–341

94. Thompson HY, Furmer RP, Schnadig VJ (1994) Metastatic squamous cell carcinoma of the tonsil presenting as multiple cystic neck masses: report of a case with fine needle aspiration findings. Acta Cytol 38:605–607

95. Thompson LDR, Heffner DK (1998) The clinical importance of cystic squamous cell carcinomas in the neck. Cancer 82:944–956

96. Hamperl H (1939) Über die "branchiogenen" Tumoren. Virchows Archiv 304:34

97. Wolff M, Rankow RM, Fleigel J (1979) Branchiogenic carcinoma – fact or fallacy? J Maxillofac Surg 7:41–47

98. Abbruzzese JL, Raber MN, Frost P (1988) An effective strategy for the evaluation of unknown primary tumors. Cancer Bull 41:157–161

99. Stoll W (1980) Laterale Halszysten und laterale Halsfisteln. Zwei verschiedene Krankheitsbilder. Laryngorhinootologie 59:585–595

100. Stoll W, Hüttenbrink KB (1982) Die laterale Halszyste. Eine Lymphknotenerkrankung. Laryngorhinootologie 61:272–275

101. Martin H, Sugarbaker EL (1941) Cancer of the tonsil. Am J Surg 52:155–196

102. Levy I, Barki Y, Tovi F (1991) Giant cervical cyst: presenting symptom of an occult thyroid carcinoma. J Laryngol Otol 105:863–864

103. Levy I, Barki Y, Tovi F (1992) Cystic metastases of the neck from occult thyroid adenocarcinoma. Am J Surg 163:298–300

104. McDermott ID, Watters GWR (1996) Metastatic papillary thyroid carcinoma presenting as a typical branchial cyst. J Laryngol Otol 100:490–492

105. Batsakis JG (1979) Metastatic neoplasms to and from the head and neck. In: Tumors of Head and Neck. Baltimore: Williams and Wilkins, 244–245

Distant Metastases

Epidemiology. The incidence of distant metastases of squamous cell carcinomas in the area of the upper aerodigestive tract is relatively low in comparison to other malignancies, e. g., those situated in the stomach, the pancreas, the lungs, the breast or the kidneys. Distant metastases of squamous cell carcinomas are mainly influenced by the location of the primary tumor and the initial T and N stage. Excluding adenoid cystic carcinoma, the occurrence of distant metastases without previous lymphogenic metastatic spread is somewhat of an anomaly [1]. Furthermore, the occurrence of distant metastases seems to be the result of a complex process that has its origin in the primary tumor in genetically predisposed tumor bearers. This results in the promotion and progression of malignant cell mutations that favor clone expansion and uncontrolled growth due to autocrine growth factors and growth factor receptors (EGF-R) [2].

In patients suffering from squamous cell carcinomas of the head and neck, clinical studies show an incidence of distant metastases that varies between 4–26 % [3]. In contrast, autopsy examinations reveal a significantly higher incidence, with values of more than 40 % [4]. The frequency of distant metastases at first presentation is between 1.5 % and 16.8 % [1]. The initial diagnosis occurs typically 9–12 months after initial tumor identification, and, in 84 % of the cases, it occurs within the first two years [1,5]. Lungs, bones, liver and brain are the only locations where distant metastases can be diagnosed by means of screening tests. However, generally all regions of the body can be affected by distant metastases of squamous cell carcinomas of the head and neck. In a retrospective analysis of 727 patients suffering from head and neck cancer, Calhoun and co-workers [5] found that the lung was the most frequent location for distant metastatic spread in 83.4 % of the cases, followed by bones (31.3 %) and the liver (6 %). Regarding this last statistic, it should be mentioned that metastases of the liver is more evident at the time of autopsy. Another retrospective examination of 101 patients showed that the lung was affected by distant metastases in 70 % of the cases, the liver in 42.5 % of the cases and the bones in 15 % of the cases [6].

The average survival in patients with distant metastatic spread is between 4.3–7.3 months [5,7]; as a result, these patients are generally considered terminally ill and only palliative treatment provided [8].

10.1 Nasopharynx

Five years after curative treatment, about 30 % of the nasopharyngeal cancer patients have developed distant metastases, with a mean diagnosis of eight months (40 % without locoregional control and 29 % with locoregional control) [9, 10]. The expected survival after the occurrence of distant metastases is about five months. Distant metastases are mainly observed in the bony skeleton (48 %), the lung (27 %) and the liver (11 %) [11].

10.2 Lips and Anterior Oral Cavity

Distant metastatic spread originating from carcinomas of the lip occurs only rarely [12]. The reason for this is that, with this kind of tumor, 93 % of the cases are detected in an early stage [13]. Accordingly, metastatic spread into regional lymph nodes is estimated to be lower than 10 %. Distant metastases are even lower, with values between 0.5 % and 2 %. Generally, these cases are seen only with advanced tumors where regional lymph node metastases have occurred [14].

10.3 Oropharynx

The patients suffering from oropharyngeal carcinomas who develop distant metastases in the further course of their disease typically have recurrences in the area of the primary tumor. The detection of pulmonary distant metastases are observed most often in patients with advanced stage disease and with initial bilateral lymphogenic metastatic spread and/or involvement of a lymph node metastasis in level IV. The frequency of pulmonary hematogenous metastatic spread is about 56 %. Distant metastatic involvement of the bone accounts for 15 % of the cases, and distant metastatic involvement of the liver occurs in 12 % of the cases [15].

10.4 Larynx and Hypopharynx

In a study performed by Spector, the total frequency of hematogenous metastatic spread in carcinomas of the larynx and hypopharynx amounted to 8.5 % [16]. There was a correlation between advanced stage of the primary tumor (T4 stage), the presence of regional lymph nodes metastases (N stage) and the location of the primary tumor in the hypopharynx. Patients with carcinomas localized in the area of the hypopharynx developed distant metastases three times more frequently than patients suffering from laryngeal carcinomas. In addition, advanced regional lymphogenic metastatic spread (N2 and N3 stage) tripled the frequency of distant metastases [16].

10.5 Cervical Esophagus

Often carcinomas of the cervical esophagus are detected late at an advanced stage. At the time of diagnosis, distant metastases are already present in 20 % of the cases [17]. Furthermore, 6–28 % of the patients reveal multiple synchronous or metachronous tumors of the trachea and esophagus. In carcinoma of the cervical esophagus, the frequency of distant metastases is generally influenced by the T and N stages [18].

10.6 Salivary Glands

The frequency of distant metastases over a 20-year period amounts to 17% for patients suffering from parotid tumors, 37% for patients with tumors of the submandibular gland and 24% for patients suffering from carcinomas of the minor salivary glands. With respect to the latter, the occurrence of distant metastases, as well as the frequency of metastatic spread to regional lymph nodes, depends on the histological type of the malignancy of the salivary glands. In particular, patients suffering from high-grade mucoepidermoid carcinoma, adenoid cystic carcinoma, squamous cell carcinoma or an undifferentiated carcinoma of the salivary glands often develop distant metastases. Distant metastases are observed occasionally in cases of basal cell carcinoma and acinic cell carcinoma [19].

10.7 Thyroid Gland

Hematogenous metastatic spread in cases of carcinoma of the thyroid gland can already be present at the time of the initial diagnosis, or it can occur in the further course of the disease after initial treatment [20]. Nevertheless, the long-term survival rate of patients with distant metastases amounts to 43% if treated appropriately [21]. The frequency of distant metastases in cases of carcinoma of the thyroid gland is directly related to the age of the patient, the size of the tumor, the presence of extracapsular extension and the histology of the cancer. For well-differentiated carcinomas of the thyroid gland, the total incidence of distant metastases at the time of first presentation amounts to an average of about 4% [21]. The individual frequency of distant metastases in cases of medullary and anaplastic carcinomas of the thyroid, however, is much higher. The total frequency of distant metastases in cases of papillary carcinoma is estimated to be about 10%, while the frequency of follicular and medullar carcinomas is between 22–33%.

Clinical Aspects. Generally, distant metastases of carcinomas of the upper aerodigestive tract present with non-specific clinical symptoms. Indications of the presence of pulmonary metastases may be an asymptomatic cough, pain, hemoptysis, labored breathing or weight loss. Pain in the area of the bony skeleton that occurs especially at night and improves with movement is common. Pathologic fractures can be observed as a result of bone metastases. Pain in the area of the liver, hepatitis and fever or weight loss is associated with liver metastases. Histochemically, liver function tests – including alkaline phosphatase – are elevated. Headache, nausea, neurologic complaints and psychic changes are symptoms indicating the presence of cerebral metastases.

Diagnosis. In view of the abovementioned considerations, the initial staging is of major importance in relation to introducing a specific therapeutic or palliative treatment strategy. Routinely applied diagnostic procedures include the CT scan, MRI, bone scintigraphy and abdominal sonography, chosen according to the organ system. Positron emission tomography (PET) cannot yet be considered a routine diagnostic procedure.

Therapy. In some cases, the surgical treatment of metastasis to the bone is appropriate. Generally, however, palliative radio(chemo)therapy is the treatment of choice. This is especially true in cases of pain that does not respond to other treatment and in cases of lytic metastases in charged areas. Here, the application of bisphosphonates has a special importance for pain reduction and for the reduction of pathologic fractures. Likewise, solitary cerebral metastases can be removed surgically, or, according to data from a phase III study, treated radiologically with life prolonging intention. A final assessment of the significance of a stereotactic radiosurgical treatment cannot be given at this time. It is primarily used to treat solitary metastases in patients who were not initially treated radiologically [12]. Surgical resection of solitary pulmonary metastases can be done with curative intent, whereas radiotherapy is generally performed only for palliative reasons. However, increased survival can be seen with a limited number of metastatic foci, smaller metastases and where locoregional control is present.

Even if patients suffering from distant metastases of head and neck carcinomas have a generally poor prognosis and the disposable treatment options are very limited, every medical effort must be made to achieve the best care possible as the disease progresses. The quality of life of these patients should be the objective of each treatment strategy performed for the purpose of palliation. Sufficient pain control therapy is of great importance. At the same time, vital functions such as respiration and nutrition must be ensured and, if necessary, elective tracheotomy or percutaneous gastrotomy should be performed. Due to the fact that it is almost impossible for the families of these patients to care for them adequately, the support of nursing services or institutions should be discussed with relatives or concerned persons.

References

1. Ferlito A, Shaha AR, Silver CE, Rinaldo A, Mondin V (2001) Incidence and sites of distant metastases from head and neck cancer. ORL 63:202–207

2. Petruzzelly GJ (2001) The Biology of Distant Metastases in Head and Neck Cancer. ORL 63: 192–210

3. Leemans CR (1992) The value of neck dissection in head and neck cancer: A therapeutic and staging procedure. Med Diss, Utrecht

4. Zbaeren P, Lehmann W (1987) Frequency and sites of distant metastases in head and neck squamous cell carcinoma. Arch Otolaryngol Head Neck Surg 113:762–764

5. Calhoun KH, Fulmer P, Weiss R, Hokanson JA (1994) Distant metastases from head and neck squamous cell carcinoma. Laryngoscope 104:1199–1205

6. Werner JA, Dünne AA, Lippert BM (2002) Indikationen zur Halsoperation bei nicht nachweisbaren Lymphknotenmetastasen. Teil I HNO 50:253–263

7. Troell RJ, Terris DJ (1995) Detection of metastases from head and neck cancers. Laryngoscope 105:247–250

8. Don DM, Anzai Y, Lufkin RB, Fu YS, Calcaterra TC (1995) Evaluation of cervical lymph node metastases in squamous cell carcinoma of the head and neck. Laryngoscope 105: 669–674

9. Kwong D, Sham J, Choy D (1994) The effect of locoregional control on distant metastatic dissemination in carcinoma of the nasopharynx: An analysis of 1301 patients. Int J Radiat Oncol Biol Phys 30:1029–1036

10. Geara FB, Sanguineti G, Tucker SL, Garden AS, Ang KK, Morrison WH, Peters LJ (1997) Carcinoma of the nasopharynx treated by radiotherapy alone: determinants of distant metastasis and survival. Radiother Oncol 43:53–61

11. Chiesa F, De Paoli F (2001) Distant metastases from nasopharyngeal cancer. ORL 63:214–216

12. Betka J (2001) Distant metastases from lip and oral cavity cancer. ORL 63:217–221

13. Greenlee RT, Murray T, Bolden S, Wingo AP (2000) Cancer Statistics, 2000. CA Cancer J Clin 50:7–33

14. de Visscher JG, van den Elsaker K, Grond AJ, van der Wal JE, van der Waal I (1998) Surgical treatment of squamous cell carcinoma of the lower lip: Evaluation of long-term results and prognostic factors – a retrospective analysis of 184 patients. J Oral Maxillofac Surg 56:814–820

15. Goodwin WJ (2001) Distant metastases from oropharyngeal cancer. ORL 63:222–223

16. Spector GJ (2001) Distant metastases from laryngeal and hypopharyngeal cancer. ORL 63:224–228

17. Marmuse JP, Koka VN, Guedon C, Benhamou G (1995) Surgical treatment of carcinoma of the proximal esophagus. Am J Surg 169:386–390

18. Bresadola F, Terrosu G, Uzzau A, Bresadola V (2001) Distant metastases from cervical esophagus cancer. ORL 63:229–232

19. Bradley PJ (2001) Distant metastases from salivary glands cancer. ORL 63:233–242

20. Shaha AR, Shah JP, Loree TR (1996) Patterns of nodal and distant metastasis based on histologic varieties in differentiated carcinoma of the thyroid. Am J Surg 172:692–694

21. Shaha AR, Ferlito A, Rinaldo A (2001) Distant metastases from thyroid and parathyroid cancer. ORL 63:243–249

Post-Therapeutic Follow-Up Principles

11.1 General Considerations

The follow-up of patients with head and neck carcinomas is a topic of repeated discussion [1–8]. The focal point of this chapter is the importance of interdisciplinary cooperation in the treatment of cancer patients, and in follow-up examinations. The intentions of tumor follow-up are manifold. They involve the early detection of recurrences, metastases and secondary carcinomas; additionally, they involve adequate pain control therapy, as well as somatic, psychic and social rehabilitation and reintegration [9–13]. The nature of the follow-up examinations varies significantly, especially in reference to the time interval between single examinations, the use of diagnostic tools and the duration of the follow-up. Interestingly, the correlation between extended tumor follow-up and longer survival is debatable [5, 14–16].

In this chapter, the current state of tumor follow-up shall be examined, in reference to time, type and extent of follow-up, as well as the costs of follow-up examinations. This overview is exclusively oriented toward the follow-up of patients suffering from squamous cell carcinomas of the upper aerodigestive tract who were treated with curative intention surgically, radio-oncologically or with combined therapy.

11.2 Follow-Up Interval

The intervals between single tumor follow-up examinations depend largely on primary tumor location, the risk of developing a secondary carcinoma and the extent of the primary therapeutic intervention, as well as on the recurrence-free interval after initial treatment. About 90% of all local recurrences or regional metastases occur within the first two years after primary treatment [17–19]. Conversely, the risk of developing a secondary carcinoma increases every year after the initial treatment. A widespread practice is to perform follow-up examinations during the first year after tumor therapy in intervals of 4 weeks, and to extend the intervals to 8 weeks during the second year, 3 months during the third year and 6 months during the fourth and fifth years [1].

In a study published by Marchant et al. [6], 290 members of the American Society for Head and Neck Surgery (ASHNS) were asked in a questionnaire to specify their recommended follow-up intervals. In the first year, they recommended a follow-up every month, in the second year, every 2 months and in the third to fifth years, every 6 months. Paniello et al. [7] also evaluated questionnaires on follow-up intervals. He found that in the first postoperative year, 7–10 follow-up examinations were performed, in the second postoperative year, 5–6 examinations, in the third year, 2–4 examinations, and in the fourth and fifth years, 2–3 examinations. In general, authors agree that with every year after primary therapy the number of follow-up examinations can be reduced.

The guidelines of the German Society of Otorhinolaryngology, Head and Neck Surgery recommend two different follow-up schedules. For tumors having a low risk of recurrence or secondary occurrence in the upper aerodigestive tract, the recommended follow-up interval is 3 months during the first year, 4–6 months during the second year, every 6 months during the third–fifth years and, after the fifth year, annually. For advanced-stage tumors, or after incomplete resection (R1- or R2 resection), control examinations are recommended at 6-week intervals during the first year, at 3-month intervals during the second year, at 6-month intervals during the third–fifth years and, after the fifth year, annually [2].

The survival time of patients with an initially advanced tumor stage can frequently not be prolonged despite intensive tumor follow-up. Critics therefore [3–5, 16] question the benefit of extended and long-term tumor follow-up. In a retrospective study, Boysen et al. [3] found that, in spite of follow-up intervals of 2 or 3 months, long-term survival could only be improved significantly within the first two years in patients suffering from laryngeal carcinomas that had been primarily irradiated.

According to the results of von Wolfensberger et al. [16], a curative secondary treatment could only be performed in patients with a low T category without cervical lymph node metastases. The patients included in the evaluation were examined during the first two years 4 times per year, and during the third through fifth years, every six months.

A second study from Boysen et al. [4] evaluated the effectiveness of an intensive tumor follow-up. The study showed that in spite of tumor detection in intervals of 2–3 months during the first two years, and in intervals of 3–4 months during the following three years, successful secondary treatment of local recurrences could only be effected in cases of laryngeal carcinoma or carcinoma of the oral cavity. These patients had either been irradiated or the primary tumor resection had been limited. In an evaluation performed by Cooney et al. [5] of patients who recurred after treatment of advanced cancer, no significant difference in survival was observed, in spite of follow-up examinations seven times during the first year, every 2–3 months during the second year and every 4–6 months during the third–fifth years.

In contrast to the abovementioned results, other authors [6, 7, 20] favor intensive follow-up. As part of the follow-up routine, Snow et al. [20] evaluate whether a secondary intervention offers the possibility of neck dissection. Patients who still have this therapeutic option are seen every month during the first year and every two months during the second year. The prognosis, however, of patients with a regional tumor recurrence after an extended surgical primary intervention with neck dissection and postoperative radiation is very poor, even when it is diagnosed early.

11.3 Type, Extent and Costs of Follow-Up Examinations

In cases of circumscribed T1 and T2 upper aerodigestive tract tumors that were not primarily treated with neck dissection, we perform follow-up examinations during the first year every month, during the second year every two months, and during the third–fifth years, every three months. In these patients, regional recurrence can still be treated by neck dissection with curative intent. Such follow-up is indicated for patients having undergone primary radiotherapy in cases of laryngeal carcinoma. Tumor recurrences with regional lymph node metastases generally have a very poor prognosis even if they are diagnosed relatively early. These patients should be seen during the first two years every 3 months, during the third year, every 4 months and, afterwards, every 6 months. Of course, the slightest suspicion of the presence of a recurrence of a secondary carcinoma warrants immediate examination using a rigorous diagnostic protocol.

Due to the fact that, in patients suffering from squamous cell carcinomas of the head and neck, about 90% of the metastases or recurrences occur within the first two years after primary treatment [21–23], frequently the expression "tumor cure" is used after 5 years of tumor-free survival. Boysen et al. [3, 4] recommend discontinuing follow-up examinations following the fifth year after primary treatment due to the fact that, according to their studies, therapy of a secondary primary carcinoma during this period does not lead to a significantly increased survival rate. In contrast, an evaluation of 428 patients performed by Visscher et al. [14] showed that the duration of the follow-up should depend on the site and stage of the primary cancer. They demonstrated that a curative secondary therapy could be performed successfully in patients with a glottic laryngeal carcinoma in stages I and II up to 10 years after primary treatment and, in stages III and IV, up to 2 years after primary treatment. With stage I or II supraglottic, laryngeal carcinoma, curative resection could be performed successfully up to 3 years after primary treatment and, with stage III and IV, up to 7 years after primary treatment. Curative secondary therapy for

subglottic cancer could be performed up to two years after primary treatment and, with a carcinoma of the oral cavity or pharynx, up to 5 years after primary therapy. The occurrence of a second primary carcinoma was not evaluated in their study. A lifelong follow-up is recommended by the majority of authors in order to detect and treat secondary carcinomas with curative intention [6, 16, 20]. This is especially important if patients use tobacco.

In the view of Warren and Gates, secondary carcinomas must be identified *histologically*, based on criteria established for secondary carcinoma; consequently, metastases of the primary tumor are not included in this category [24]. The chances of developing a secondary carcinoma, according to the literature, are between 10 and 20% in patients suffering from malignant tumors of the head and neck [15, 25–27]. The yearly incidence amounts to 3–7% [27–29]. There is a clear tendency for secondary carcinoma to manifest in the aerodigestive tract if the primary tumor was located in the area of the oral cavity, the oropharynx or the hypopharynx [30]. These patients develop a secondary carcinoma in about 16–18% of the cases. In contrast, the probability of developing a secondary carcinoma in cases of nasopharyngeal carcinoma is only about 8% [31]. The follow-up examinations of oncologic patients should be performed from a long-term perspective, due to the relatively high risk of developing a secondary carcinoma in the abovementioned tumor locations (oral cavity, oropharynx, hypopharynx and, also, larynx).

The decisive factor for the chances of surviving a secondary carcinoma is site. Secondary carcinomas located in the lung or esophagus nearly always have a very unfavorable prognosis. In contrast, secondary carcinomas in the region of the oral cavity or the larynx can often be cured, if they are diagnosed and treated at an early stage.

The type and extent of the oncologic follow-up vary from hospital to hospital. Careful history, local inspection and palpation of the neck are essential for every follow-up examination. In patients with a low risk of recurrence, each examination should include a comprehensive otolaryngologic examination with indirect mirror examination – or even flexible fiberoptic examinations – as well as palpation of the neck. Patients with a higher risk of developing recurrences should additionally be examined every three months after primary intervention with CT or MRI scans with imaging of the tumor region, including the lymphatic vessels. Sonography of the lymphatic drainage region is also indicated at short intervals. A second control CT scan may be indicated at the second year follow-up exam [2].

The diagnostic tools used during the follow-up examinations after treatments for cancer of the upper aerodigestive tract, neck, thorax, abdomen and bony skeleton are described below.

11.3.1 The Upper Aerodigestive Tract

Without indicating explicitly the location of the primary tumor or the respective tumor stage, Bier et al. [1] recommend a yearly routinely-performed panendoscopy as the most reliable diagnostic procedure for detection of secondary carcinomas, as well as recurrences or metastases, of the upper aerodigestive tract. In contrast, yearly panendoscopy is not part of the standard follow-up for most authors [4, 7, 16, 20]. Furthermore, panendoscopy has traditionally been performed only with general anesthesia in cases of obligatory hypopharyngoscopy, which, as a result, creates an additional risk for patients due to co-morbidities. Using panendoscopy, esophageal carcinomas can be identified in an early stage. However, the 5-year-survival rate is only 15–20%, even in cases of operable esophageal carcinoma [32, 33]. The recently described technique of using ultra-thin transnasal esophagoscopy in a clinic setting with topical anesthesia will likely render panendoscopy under general anesthesia unnecessary.

11.3.2 Neck

In Europe, B-mode sonography is still considered the most important pre-therapeutic procedure for the diagnosis of lymph node metastases of the head and neck. It has a sensitivity of more than 70% and a specificity of nearly 100%, and it can be accompanied by ultrasound-assisted aspiration cytology [31, 34].

When neck dissection is performed as a secondary curative intervention, some authors recommend a sonographic examination of the neck at each follow-up visit during the first two years [1, 20]. Other studies, however, do not use sonography as a diagnostic tool [3, 4, 16]. American Head and Neck surgeons should familiarize themselves with this tool and develop expertise using it so that they can add it to their diagnostic regimen.

11.3.3 Thorax

The purpose of the yearly chest x-ray performed routinely by many authors is to diagnose secondary carcinomas or metastases from a head or neck primary cancer to the lungs [1, 6, 14]. However, conventional chest x-rays often do not detect carcinoma of the lung at an early stage [12, 35]. A prospective study evaluated by Reiner et al. [36] showed that only 29% of pulmonary metastases or secondary carcinomas diagnosed in a thoracic CT scan could also be detected with ordinary chest AP and lateral x-rays. In a comparison of chest x-ray to CT scanning of the thorax for the purpose evaluating pulmonary masses, the sensitivity was shown to be 21% and the specificity, 99% [37]. The vast majority of pulmonary metastases or second primary lung carcinomas detected by conventional chest x-ray are of advanced tumor stage when only palliative therapy is possible. Unfortunately, the 5-year-survival rate of patients with malignant processes diagnosed early amounts to only 20% in cases of pulmonary metastases [38], and to only 8% [39] in cases of a second, primary lung carcinoma. Because survival is not increased significantly in their studies, some authors do not perform yearly chest x-rays in oncologic follow-up examinations [3–5]. A study performed by de Visscher et al., however, showed that the yearly chest x-ray could be used successfully in oncologic follow-up. In their study of 301 patients suffering from laryngeal carcinoma, fifteen secondary carcinomas were diagnosed by chest x-ray, and six of these cases were treatable with curative intent.

11.3.4 Abdomen and Scintigraphy of the Skeletal Bones

Distant metastases of squamous cell carcinomas of the upper aerodigestive tract are localized in the lung, the mediastinum, the bony skeleton and the liver [40–42]. For oncologic follow-up from the first to the fifth year, Bier et al. [1] recommended routine performance of yearly sonography of the abdomen. In a study by Dost et al. [41], 367 patients with diagnosed head and neck tumors underwent sonography of the epigastric region. Three of these patients were suspected of having metastases in the liver, which was confirmed in two cases. Often, abdominal masses can be readily detected sonographically and then biopsied under sonographic control [43, 44]. At the time of diagnosis, a suspicion of an abdominal distant metastasis is present in only 0.8 % of the examined patients suffering from a manifest squamous cell carcinoma of the head and neck [45]. Given the course of the disease, abdominal distant metastases occur very rarely and, when they do occur, offer few therapeutic options. Because of this, the usefulness of a routinely performed abdominal sonography in asymptomatic patients must be questioned. We do not recommend routine sonography of the epigastric region; nor do we recommend abdominal CT or MRI scans.

By means of scintigraphy of the skeleton (bone scans) it is possible to identify bony neoplasms smaller than 1cm earlier than with conventional x-rays [46–48]. The procedure, however, is relatively nonspecific. In addition to metastases, it reveals arthritis, osteoporosis, fractures and inflammatory bony processes [41, 49–53]. Due to the high number of false-positive results, further diagnostic clarification is necessary using ordinary x-rays, CT or MRI scans.

Due to the fact that the therapeutic options are limited with abdominal or bony distant metastases, most authors do not perform routine imaging studies of the epigastric region or scintigraphy of the skeleton in oncologic follow-up [16, 20]. In contrast, when patients develop loco-regional recurrence of head and neck cancer, distant work-up is important in order to exclude metastases, which would render any loco-regional therapy only palliative. PET scanning done in patients with loco-regional recurrence is very useful in determining the need for subsequent CT, MRI or ordinary x-rays of suspicious skeletal areas.

11.3.5 Possible Strategies

Color-coded duplex sonography of cervical soft tissues and ultrasound- guided aspiration cytology should generally be performed at each follow-up examination and for as long as a curative treatment option is possible. Due to its limited significance, and to the extremely poor prognosis in cases of pulmonary metastases, the yearly chest x-ray can be dispensed with. If chest imaging is indicated, we perform a CT scan of this area. In cases of suspected tumor, decisions concerning the use of panendoscopy, scintigraphy of the skeleton, sonography of the epigastric region and CT or MRI scanning, must be made on a case-by-case basis. The role of PET scanning was addressed in the chapter on examination methods.

Many patients today are treated in a multidisciplinary manner, where the patient follow-up is shared between the head and neck surgeon and the radiation oncologist. Immediately after surgery, of course, the surgeon must perform the follow-up. Once the patient is through the period of potential postoperative complications or other postoperative management requirements, however, other specialists can check for cancer recurrence. Typically, in the first year after surgery, at approximately the third follow-up month, subsequent visits can be rotated on a one-month basis between the radiation therapist and the head and neck surgeon. This decreases the number of visits a patient must make, while, at the same time, providing excellent surveillance when the risk of cancer recurrence is highest. The approach, of course, depends on the ability of the radiation oncologist to adequately visualize the areas of possible cancer recurrence, which today is much easier, due to flexible nasopharyngoscopes and other modern instrumentation. If the radiation oncologist in uncomfortable using these diagnostic tools, then more of the follow-up will need to be done by the head and neck surgeon.

When patients with advanced cancer receive radiochemotherapy as part of their treatment, medical oncologists will also be involved. Their role, however, is different from that of either the surgeon or the radiation oncologist, in that they are not trained to see the deeper aerodigestive tract sites. Conversely, their expertise is often better when it comes to the evaluation and treatment of distant metastases. The involvement of medical oncologists in the follow-up process will vary for each patient.

It is very important that the patients have at least one member of the interdisciplinary cancer team as their main physician. If most of the therapy has been surgical, which is generally the case, then the main physician will be the head and neck surgeon. Occasionally, the radiation therapist will be the primary physician. It is especially important for the key physician to maintain patient contact throughout the patient's life, even if the patient, who has been treated primarily by surgery or by radiation, develops distant metastatic disease. It is emotionally very difficult for a patient if the primary physician drops out of the follow-up and totally defers patient care to the medical oncologist. Additionally, the key physician will usually have the best relationship with the patient and his family when issues of death and dying become necessary to discuss. Further, the primary physician is often best able to deal with metabolic issues, wound debridement and other patient concerns, which medical oncologists are usually less familiar with. Finally, the medical oncologist will greatly appreciate the close cooperation of both of the other specialists if a patient faces these difficult issues.

References

1. Bier H, Schultze M, Ganzer U (1993) Anmerkungen zur Nachsorge von Tumorpatienten. HNO 41:47–54
2. Bootz F (2000) Leitlinien der Deutschen Gesellschaft für Hals-Nasen-Ohren-Heilkunde, Kopf und Hals-Chirurgie: Onkologie des Kopf-Hals-Bereiches. HNO 48:104–118
3. Boysen M, Natvig K, Winther FÖ, Tausjö J (1985) Value of routine follow-up in patients treated for squamous cell carcinoma of the head and neck. J Otolaryngol 14:211–214
4. Boysen M, Lövdal O, Tausjö J, Winther F (1992) The value of follow-up in patients treated for squamous cell carcinoma of the head and neck. Eur J Cancer 28:426–430
5. Cooney TR, Poulsen MG (1999) Is routine follow-up useful after combined-modality therapy for advanced head and neck cancer? Arch Otolaryngol Head Neck Surg 125:379–382
6. Marchant FE, Lowry LD, Moffit JJ, Sabbagh R (1993) Current national trends in the posttreatment follow-up of patients with squamous cell carcinoma of the head and neck. Am J Otolaryngol 14:88–93
7. Paniello RC, Virgo KS, Johnson MH, Clemente MF, Johnson FE (1999) Practice patterns and clinical guidelines for posttreatment follow-up of head and neck cancer. Arch. Otolaryngol. Head Neck Surg 125:309–313
8. Weymuller EA, Yueh B, Deleyiannis FW, Kuntz AL, Alsarraf R, Coltrera MD (2000) Quality of live in patients with head and neck cancer: lessons learned from 549 prospectively evaluated patients. Arch Otolaryngol Head Neck Surg 126:329–336
9. Chua KS, Reddy SK, Lee MC, Patt RB (1999) Pain and loss of function in head and neck cancer survivors. J. Pain Symptom Manage 18:193–202
10. Dropkin MJ (1999) Body image and quality of life after head and neck cancer surgery. Cancer Pract 7:309–313
11. List MA, Siston A, Haraf D, Schumm P, Kies M, Stenson K, Vokes EE (1999) Quality of life and performance in advanced head and neck cancer patients on concomitant chemoradiotherapy: a prospective examination. J Clin Oncol 17:1020–1028
12. Mathieson CM, Logan-Smith LL, Phillips J, MacPhee M, Attia EL (1996) Caring for head and neck oncology patients. Does social support lead to better quality of life? Can Fam Physician 42: 1712–1720
13. Terrell JE (1999) Quality of life assessment in head and neck cancer patients. Hematol Oncol Clin North Am 13:849–865
14. de Visscher AVM., Manni JJ (1994) Routine long-term follow-up in patients treated with curative intent for squamous cell carcinoma of the larynx, pharynx and oral cavity. Arch Otolaryngol Head Neck Surg 120:934–939
15. Snow GB (1992) Follow-up in patients treated for head and neck cancer: how frequent, how thorough and for how long. Eur J Cancer 28:315–316

16. Wolfensberger M (1988) Aufwand und Nutzen regelmäßiger Nachkontrollen bei Patienten mit Pflasterzellkarzinomen des Larynx, der Mundhöhle und des Pharynx. HNO 36:28–32

17. Leemans ChR, Tiwari RM, van der Waal I, Nauta JJP, Snow GB (1990) The efficacy of comprehensive Neck dissection with or without postoperative radiotherapy in nodal metastases of squamous cell carcinoma of the upper respiratory and digestive tracts. Laryngoscope 100:1194–1198

18. Mantravadi RVP, Skolnik EM, Haas EL, Applebaum EL (1983) Patterns of cancer recurrence in the postoperatively irradiated neck. Arch Otolaryngol 109:753–756

19. Pitman KT, Johnson JT (1999) Skin metastases from head and neck squamous cell carcinoma: incidence and impact. Head Neck 21:560–565

20. Strauss RP (1998) Psychosocial responses to oral and maxillofacial surgery for head and neck cancer. J Oral Maxillofac Surg 47:343–348

21. Brandenburg JH, Rutter SW (1977) Residual carcinoma of the larynx. Laryngoscope 87:224–236

22. Vikram B, Strong EW, Sha JP, Spiro R (1984) Failure at the primary site following multimodality treatment in advanced head and neck cancer. Head Neck Surg 6:720–723

23. Vikram B, Strong EW, Sha JP, Spiro R (1984) Failure in the neck following multimodality treatment for advanced head and neck cancer. Head Neck Surg 6:724–729

24. Warren S, Gates O (1932) Multiple malignant tumors: a survey of literature and statistical study. Am J Cancer 51:1358–1414

25. Hordijk GJ, de Long, JMA (1983) Synchronous and metachronous tumours in patients with head and neck cancer. J Otol Laryngol 97:619–621

26. Nikolaou AC, Markou CD, Petridis DG, Daniilidis IC (2000) Second primary neoplasms in patients with laryngeal carcinoma. Laryngoscope 110:58–64

27. Sturgis E, Miller R (1995) Second primary malignancies in the head and neck cancer patient. Ann Otol Rhinol Laryngol 104:946–954

28. Cooper JS, Pajak TF, Rubin P (1989) Second malignancies in patients who have head and neck cancer: incidence, effect on survival and implications based on the RTOG experience. Int J Radiat Oncol Biol Phys 17:449–456

29. Vikram B, Strong EW, Sha JP, Spiro R (1984) Second malignant neoplasms in patients successfully treated with multimodality treatment for advanced head and neck cancer. Head Neck Surg 6:734–737

30. Boysen M, Loven JÖ (1993) Second malignant neoplasms in patients with head and neck squamous cell carcinomas. Acta Oncol 32:283–288

31. Leon X, Quer M, Diez S, Orus C, Lopez-Pousa A, Burgues J (1999) Second neoplasm in patients with head and neck cancer. Head Neck 21:204–210

32. Thum P, Frey E, Schefer H (1999) Multimodale Behandlungskonzepte beim Ösophaguskarzinom: Stellenwert der Radio- und Chemotherapie. Schweiz Med Wochenschr 129:1224–1229

33. Wind P, Roullet MH, Quinaux D, Laccoureye O, Brasnu D, Cugnenc PH (1999) Long-term results after esophagectomy for squamous cell carcinoma of the esophagus associated with head and neck cancer. Am J Surg 178:251–255

34. van den Brekel MWM, Castelijns JA, Stel HV, Luth WJ, Valk J, van der Waal I (1991) Occult metastatic neck disease: Detection with US and US-guided fine-needle aspiration cytology. Radiology 180:457–461

35. Buwalda J, Zuur CL, Lubsen H, Tijssen JG., Koole R, Hordijk GJ (1999) Annual chest X-ray in patients after treatment for laryngeal or oral cancer: only a limited number of second primary lung cancers detected. Ned Tijdschr Geneekd 143:1517–1522

36. Reiner B, Siegel E, Sawyer R, Brocato RM, Maroney M, Hooper F (1997) The impact of routine CT of the chest on the diagnosis and management of newly diagnosed squamous cell carcinoma of the head and neck. Am J Roentgenol 169:667–671

37. Houghton DJ, Hughes ML, Garvey C, Beasley NJP, Hamilton JW, Gerlinger I, Jones AS (1998) Role of chest CT scanning in the management of patients with head and neck cancer. Head Neck 20:614–618

38. Koong HN, Pastorino U, Ginsberg RJ (1999) Is there a role for pneumonectomy in pulmonary metastases? International Registry of Lung Metastases. Ann Thorac Surg 68:2039–2043

39. Jones AS, Morar P Phillips DE, Field J, Husband D Helliwell TR, Path MRC (1995) Second primary tumors in patients with head and neck squamous cell carcinoma. Cancer 75:1343–1353

40. Abramson AL, Parisier SC, Zamansky MJ, Sulka M (1971) Distant metastases from carcinoma of the larynx. Laryngoscope 81: 1503–1511

41. Dost Ph, Schrader M, Talanow D (1994) Nutzen der Abdomensonographie und der Skelettszintigraphie bei der TNM-Einteilung von Tumoren im Kopf-Hals-Bereich. HNO 42:418–421

42. Merino OR, Lindberg RD, Fletcher GH (1977) An analysis of distant metastases from squamous cell carcinoma of the upper respiratory and digestive tracts. Cancer 40:45–151

43. Halvorsen RA, Thompson WM (1991) Primary neoplasms of the hollow organs of the gastrointestinal tract. Staging and follow-up. Cancer 67:1181–1188

44. Memel DS, Dodd GD, Esola CC (1996) Efficacy of sonography as a guidance technique for biopsy of abdominal, pelvic and retroperitoneal lymph nodes. Am J Roentgenol 167:957–962

45. Probert JC, Thompson RW, Bagshaw MA (1974) Patterns of spread of distant metastases in head and neck cancer. Cancer 33:127–133

46. Brauneis J, Schröder M, Laskawi R, Wild L., Schicha H (1988) Szintigraphische Metastasensuche bei Patienten mit Malignomen des Kopf-Hals-Bereichs. HNO 36:445–451

47. O'Mara RE (1976) Skeletal scanning in neoplastic disease. Cancer 7:480–486

48. Troell RJ, Terris DJ (1995) Detection of metastases from head and neck cancers. Laryngoscope 105:247–250

49. Belson TP, Lehman RH, Chobanin SL, Malin TC (1980) Bone and liver scans in patients with head and neck carcinoma. Laryngoscope 90:1291–1296

50. Brown DH, Leakos M (1998) The value of a routine bone scan in a metastatic survey. J Otolaryngol 27:187–189

51. de Bree R., Deuerloo EE, Snow GG, Leemans CR (2000) Screening for distant metastases in patients with head and neck cancer. Laryngoscope 110:397–401

52. Tiedjen KU, Hildmann H (1984) Der Stellenwert der Isotopendiagnostik bei Erkrankungen im HNO-Bereich. Laryngorhinootologie 63:498–510

53. Watkinson JC (1990) Nuclear medicine in otolaryngology. Clin Otolaryngol 15:457–469

Subject Index